THE USE OF DRUGS IN FOOD ANIMALS

BENEFITS AND RISKS

Committee on Drug Use in Food Animals
Panel on Animal Health, Food Safety, and Public Health

Board on Agriculture
National Research Council

Food and Nutrition Board
Institute of Medicine

NATIONAL ACADEMY PRESS
Washington, D.C. 1999

NATIONAL ACADEMY PRESS · 2101 Constitution Avenue, NW · Washington, D.C. 20418

NOTICE: The project that is the subject of this report was approved by the Governing Board of the National Research Council, whose members are drawn from the councils of the National Academy of Sciences, the National Academy of Engineering, and the Institute of Medicine. The members of the committee responsible for the report were chosen for their special competences and with regard for appropriate balance.

This report has been reviewed by a group other than the authors according to procedures approved by a Report Review Committee consisting of members of the National Academy of Sciences, the National Academy of Engineering, and the Institute of Medicine.

This material is based upon work supported by the U.S. Department of Agriculture, Agricultural Research Service, under Agreement No. 59-0700-1-141, the Department of Health and Human Services, Food and Drug Administration under Agreement No. 1-R13-FDO1495-01, and the Pew Charitable Trusts under Agreement No. 90-02372-000. Partial support was provided by the American Veterinary Medical Association and the American Feed Industry Association. Any opinions, findings, conclusions, or recommendations expressed in this publication are those of the author(s) and do not necessarily reflect the view of the organizations or agencies that provided support for this project.

Library of Congress Cataloging-in-Publication Data

The use of drugs in food animals : benefits and risks / Committee
on Drug Use in Food Animals, Panel on Animal Health, Food Safety,
and Public Health, Board on Agriculture, National Research Council.
    p. cm.
   Includes bibliographical references and index.
   ISBN 0-309-05436-6 (hardcover : alk. paper)
   1. Veterinary drugs. 2. Antibiotics in veterinary medicine. 3.
Food animals—Diseases—Chemotherapy. 4. Veterinary drug residues.
5. Food of animal origin—Contamination. I. National Research
Council (U.S.). Board on Agriculture. Panel on Animal Health, Food
Safety, and Public Health. Committee on Drug Use in Food Animals.
   SF917 .U74 ~~1998~~ 1999
   363.19′2—dc21

                             98-58111

About the cover: The background of the cover is an electron micrograph of *Staphylococcus aureus* and its secretion of a polysaccharide that increases the virulence of this microbe. When these bacteria secrete this matrix, they can decrease the ability of immune cells like neutrophils to attack and destroy them. Credit for the picture is given to Dr. Albert Guidry, Dr. William Wergin, and Mr. Eric Erbe, all associated with the U.S. Department of Agriculture, Agricultural Research Service at Beltsville, Maryland.

Printed in the United States of America.

v

Preface

The raising of livestock for meat, milk, and eggs has been an integral component of the food production system in this country since its first settlement in the 1600s. The U.S. capacity for food production is tremendous and remarkable, considering that now less than 2 percent of the population is genuinely vested in the raising of food for the rest of the country. Pressures for land development and the vast increase in population have commanded a shift in food-raising practices and the efficiency of food-animal production is testimony to the successful implementation of scientific discoveries in breeding, genetics, nutrition, and animal health on the farm.

Veterinary drugs are a critical component of food-animal production. They provide many benefits related to animal health, animal welfare, and economic return for the industry. Since the benefits of subtherapeutic use of antibiotics in enhancing growth and feed efficiency in animals were first observed almost half a century ago, the number and use of these products has increased. In fact, the discovery of the benefits of subtherapeutic use of antibiotics is often credited with the move toward more intensive animal production management systems, thereby allowing fewer people to produce greater quantities of food.

For decades, the quality, efficiency, value, and safety of food production in the United States has been exceptional; it has served as a model for the rest of the world. However, the U.S. food production system must continuously improve if our country expects to be successful in today's highly competitive global market and if producers hope to deliver animal-derived foods that meet the ever-increasing expectations of the consuming public.

A totally risk-free system of food production is an unreasonable and fundamentally unattainable goal. Actual human health risks associated with food-producing animals are most immediately brought into focus in reviewing the number of cases of human illness that occur from food contamination with micro-organisms of animal origin. The magnitude of this risk is somewhat difficult to assess. In terms of tracing the origin of an illness directly back to the animal, a complicated intertwining of farm, wholesale–retail, and consumer practices exists that create opportunities for disease to emerge. However, because many aspects of the risk are known and acknowledged, it could be thought of as manageable, because logical courses of action can be applied. The potential risk to human health directly associated with the use of antibiotic drugs in food animal production is a more nebulous issue but still of great concern because of what is not known, what *could* occur, and a general attitude that control and management of the situation need to be improved.

The gains that have been made in food production capacity would not have been possible were it not for the ability of reliable agricultural chemicals to contain the threat of disease to crops and animals. The health of food-producing animals is intrinsically linked to human health. That is to say, factors that affect food-animal health will, in turn, affect human health. The logic is, if you improve the health of our animals, the health of the human population should not be compromised. The use of animal drugs, antibiotics in particular, is considered by some to pose an increased health risk to the people who consume the products from those animals. The use of all drugs (in humans as well as animals) creates both benefits and risks. With proper controls, the benefits should exceed the risks, and "new" risks will replace the "old" risks at a lower level of threat. For example, the risk of suffering from an antibiotic-resistant bacterial infection is considered acceptable when compared with the risk of dying from the bacterial infection left untreated.

Public attention today focuses primarily on the favorable and unfavorable effects of animal drug use on human health. For livestock producers and veterinarians, attention also is focused on the favorable and unfavorable effects of animal drug use on animal health and on the consequences of the inadequate numbers of approved drugs available for use. Antibiotic agents are one class of drugs used extensively in food-animal production therapeutically and subtherapeutically. By far the most important concerns among stakeholders today are microbial resistance to these compounds and residues of these compounds in the food supply. In addition, significant concerns have come to the forefront from manufacturers, producers, and veterinarians that the ever-increasing cost and length of time to approve new drugs have produced a crisis in drug availability. These issues have already generated legislative activity on two occasions, in the Animal Medicinal Drug Use Clarification Act, which was passed in 1994, and in the Animal Drug Availability Act, which was signed into law October 9, 1996. There is reason to believe that, in the near future, these issues will be joined by others, particularly those related to genetic engineering technology.

As a result of these concerns and the conflicting interests surrounding them, the Panel on Animal Health, Food Safety, and Public Health, jointly sponsored by the National Research Council's Board on Agriculture and the Institute of Medicine's Food and Nutrition Board, initiated a project to contemporize the understanding of the issues and relevant information concerning use of drugs in food animals and to establish recommendations regarding a new approach to addressing the problems pertaining to availability and the effective and safe use of drugs in food animals. The Panel on Animal Health, Food Safety, and Public Health convened the Committee on Drug Use in Food Animals to address these issues. Specifically, the committee was charged with examining the benefits and risks associated with drug use in food animal production and to prepare a report with recommendations that:

- review the role of drugs in food-animal production, including accessibility and accountability in their use;
- summarize available knowledge on human health effects of drug use in food animals;
- evaluate the approval and regulatory process and delivery systems for animal drugs; and
- assess emerging trends, technologies, and alternatives to drug use in food animal production.

The committee commissioned background papers to provide an historical perspective on the role of drugs in animal production, a status report of the animal health industry, and an historical perspective on the regulatory approval process for animal drugs. The committee met four times and, on two of these occasions, held open sessions and a workshop to gather detailed information from federal regulatory agency personnel concerning the new drug approval process, procedures for setting residue tolerance levels, and drug residue testing. Representatives of the various livestock, poultry, and aquaculture organizations provided information concerning current husbandry and production practices and quality-assurance programs.

During the evaluation process, it became evident that the existing system that encompasses the total spectrum of drug development, regulation, and use is in part paralyzed by politics and perceptions. The need for a more coordinated, flexible system for tactical decision making and for strategic planning related to policies affecting animal drug use is striking. Issues attendant to drug use in food animals will continue to evolve. Thus, there is a need for a process for evaluating needs and risks in the uses for human and animal drugs that continuously updates the issues and restructures decisions rather than one that periodically resolves crises.

As the committee pursued its work, four primary objectives were identified. The unifying theme among these goals is to offer to policy makers, consumers, the communications industry, food producers, drug manufacturers, and other audiences our recommendations for needed improvements related to:

- drug resistance monitoring;
- drug residue monitoring;
- drug use and alternative strategies; and
- an integrated, continuous, decision-making process with shared responsibilities of all stakeholders to enhance availability of needed drugs and to move toward global harmonization of this process.

In addressing its charge, through these four areas, the committee developed a line of logic, which guides the elaboration of this report, as follows:

- The residue-monitoring process is critical to the protection of the consumer's health—it must be effective and match the patterns of use for *all* classes of drugs in animal production systems.
- The drug approval process is critical to the availability and accountable use of *all* classes of drugs used in animal production systems, and in the future this will include emerging issues such as genetic design strategies.
- If the drug-residue-monitoring system is effective, then the remaining risk–benefit issue of major proportion is microbial resistance to antibiotics. Based on this line of logic, and because of the urgent nature of this matter, it is treated more extensively than any other topic in this report.

Chapter 1 provides an overview of the use of drugs in food animals and some of the controversy that has existed concerning this practice for the past 30 years. It also sets the stage for examining the perceptions of the risks associated with antibiotic use in food animals and the complexity of the intertwining of food production economics, animal health, industry drug development, and consumer preferences. Chapter 2 provides an overview of current production practices in the major food-animal species and describes the industry-initiated quality-assurance programs in place for cattle (beef and dairy), swine, and poultry producers. Chapter 3 discusses the primary benefits and hazards to human health of the use of drugs in food-animal production. Chapter 4 presents issues related to development of new drugs, the current approval process, and issues related to new developments in the approval process that are attempting to relieve some of the time lag and expense of developing new drugs. Antibiotic approval is the most pressing aspect of this process. Recommendations are offered to focus resources on public health risks. Chapter 5 summarizes the pertinent features of the drug-residue-monitoring program in the United States, explaining that an effective system is the critical assumption upon which all other strategies rest. In recent years significant interest has emerged, as has fear, in the development of antibiotic resistance in human and veterinary health arenas. The importance of this area of concern cannot be understated, and the specifics of this topic are presented in Chapter 6. The effects of therapeutic and subtherapeutic use of antibiotics on resistance in animals are discussed, as are the mechanisms through which resistance can develop. Finally, new data are presented that underscore much of the controversy in views regarding the approval of new antibiotics for general use in food animals with particular reference to the class of antibiotics called fluoroquinolones targeted to the development of resistance in *Salmonella*. Chapter 7 describes the economic implications of eliminating subtherapeutic drug use in food animals, and Chapter 8 discusses alternative strategies to reduce the need for drug use and highlights promising areas for further research.

Successful food-animal production management systems are continuously changing as advances are made in biomedical and agricultural science. Furthermore, consumer trends shift, and multiple factors alter the priorities and practices of the food production and pharmaceutical industries as well as of public health and health care policy makers.

Capitalizing on opportunities and solving problems pertaining to food-animal production systems now and in the future will be best accomplished through an integrated process that continuously assesses the strengths and weaknesses of the total system, rather than the various components separately, and uses the expertise of all stakeholders. This will be successful only if the various stakeholders define the best long-term solutions instead of short-term wins and losses and have access to information that is relevant, comprehensive, and accurate.

Since the committee began its deliberations, movement has indeed begun in this direction, as indicated by the alliance of food-animal producers, veterinarians, the animal pharmaceutical industry, and the Center for Veterinary Medicine of the Food and Drug Administration to work out a solution to accelerate the approval process for needed new animal drugs.

James R. Coffman, *Chair*
Committee on Drug Use in Food Animals

Acknowledgments

The committee would like to acknowledge the generous support for this study provided by the U.S. Department of Agriculture Agricultural Research Service, the Department of Health and Human Services Food and Drug Administration, and the Pew Charitable Trusts. In addition, the committee appreciates the support provided by the American Veterinary Medical Association and the American Feed Industry Association.

The committee wishes to thank Theodore H. Elsasser and Michael J. Phillips for their dedication and untiring efforts in seeing this project through to completion. In addition, the committee thanks Lester Crawford, Harold Hafs, and John Welser for the preparation of commissioned papers important to the committee's deliberations. Appreciation is also given to Juliemarie Goupil, Shirley Thatcher, Lucyna Kurtyka, Melinda Simons, Charlotte Kirk Baer, Suzanne Patrick, and Anne Kelly for their assistance with the report preparation, and to Mary Poos for her work in the early stages of the project.

This report has been reviewed by individuals chosen for their diverse perspectives and technical expertise, in accordance with procedures approved by the National Research Council (NRC) Report Review Committee. The purpose of this independent review is to provide candid and critical comments that will assist the authors and NRC in making the published report as sound as possible and to ensure that the report meets institutional standards for objectivity, evidence, and responsiveness to the study charge. The content of the review comments and draft manuscript remain confidential to protect the integrity of the deliberative process. We wish to thank the following individuals for their participation in the review of this report: Dale Bauman, Cornell University; Charles Carpenter, Brown

University; H. Russell Cross, IDEXX; John Dowling, Harvard University; Johanna Dwyer, New England Medical Center; D. Mark Hegsted, Southborough, MA; Larry Katzenstein, Bronx, NY; Kirk Klasing, University of California; James Peters, Alpharma, Inc.; Eileen van Ravenswaay, Michigan State University; H.E. Umbarger, West Lafayette, IN; and Judi Weissinger, Weissinger Solutions Inc. While these individuals listed above provided many constructive comments and suggestions, responsibility for the final content of this report rests solely with authoring committee and with NRC.

During the course of the study, committee member R. Gregory Stewart changed employment to became affiliated with a pharmaceutical firm that has a drug approval application pending before the Food and Drug Administration for a fluoroquinolone antibiotic. As a result, Dr. Stewart has excused himself from the committee discussion and deliberations pertaining to this class of antibiotics.

Contents

EXECUTIVE SUMMARY   1
   The Committee Process, 3
   Food-Animal Drug Use, 4
   Approval and Oversight of Food-Animal Drugs, 5
   Monitoring of Drug Residues, 6
   Resistance to Antibiotic Drugs, 6
   Conclusions, 9
   Major Recommendations, 10
      Development, Approval, and Availability of Food-Animal Drugs, 10
      Resistance to Antibiotic Drugs, 11
      Alternatives to Drug Use in Food Animals, 11

1 DRUGS USED IN FOOD ANIMALS: BACKGROUND AND PERSPECTIVES   12
   The Role of This Report, 13
   Review of Previous Reports, 15
   The Antibiotic Issue, 19
      A Possible Scenario, 20
      The Emergence of Antibiotics in Our Lives, 20
      Food-Animal Antibiotic Resistance and Human Health, 22

2 FOOD-ANIMAL PRODUCTION PRACTICES AND DRUG USE   27
   Overview, 27
   The Poultry Industry, 29
      An Integrated Industry, 30
      History and Trends in Drug Use, 31

Routes of Drug Administration, 34
   Feed, 34
   One-Day-of-Age Injection, 34
   Water Medication, 34
Growth Promotion, 38
Disease Control, 38
   Salmonella Control, 38
   Escherichia coli Control, 39
   Clostridium Control, 39
The Swine Industry, 40
   Disease Control and Use of Drugs and Chemicals, 41
   Growth and Metabolic Performance, 42
The Dairy Industry, 44
   Disease Control and Prophylactic Treatments, 45
   Therapeutic Treatment of Disease, 45
   Antibiotic Drug Use, 47
   Production Enhancers, 48
The Beef Industry, 48
   Disease Prevention, 50
   Trends in Drug Use, 50
   Therapeutic Drug Use, 51
   Vaccinations, 53
The Veal Industry, 53
The Sheep Industry, 54
Minor Species, 56
The Aquaculture Industry, 56
Quality-Assurance Programs and Animal Health Maintenance, 60
   Poultry Quality-Assurance Programs, 60
   Pork Quality-Assurance Programs, 61
   Dairy Quality-Assurance Programs, 63
   Beef Quality-Assurance Program, 67
Summary of Findings, 68

3 BENEFITS AND RISKS TO HUMAN HEALTH   69
Overview, 69
Prevention, 71
Treatment, 72
Benefits of Antibiotic Use, 73
Possible Hazards of Antibiotic Use, 75
   Antibiotic Resistance as a Human Health Risk, 76
   Antibiotic Resistance Trends, 78
Human Health Risks from Drug Residues in Foods, 81
   Antibiotic Toxicities, 83
   Allergenicity, 84

Relative Risks: Residues versus Microbial Contamination, 85
Summary of Findings, 86

4   DRUG DEVELOPMENT, GOVERNMENT APPROVAL, AND THE
    REGULATORY PROCESS   88
    Overview, 88
    Restructuring the Regulatory and Approval Process, 91
        Reforming the Regulatory Process, 95
        The Animal Medicinal Drug Use Clarification Act, 96
        The Animal Drug Availability Act, 99
    Human Health Risk, Residues, and Approval, 100
        Perspectives on Developing Drugs, 101
    Worldwide Harmonization of the Animal Drug Approval Process, 104
    Summary of Findings and Recommendations, 106
        Recommendations, 107

5   DRUG RESIDUES AND MICROBIAL CONTAMINATION IN FOOD:
    MONITORING AND ENFORCEMENT   110
    Drug Residue Standards and Screening, 111
    Tracking Drug Residues in Food, 113
    Drug Residues in Meat and Poultry, 115
    Drug Residues in Fish and Seafood, 119
    Drug Residues in Milk, 119
        The Grade A Pasteurized Milk Ordinance, 121
        Drug Residue Testing in Milk, 122
        Drug Monitoring in Milk, 124
        Unresolved Dairy Testing Issues, 125
    Food-Borne Pathogens and Contamination of Food, 126
        Determination of Pathogens, 127
        A Nine-Year Survey of Reported Food-Borne Illness, 133
    Integrating Issues of Residues and Microbial Contamination, 137
    Summary of Findings and Recommendations, 140
        Recommendations, 141

6   ISSUES SPECIFIC TO ANTIBIOTICS   142
    Development and Functionality of Antibiotic Drugs, 143
    Identifying and Screening Antibiotics, 145
    Bacterial Resistance, 148
    Antibiotic-Resistant Bacteria and Animal Management, 150
    Subtherapeutic versus Therapeutic Use of Drugs, 153
    Human and Veterinary Clinical Implications of Antibiotic Resistance, 161
    Cases to Test the System, 166
        The Fluoroquinolones Issue, 168
        The Virginiamycin Issue, 175

Summary of Findings and Recommendations, 176
Recommendations, 177

7   COSTS OF ELIMINATING SUBTHERAPEUTIC USE OF ANTIBIOTICS   179
Considerations in Determining the Effect of a Ban, 180
Definition of Subtherapeutic Use, 180
Measurement Choice, 180
Viable Antibiotic Substitutes, 182
Total Versus Partial Ban, 182
Consumer Behavior, 183
Results of Economic Analysis and Conclusions, 184
Appendix, 186
Technical Notes for Table 7–1, 186
Chicken Data, 186
Turkey Data, 187
Beef Data, 187
Pork Data, 187

8   APPROACHES TO MINIMIZING ANTIBIOTIC USE IN FOOD-ANIMAL
PRODUCTION   188
Animal Management, 190
Ambient Temperature and Heat Stress, 190
Overcrowding and Behavioral Stress, 193
Vaccination Strategies to Prevent Disease, 193
DNA Vaccination, 195
Beneficial Microbial Cultures, Probiotics, and Competitive-
Exclusion Alternatives, 195
Biosecurity, 197
Fly Control, 199
Moisture, Mud, and Manure, 199
Enhancing Natural Mediators of Immune Function, 200
Killed Bacterial Adjuvants: Biomodulation of Cytokine
and Immune Function, 202
Nutrition, 202
Disease Eradication 206
Genetics, 207
Recommendations, 208

REFERENCES   210

ABOUT THE AUTHORS   235

INDEX   239

Tables and Figures

TABLES

1–1   Summary of Previous Major Reports on Food-Animal Antibiotics, 16

2–1   Coccidiostats Approved for Use in Broilers, Turkeys, and Layers, 32
2–2   Major Claims of Antibiotics Approved for Use in Chickens and Turkeys, 32
2–3   Cost of Drug and Vaccine Use in Broilers from 1989 to 1994, 35
2–4   Turkey Medication and Vaccine Cost Analysis, 36
2–5   Cost of Medication and Vaccination Used for Turkeys and Broilers in the United States, 37
2–6   Major Claims of Antibiotics Approved for Use in Hogs, 42
2–7   Major Claims of Chemotherapeutics Approved for Use in Hogs, 43
2–8   Intramammary Antibiotics Approved for Dairy Cattle, 45
2–9   Distribution of Health Costs per Cow by Functional Category, 46
2–10   Estimated Annual Losses Caused by Mastitis, 47
2–11   Major Claims for Systemic Antimicrobials Approved for Use in Beef and Dairy Cattle, 52
2–12   Steroid Products Labeled for Improved Growth and/or Feed Efficiency in Cattle, 53
2–13   Major Claims of Antibacterials Approved for Use in Sheep, 55
2–14   Major Claims for Drugs Approved for Use in Minor Species, 57
2–15   FDA-Approved New Drugs for Use in Aquaculture, 59

xix

3–1   The Effect of Implementation of a Veterinary Preventive-Medicine Scheme on Offal and Carcass Rejections from 12 Finishing Farms, 76

4–1   Food-Animal Populations in the United States, 102
4–2   Comparative Value of FDA-Regulated Industries, 102
4–3   Annual Sales of Animal Drugs, 103

5–1   FSIS Animal Drug Residue Test Results, 118
5–2   Drug Residue Analysis Results for Grade A and Non-Grade-A Milk, 121
5–3   Survey Report of Microbiological Hazards in Swine, 128
5–4   Survey Report of Microbiological Hazards in Cattle, 130
5–5   Survey Report of Microbiological Hazards in Lamb, 132
5–6   Survey Report of Microbiological Hazards in Poultry, 134

6–1   *E. coli* Resistance to TMP-SMX, 163
6–2   Resistance of TMP-SMX-Resistant *E. coli* Isolates to Other Antimicrobial Agents, 164
6–3   Antimicrobial Resistance of *E. coli* Strains Isolated from Enteritis in Calves in the United States, Canada, and France, 165
6–4   Antibiotic Resistance in *Salmonella* from Animals, Percentage of Cultures Showing Resistance, 165
6–5   Antibiotic Resistance in *Salmonella typhimurium* from Animals, Percentage of Cultures Showing Resistance, 167

7–1   Approximate Annual Costs of a Ban on Subtherapeutic Antibiotic Use in Four Domestic Retail Markets, 185

8–1   Efficacy of Recombinant Bovine IFN-γ against *E. coli* Mastitis, 201
8–2   Effect of GCSF on Blood and Milk Leukocyte Profiles and Efficacy against *Staphylococcus aureus* Mastitis, 201
8–3   Blood Selenium, GSH-Px, and Serum Vitamin E of Cows from Low- and High-SCC Herds, 204

FIGURES

4–1   CVM Organizational Structure, 90
4–2   Comparison of the Traditional and Re-Engineered Approval Processes, 92
4–3   Effect of Re-Engineering the Approval Process on the Time to Approve New Animal Drug Applications, 93
4–4   Trends in Animal Drug Approvals since 1990, 94

5–1   Seasonality of Reported Cases of Food-Borne Disease as Monitored
       Across the Seven Sentinel Organisms at All Locations, 137

6–1   *Salmonella* DT-104 Ciprofloxacin-Resistant Human Isolates Confirmed
       in the United Kingdom, 173

Executive Summary

Americans cherish the availability and affordability of a vast food supply. At the same time, we expect the foods we choose to buy and eat to be clean, fresh, and not contaminated with debris, chemicals, or organisms that cause sickness or discomfort. Many of our foods come from "food animals" or "food-producing" animals raised specifically to provide meat, milk, and eggs. These animals serve primarily as a rich source of protein and protein-related products, vitamins, and minerals, some of which are not readily available from nonanimal sources.

Food animals convert one form of nutrient (usually grain or lignocellulosic feed such as grass, hay, or silage) to another form that differs in amino acid content, nutrient composition, and general nutritional benefit. Chickens can be raised at remarkable rates of weight gain and great metabolic efficiency to yield lean white meat. Laying hens provide a useful protein source in the eggs they produce. It takes longer for a steer to mature to a size that is marketable for beef or for a cow to mature to the point of providing milk. However, ruminants are unique in the human food chain in that they convert low-quality protein and plant-derived feed that is fundamentally indigestible by humans into meat and milk that are readily used by humans. Similarly, swine, fish, and minor species contribute to the supply of available and affordable animal-derived food.

In current agricultural practice, raising animals for food depends heavily on the use of pharmacologically active compounds: drugs. The use of drugs in food animals is fundamental to animal health and well-being and to the economics of the industry. However, their use also is associated with human health effects. There are two sides to the issue of how drug use in food animals affects the health of humans: Reported benefits are derived largely from the maintenance of good animal health and, therefore, the reduced chance that disease will spread to humans from animals. But drugs used in food-animal production and residues of those drugs could enter human food and increase the risk of ill-health in persons who consume products from treated animals. Moreover, the use of antibiotics in food animals could contribute to the emergence of antibiotic-resistant microorganisms in animals that could be transmitted to humans and result in infections that could be difficult to treat.

There are five major classes of drugs used in food animals:

- topical antiseptics, bactericides, and fungicides used to treat skin or hoof infections, cuts, and abrasions;
- ionophores, which alter stomach microorganisms to provide more favorable and efficient energy substrates from bacterial conversion of feeds and to impart some degree of protection against some parasites;
- hormone and hormonelike production enhancers (anabolic hormones for meat production and bovine somatotropin for increased milk production in dairy cows);
- antiparasite drugs; and
- antibiotics used to control overt and occult disease and to promote growth.

There are also compounds used to modify gastrointestinal environments to reduce the likelihood of rumen foaming and bloat in cattle, organic and inorganic water treatments that reduce the chances of infection in aquaculture, and miscellaneous substances used with the advice of veterinarians to treat specific conditions. Noticeably absent from the list is a specific class of drugs for treating pain and discomfort in food animals.

In response to growing public concern over food safety in relation to the use of drugs in food animals, the U.S. Department of Agriculture (USDA) and the Center for Veterinary Medicine (CVM) of the Food and Drug Administration (FDA) asked the National Research Council to form a committee to examine and review the benefits and risks associated with drug use in the food-animal industry. The National Research Council assigned the task to the Board on Agriculture, which, through the Panel on Animal Health, Food Safety, and Public Health—a joint panel with the Institute of Medicine—convened the Committee on Drug Use in Food Animals. The committee was charged with reviewing, evaluating, and making recommendations related to the need for drugs and their availability and accountability in agriculture, the benefits and risks to human health and food safety associated with food-animal drugs, the development of food-animal drugs and the process of approval of their use, and the emerging trends in animal health care and the availability of alternative management practices for raising food animals. In particular, the sponsors stressed the importance of evaluating the class of drugs known as antibiotics.

The committee's report summarizes the current state of the science concerning the relationship between food-animal drug use and public health, reviews the rationale and process under which food-animal drugs are developed by industry and approved by the federal government for use, addresses alternative measures that might be considered in food-animal production strategies to lower use of and dependence on drugs—specifically antibiotics—and summarizes the basic strategies and practices used in modern animal production. Risks and benefits to human and animal health and to animal production economics and efficiency are identified but because quantitative information was insufficient or confounding, not objectively ranked.

THE COMMITTEE PROCESS

The committee reviewed the major classes of drugs used in food animals, focusing on the potential effect of drugs used both for human and for animal health. The committee conducted a review of the scientific literature; heard testimony on animal-drug-related issues; and reviewed federal regulations that provide guidelines and list mandatory practices for drug use, monitoring capabilities for drugs and residues in foods, veterinary oversight in prescription drug use, rates of violations, and instances of documented health problems. The committee concluded that most drugs used and most drug residues found in animal-derived foods pose a relatively low risk to the public so long as the drugs are used responsibly and in keeping with label instructions.

There were, however, concerns about the effects of antibiotic use in food animals. Effects on human health were not related to food contamination from the use of antibiotics or from antibiotic residues. Rather, the concern was narrowed to the effect of antibiotic use on the emergence in food animals of populations of microorganisms that become resistant to the biochemical mechanism by which an antibiotic drug kills or severely restricts the proliferative capability of microorganisms. For example, a review of the scientific literature found that studies focused on antibiotic resistance in human health outnumber those related to drug and chemical residues by almost 10 to 1. In addition, there has been a notable increase in reported cases of human illness associated with antibiotic resistance and an increase in documented resistance patterns from veterinary microbiological surveillance data.

Based on that information, the committee decided to focus on the potential for antibiotic resistance as the main food-animal drug issue. The committee updated and consolidated the most recent findings and opinions that address the human health risk or shape perceptions of the risk. It also summarized the science behind the process by which bacteria become resistant to antibiotic drugs and the ramifications for animals and humans.

FOOD-ANIMAL DRUG USE

Intensive production practices in the modern farming industry have created a new set of management concerns and interactions. Animal-to-animal contact is often closer, less space is available, and preventive-health measures are much more important than are therapeutic ones. Antibiotic use with prescription or veterinary oversight is assumed to be, in general, highly accountable. As with many human drugs for which adequate directions can be written for the lay user, some food-animal drugs can be purchased over the counter without a prescription, usually from distributors of animal feed and other animal production supplies. Accountability of use is improved when producers follow industry quality-assurance guidelines and, with the assistance of veterinarians, document the instances of drug use and the practices associated with drug use.

Most drugs used in food animals have a specific purpose: to treat cuts and abrasions, to enhance growth, to fight parasites. Antibiotics are among the few classes of drugs used in food animals both therapeutically to treat disease and subtherapeutically to increase production performance, to increase efficiency of use of feed for growth or product output, and to modify the nutrient composition of an animal product. Therapeutic use generally occurs after diagnosis of disease, and treatment is governed by label instructions. Subtherapeutic use, defined in the United States as the use of an antibiotic as a feed additive at less than 200 g per ton of feed, delivers antibiotics that have therapeutic effects but at dosages below those required to treat established infections. In most cases, subtherapeutic drugs are given to animals in feed or water.

Antibiotics used to improve the health of animals can increase growth rates and thus offer an economic benefit. When antibiotics stabilize animal health, food animals are able to use nutrients for growth and production rather than to fight infection. Subtherapeutic drugs are used in a range of concentrations, which vary with the type of antibiotic, the food-animal species, and the purpose of treatment. The bacterial species affected also vary with the drug used, so the potential for drug use to affect resistance and human disease varies from drug to drug, from dose to dose, and from animal species to animal species.

There is substantial food-animal industry concern that the unavailability of approved antibiotics compromises food-animal production practices in the United States. Many producers believe that, without more antibiotic choices, current production capacity and economic return might not be maintained, animal well-being could decline, and human health could be affected. The human medical community has the same concern about the lack of development of newer antibiotics to treat antibiotic-resistant bacterial infection in people. The human health care community also calls the use of these drugs in food animals into question because of the possibility that drugs used in animals will become ineffective in treating human diseases as a result of drug resistance in pathogens.

APPROVAL AND OVERSIGHT OF FOOD-ANIMAL DRUGS

New developments and FDA regulations have begun to offset the perceived shortage of drug choices for veterinarians to treat food animal diseases and other problems. CVM has authority for approving new food-animal drugs and feed additives and for regulating, tracking, and monitoring their use and their residues. A considerable portion of the monitoring activity, particularly for detecting drug residue violations, is done by FDA in cooperation with the Food Safety Inspection Service of USDA. CVM's mandate, through the Food, Drug and Cosmetic Act, is to make public health its paramount responsibility.

In the opinion of several organizations, regulatory decisions aimed at protecting people, animals, and the environment from harmful food-animal drugs have also produced delays in the approval of effective new drugs. The cost of production has increased for drug developers and frustration with the process has increased as communication between CVM and drug developers has become strained. Some organizations have used the term "crisis" to describe the present lack of choice of pharmaceuticals to administer to food animals when traditional therapies prove ineffective. The crisis reflects the fears inherent in conflicting concerns and the fears that arise when the choices and practices of one stakeholder are restricted by those of other stakeholders.

CVM has responded to industry concerns and to the enactment of new laws by reorganizing many of its operations and streamlining procedures to expedite drug approval even as it continues to meet the federal mandate to protect the public health. When no approved drug is available or when higher-than-approved dosages of approved drugs are needed, veterinarians must use their professional judgment regarding the benefits and risks to sick animals associated with extra-label use of drugs. Extra-label use for analgesic purposes is common because few animal-specific drugs have been approved for the relief of pain and suffering. Extra-label use also is common in the therapeutic treatment of minor species (goats, deer, llamas, fish, exotic pets) of food and companion animals of which the per capita use or consumption is relatively low; drugs approved for common food-animal species are typically used.

Legislative reform occurred in 1996 with the passage of the Animal Medicinal Drug Use Clarification Act (AMDUCA). AMDUCA legalized some aspects of extra-label drug use by giving veterinarians latitude in prescribing drugs for nonapproved species or dosages. Extra-label drug use is allowed only when a well-defined veterinarian–client–patient relationship is established, when drug use is accurately documented, and when accountability is ensured. A national database called the Food Animal Residue Avoidance Databank (FARAD) provides a valid and needed reference for practicing veterinarians with regard to the implementation and success of AMDUCA. Through FARAD, veterinarians can obtain information on specific veterinary and nonveterinary drugs for treating sick animals and recommend appropriate dosing and withdrawal times.

A second law aimed at streamlining the approval process is the Animal Drug Availability Act (ADAA), which was also signed into law in 1996. ADAA was developed to remove barriers in the drug approval process by reducing the stringency of requirements for proof of efficacy, by making clear early in the process which data CVM would require for approval, and by providing more flexible labeling to permit a range of dosages within a given species. Final FDA regulations based on ADAA are anticipated to be available by 1999.

There is still a need in the food-animal industry for FDA to approve more drugs for specific uses, but progress has been made in legalizing the use of medications for food animals under the guidance of veterinarians.

MONITORING OF DRUG RESIDUES

Drug residues in animal-derived food products are an important consideration for consumers. Residues of drugs used in the food-animal industry threaten human health by being acutely or cumulatively allergenic, toxic, mutagenic, teratogenic, or carcinogenic. There is inconclusive evidence that antibiotic residues transferred to humans through food might set up a biological milieu that favors the emergence of microbial strains within a host.

The processes for identifying drug residues and stopping their entry into the food chain were evaluated by the committee on the basis of drug-residue-screening data. There is always a need to increase the specificity and accuracy of screening and testing, and increased research in this regard would facilitate improvements in the monitoring process. Erring on the conservative side, regulatory agencies do find some degree of false-positive drug residue infractions. Food-animal producers generally use drugs responsibly and in keeping with manufacturers' labels. In the view of the committee, residue-monitoring procedures must be and are deployed effectively to protect consumers against possible adverse effects of ingesting small or trace amounts of drug residues. With an effective monitoring and enforcement system in place, an efficient and accountable regulatory system is freer to provide more rapid approvals and greater availability of drugs. However, only the legal use of food-animal drugs can be accounted for; with the availability of some food-animal drugs as over-the-counter preparations, prescription drug use offers the greatest accountability. (Illegal drug use in food animals and its inherent problems were largely outside the charge to this committee.) To judge by the few detected incidents of illegal drug residues in milk, eggs, or meat, the health risk posed by drug residues in foods is minimal and specific.

RESISTANCE TO ANTIBIOTIC DRUGS

With an effective residue-monitoring system in place, the dominant issue in the use of drugs in food animals is the microbial acquisition of resistance to antibiotics. This issue dominates both the drug approval process and the risk–benefit aspect of drug use in food animals, and therefore it was central to the committee's response to its charge.

Microorganisms can mutate to develop or acquire resistance to antibiotic drugs. Several questions determine whether this resistance will result in an increased hazard for humans: First, is the microorganism zoonotic; that is, can it cause a human disease by moving from the animal to a human? Second, are there missteps in the normal safety procedures for processing and handling animal-derived foods that are intended to reduce the risk of transmission of zoonotic microorganisms to humans, whether they are resistant to antibiotics or not? Third, if transmitted to humans from an animal source, is the microorganism more virulent than in its less-antibiotic-resistant form? Fourth, if the microorganism is zoonotic, is the zoonosis treatable with other antibiotics? Finally, are there enough new antibiotics in development to substitute for antibiotics to which microorganisms have become resistant? How these questions are answered determines the extent of hazard to humans.

The committee's findings on antibiotic resistance for food animals are as follows:

• Use of antibiotics increases the risk of emergence of microorganisms that are resistant to specific, and perhaps other, antibiotics. Development of this kind of resistance is not restricted to antibiotic use in food animals; it is far more prevalent because of misuses in human medicine. Issues concerning antibiotic use in food animals and humans should be coordinated—with regard to use patterns, resistance trends, surveillance data, and recommendations for use—in a partnership of regulatory agencies, pharmaceutical companies, the food-animal industry, and animal and human health care professionals.

• The emergence of resistance in bacteria in animals that receive antibiotics is related to the concentrations of the drugs to which bacteria are exposed and also to the duration of treatment or exposure. There are no clear definitions of the duration or dosage at which resistance develops. The FDA definitions of therapeutic and subtherapeutic uses of animal antibiotics are oversimplified; this is important because the extent of drug use affects the propensity for resistance. Generalized assumptions and conclusions pertaining to the risk posed by therapeutic or subtherapeutic use are also oversimplified in evaluations of the human health risk associated with antibiotic use in food animals. Resistance emergence should be classified with regard to each antibiotic used, the concentration and dosage administered, the blood and tissue concentrations attained, the bacterial species or strain affected, and the animal species in which the drug is used. A specific data-driven link should be available to substantiate that the use of an antibiotic at a particular dosage not only promotes resistance but also poses a disease threat to other animals or humans. The definition of resistance is central to documenting changes in patterns and magnitudes of resistance emergence associated with the use of antibiotics in food-animal production.

• A link can be demonstrated between the use of antibiotics in food animals, the development of resistant microorganisms in those animals, and the zoonotic spread of pathogens to humans. The incidence of the spread of human disease in that way is historically very low, but data are seriously inadequate to ascertain whether the incidence is changing. It is difficult to establish whether resistance detection has increased because more antibiotics are needed in food animals or because of the perpetuation of resistant species in food animals, the environment, or other reservoirs. Furthermore, care should be used in evaluating the likelihood of disease spread of this kind because disease incidence is not uniform throughout the human population. Infants, the elderly, and the immunocompromised constitute population groups at greater-than-average risk for infection. Farm workers and pharmaceutical technicians who work with antibiotic compounds, feeds, feed premixes, and concentrates, and people who work with sick and therapeutically treated animals also could be at greater risk for clinical resistance. Resistance in bacteria in farm workers might arise either from contracting an infection with resistant bacteria from a treated animal or from developing resistance in an endogenous pathogen through increased exposure to the food-animal drug.

• A major impediment to determining the effect of antibiotic use in food animals on human health risk is the complexity of food-animal drug treatment and subsequent food-processing and handling interactions. Data suggest that most human disease scenarios associated with food-animal pathogens are related to enteric diseases contracted principally through consumption of pathogen-contaminated foods. The initial event that facilitated the emergence of an antibiotic-resistant microorganism might have been the use of an antibiotic on a farm. Post-farm food processing, storage, and improper handling and cooking are major contributors to the chain of events that allows the pathogen to contaminate the product, proliferate on or in the food, and attain the large numbers that cause disease.

• Substantial information gaps contribute to the difficulty of assessing the effect of antibiotic use in food animals on human health. First, it is unclear that the observed or perceived increases in transference of antibiotic resistance to humans are associated with the use of antibiotics in the food-animal industry. Second, there are no scientific data on resistance emergence and pathogen transfer in situations in which a therapeutic drug intervention is prescribed during subtherapeutic drug use for growth promotion that began in the absence of disease and when no prior disease state existed. Third, there are only sparse data to relate the dosages of a drug necessary to foster resistance to those dosages used and the observed degree of resistance. Fourth, antibiotic use is an integral part of the food-production system in the United States, and it is effective in enhancing growth. Fifth, the detection of antibiotic-resistant microorganisms in treated animals does not automatically imply the presence of disease; many drug-resistant bacteria are not pathogens. Sixth, human oral antibiotic use might predispose some parts of the population to increased susceptibility to enteric clinical infection with food-animal enteric pathogens; there are few data for assessing how genes that code for resistance in bacteria move among and between bacterial species, and there is no concrete information on whether or how nonpathogenic bacteria exposed to antibiotics participate in the resistance emergence phenomenon. Finally, although conservative measures in the food-animal drug approval process might be prudent, until these questions are answered definitely, the quest for new antibiotics for use in food animals must continue. Mechanisms must be instituted to increase research funding to discover new mechanisms of antibiotic drug action; to increase and expedite FDA approvals of new drugs; to provide base funding for the aspects of long-term experimental resistance emergence research and surveillance research that are not likely to be funded by short-term competitive grants; and to develop more precise, accurate, and rapid tests of microbial, pathogenic, and antibiotic-resistant organisms for monitoring purposes.

• Alternatives to antibiotic use for maintaining animal health and productivity—such as new vaccination techniques, improved animal nutrition, and genetic strategies—must be sought. Existing alternatives should be implemented in a practical manner so that the appropriate uses of antibiotics and their effectiveness are maintained. Furthermore, risk factors in the development of resistance other than antibiotic use need to be better understood through increased research.

CONCLUSIONS

The committee concludes that the use of drugs in the food-animal production industry is not without some problems and concerns, but it does not appear to constitute an immediate public health concern; additional data might alter this conclusion. The greatest concern is associated with the use of antibiotics in food animals in such a way that there is a potential for antibiotic resistance to develop in or be transferred to pathogens that can cause disease in humans. This report acknowledges that there is a link between the use of antibiotics in food animals, the development of bacterial resistance to these drugs, and human disease—although the incidence of such disease is very low. A substantial change in the human health risk posed by antibiotic use would affect not only how animal drugs are reviewed, approved, and used, but also how food animals are produced. It should be noted that antibiotics are still effective for their intended purposes at the recommended dosages.

Bacterial resistance to antibiotics will be the most important motivating factor in the development of new drugs to fight infections and in the modification of processes by which drugs are approved. Regulatory agency approval practices have improved in recent years and continue to do so. Reasonable balance in accountability, oversight, and veterinarians' access to alternative drugs has increased with the passage of ADAA and AMDUCA. However, those are only temporary solutions to a continuing problem. Unless new antibiotics become available, even the extra-label use of antibiotics is expected to become ineffective. There is a great need to understand better both the magnitude of the risk and the options available to minimize the risk while maintaining the benefits these drugs confer on agriculture. Constant vigilance in monitoring trends in antibiotic resistance in farm animals and humans is strongly encouraged.

New antibiotic drugs are needed to combat emerging animal diseases that do not respond to traditional drugs and so threaten public confidence in animal agriculture and human medicine. Professionals in human health care should be concerned that they do not have enough specialty antibiotics to treat resistant and emerging infections in humans, as should veterinarians. The question is, should newly discovered medications be held in reserve for human or animal use only? Antibiotics should be available to treat specific human and animal diseases with proper accountability and oversight of the drugs used.

Information gaps hinder the decision- and policy-making processes for regulatory approval and antibiotic use in food animals. A data-driven scientific consensus on the human health risk posed by antibiotic use in food animals is lacking.

MAJOR RECOMMENDATIONS

Development, Approval, and Availability of Food-Animal Drugs

• *The committee recommends that the Center for Veterinary Medicine continue procedural reform to expedite the drug approval review process and broaden its perspective on efficacy and risk assessment to encompass review of data on products already approved and used elsewhere in the world.*

• *The committee recommends that, to improve drug availability, worldwide harmonization of requirements for drug development and review be considered and further enhanced among the federal agencies that are responsible for ensuring the safety of the food supply.*

• *The committee recommends that the Center for Veterinary Medicine base drug use guidelines on maximal safe dosage regimens for specific food animals, consider greater emphasis on the pharmacokinetics of drug elimination from tissues that are consumed in large quantity, and set drug withdrawal times accordingly.*

• *The committee recommends increased funding for basic research that explores and discovers new or novel antibiotics and mechanisms of their action, including the development of more rapid and wide-screen diagnostics to improve the tracking of emerging antibiotic resistance and zoonotic disease.*

Resistance to Antibiotic Drugs

- *The committee recommends establishment of integrated national databases to support a rational, visible, science-driven decision-making process and policy development for regulatory approval and use of antibiotics in food animals, which would ensure the effectiveness of these drugs and the safety of foods of animal origin.*
- *The committee recommends that further development and use of antibiotics in both human medicine and food-animal practices have oversight by an interdisciplinary panel of experts composed of representatives of the veterinary and animal health industry, the human medicine community, consumer advocacy, the animal production industry, research, epidemiology, and the regulatory agencies.*

Alternatives to Drug Use in Food Animals

- *The committee recommends increased public- and private-sector research on the effect of nutrition and management practices on immune function and disease resistance in all species of food animals.*
- *The committee recommends increased public- and private-sector research on strategies for the development of new vaccination techniques, on a better understanding of the biochemical basis of antibody production, and on genetic selection and molecular genetic engineering for disease resistance.*

1

Drugs Used in Food Animals: Background and Perspectives

Today's society challenges the industries that make goods and products purchased by consumers to be open and accountable in their practices. Failure to do so raises questions, concerns, and, ultimately, fears about the decision-making processes that affect public health and public confidence. Public education and mass media communication has led the public to object to practices it perceives as threatening to human health. With a vast amount of data and rapid access to it (for example, through the Internet), some health professionals and consumers are asking legitimate questions about issues that range from environmental pollution to microwave radiation from recreational electronic devices. Agriculture and its food production practices are not immune to public scrutiny. On the one hand, consumers want a wide variety of products at reasonable prices. On the other hand, they demand safe, wholesome, and nutritious food products, and they question agricultural practices that are intended only to increase productivity and economic return for the farm.

In current agricultural practice, raising animals for food depends heavily on the use of pharmacologically active compounds: drugs. The use of drugs in food animals is fundamental to animal health and well-being and to the economics of the industry. However, drug use also is associated with human health effects.

There are five major classes of drugs used in food animals: (1) topical antiseptics, bactericides, and fungicides used to treat surface skin or hoof infections, cuts, and abrasions; (2) ionophores, which alter rumen microorganisms to provide more favorable and efficient energy substrates from bacterial conversion of feed and to impart some degree of protection against some parasites; (3) steroid anabolic growth promoters (whose mechanism of action resides in the interaction

12

of estrogen-, progesterone-, or testosterone-like compounds with specific classes of hormone receptors in animal cells) and peptide production enhancers (recombinant bovine somatotropin for increased milk production in dairy cows); (4) antiparasite drugs; and (5) antibiotics as used to control overt and occult diseases, and to promote growth. There are other drugs that modify the gastrointestinal environment to reduce the likelihood of rumen foaming and bloat in cattle, organic and inorganic water treatments that reduce the chances for water or fish infection in aquaculture, and miscellaneous drugs and compounds used with the advice of veterinarians to treat specific conditions.

There are different ways to view the issue of how animal drug use affects health. Reported benefits are derived largely from the maintenance of good animal health, which lowers the chance that disease will spread to humans from animals. However, drugs used in food-animal production and drug residues in food products could increase the risk of ill health in persons who consume products from treated animals. The use of one class of drugs, antibiotics, could contribute to the emergence of antibiotic-resistant microorganisms in animals that could be transmitted to humans, causing infections that could be difficult to treat.

The public has been concerned about the use of drugs in food animals for a long time. For example, in 1987, three out of five consumers viewed antibiotics in poultry and livestock as a serious health hazard, and an additional one-third of the people asked had some degree of concern about the hazard (Scroggins 1988). Using an historical database derived from frequency of specific topics in news articles and the amount of media attention paid to food safety between 1937 and 1991, the Economic Research Service (ERS) of the United States Department of Agriculture (USDA) reported that concern about pathogens in food was the issue most frequently cited (ERS 1994). The issue was of greater concern than others, including the effects of excess consumption of a food product, pesticide residues, toxic-waste residues, animal hormones, and "unsafe practices."

THE ROLE OF THIS REPORT

The U.S. Congress instructed USDA, through authorizing legislation in the 1990 Farm Bill, to commission a study by the National Academy of Sciences to summarize use of drugs in food-animal production, the practices used to administer these drugs to animals, and the processes for monitoring the drug use and residues in the food chain. In 1992, with funding support from USDA, the Center for Veterinary Medicine of the Food and Drug Administration (FDA), the Pew Charitable Trust, the American Veterinary Medical Association, and the American Feed Industry Association, the National Research Council (NRC) established the Panel on Animal Health, Food Safety, and Public Health under the joint auspices of the Board on Agriculture and the Institute of Medicine's (IOM) Food and Nutrition Board. The panel convened the Committee on Drug Use in Food

Animals.   The committee was composed of private, public, and institutional stakeholders and experts in agriculture, veterinary medicine, human medicine, epidemiology, and economics.   It was responsible for developing a strategy to identify the risks and benefits associated with the use of pharmaceutical products in food animals and for providing a report on these issues that included the following:

- Review of the role and uses of drugs in food-animal production.
- Summary of mechanisms of drug availability, accountability, and monitoring.
- Summary, evaluation, and progress report of the regulatory approval process for animal drug use.
- Summary of data regarding the effects of drug use in food animals on human health.
- Summary of mechanisms of antibiotic availability, accountability, and monitoring.
- Identification of emerging trends and technologies in food-animal production, and alternatives to antibiotic-drug use in food animals.
- Recommendations for research needs and priorities in animal health and drug use.
- Recommendations regarding antibiotic use, availability, and accountability and a strategy for the future.

The issues surrounding the benefits and risks to human health attendant to the use of drugs, particularly antibiotics, in food animals have been the focus of many reports. The committee was faced with assessing risk for a large number of drugs and compounds in food-producing animals and with evaluating drug use and availability, accountability, and regulatory approval.

To help accomplish the task, the committee conducted a review of the scientific literature to identify sources of problems.   A search of scientific databases (AGRICOLA, maintained through the USDA National Agriculture Library, Beltsville, Maryland, 1970 to present; BIOSIS, Biological Abstracts, Inc., Philadelphia, Pennsylvania, 1980 to present) revealed that citations focused on antibiotic resistance to human health outnumbered by almost ten-to-one those related to drug and chemical residues and their effect on human health. For example, within these categories, 1,649 papers were published on antibiotic residues, topical antiseptics, steroid and nonsteroid growth promoters, antiparasitic drugs, animal-directed chlorinated hydrocarbons, sulfa drugs, and arsenical compounds as follows: (AGRICOLA) 585, 3, 110, 8, 48, 7, and 29, respectively; (BIOSIS) 490, 3, 90, 77, 51, 15, and 33, respectively. In contrast, there were 5,755 cited papers in BIOSIS that concerned antibiotic resistance and human health. These results strongly suggest that the greater public health concern with regard to drugs and health risk clearly resides with the use of antibiotics.

The committee also heard testimony on issues related to animal drug use, and it reviewed federal regulations that provide guidelines and list mandatory practices for drug use, monitoring capabilities for drugs and residues in foods, veterinary oversight in prescription drug use, rates of violations and incidences of documented human health problems. The committee concluded that most drugs and drug residues in animal-derived foods pose a relatively low risk to the general public when the drugs are used in a responsible manner consistent with labeling instructions. However, there were mixed concerns about the overall consequences of antibiotic use in food animals. These concerns were centered in conflicting data and views on the influence of antibiotic use on human health, the consequences of their use on animal health, and the economics of food animal production. Health experts expressed concern that animal and human health would be challenged in the future by a growing shortage of antibiotics to treat emerging pathogens that have acquired resistance to the killing effects of many antibiotics in common use today.

After a brief overview of general practices of drug use in food animal agriculture, a summary of the processes through which drugs are approved and made available for use in animals, and a review of the drug residue-monitoring process, the report focuses mainly on the issue of antibiotic drug use in food animals. In later chapters, the potential economic effects of reducing use or banning some antibiotics are presented and alternative management practices to reduce the use of antibiotics in food-animal production are reviewed.

REVIEW OF PREVIOUS REPORTS

Major reports issued on antibiotic drug use in food animals and related topics have been somewhat inconclusive in their findings or are currently outdated. It has been 30 years since the Swann Committee Report (Swann 1969), 17 years since the Council on Agriculture and Science Technology (CAST) report (CAST 1981), and almost 10 years since the IOM report (IOM 1989). For one reason or another, the basic answer to the question of human health consequences of antibiotic drug use in food animals is still not known for certain.

A summary of these and other reports is presented in Table 1–1. The Swann report recommended a ban on the subtherapeutic[1] use of antibiotics in food-producing animals. The results of implementing the Swann report recommendations (where the definition of antibiotic class uses was established along with many of the subtherapeutic applications) on human health and antibiotic resistance (reviewed later in this report) are questionable (Dupont and Steel 1987). There does not appear to be any overall reduction in the rate of emergence of

---

[1]Subtherapeutic concentration of antibiotics in the United States is defined as an amount added to feed at a concentration of <200 g/t (NRC 1980, IOM 1989).

TABLE 1–1 Summary of Previous Major Reports on Food-Animal Antibiotics

Title	Source	Date	Recommendation
The Report to Parliament by the joint Committee on Antibiotic Uses in Animal Husbandry and Veterinary Medicine	English Parliament	1969	Reclassification and use restriction of antibiotics into therapeutic (prescription) and nonprescription feed additives. Nutritional use banned.
The Effects on Human Health of Subtherapeutic Use of Antimicrobials in Animal Feeds	National Research Council	1980	". . . literature . . . is insufficient for assessing the direct relationship between the use of subtherapeutic levels of antimicrobials in animal feeds and the health of humans." ". . . data gathered in the U.K., Germany and the Netherlands do not indicate clearly [that the restrictions placed on these uses in these countries] reduced or averted the postulated hazards to human health."
Antibiotics in Animal Feeds	Council for Agricultural Science & Technology, Report 88	1981	"Studies of long-term administration of antibiotics to humans indicate that infections due to bacteria resistant to antibiotics are dose-related. The literature reviewed showed no such infections with subtherapeutic dosages, but occasional infection with therapeutic doses. Thus it would be irrational to ban subtherapeutic use . . . without also banning therapeutic use."

Human Health Risks with the Subtherapeutic Use of Penicillin or Tetracyclines in Animal Feed	Institute of Medicine	1989	Results demonstrate the selection for resistance to develop with the use of antibiotics on the farm in therapeutic and nontherapeutic dose applications. "[T]he committee was unable to find a substantial body of direct evidence that established the existence of a definite human health hazard in the use of subtherapeutic concentrations of penicillins and tetracyclines in animal feeds." Likeliest estimates for mortality were formulated.
The Medical Impact of the Use of Antimicrobials in Food Animals	World Health Organization	1997	"The use of any antimicrobial agent for growth promotion in animals should be terminated if it is used in human therapeutics or known to select for cross-resistance to antimicrobials used in human medicine."

Sources: Swann, 1969; NRC, 1980; CAST, 1981; IOM, 1989; WHO, 1997.

antibiotic resistance in the United Kingdom from the banning of subtherapeutic use of antibiotics. However, Wegener (Muirhead 1998), in a report to FDA, suggested that, in some European countries, there could be a decline in the occurrence of specific antibiotic resistance (vancomycin-like resistance) in chickens and humans attendant to the ban on avoparcin (a related antibiotic).

Critics of the Swann report cite problems that could help explain the continued persistence of resistance after the ban on subtherapeutic antibiotic use in food animals. Some argue that the recommendations were not systematically and uniformly implemented as intended, and that instances of failure to comply with the recommendations allowed the rates of resistance emergence to continue. Others contend that the real problem resides in the therapeutic use of antibiotics in animals and that, unless there is a total ban on antibiotics in food animals, there will be no reduction in the emergence of resistance. Still others argue that effects do occur, but the use of antibiotics in food animals is largely insignificant in terms of their consequences for human health.

The 1981 CAST report suggested that problems could be identified with the use of antibiotics in food animals (such as resistance development and zoonotic disease transfer in general), but the problems had so little effect on human health (the number of reported clinical cases versus the number of food animals in which antibiotics were used) that they were largely insignificant.

The 1989 IOM report focused on the human health risks of penicillin and tetracyclines used subtherapeutically in animal feed. Several cases of human illness attributable to antibiotic-resistant pathogens that originated in livestock receiving antibiotics were discussed. However, the IOM (1989) committee could find no direct evidence to link subtherapeutic use of antibiotics to a definite human hazard. The report made some mathematical predictions of impact of human health consequences. Its model relied on several assumptions, and the committee that drafted the report readily acknowledged that estimates derived from these assumptions could be further refined, but that relevant data needed to be compiled to accomplish this task.

In 1997 the World Health Organization (WHO) released findings that focused on the subtherapeutic use of antibiotics. Based on the report, WHO concluded that resistance to animal microbes arising from the subtherapeutic use of antibiotics is a high-priority issue. WHO would phase out the subtherapeutic use of antibiotics, particularly those used to treat humans, in food animals.

The present report updates relevant information on the following three issues: (1) patterns of antibiotic use in food animals, (2) mechanisms underlying antibiotic resistance in bacteria, and (3) differentiation of relevant data from opinions that support or refute perceptions of health risks associated with the use of antibiotics in animals as well as particular aspects of antibiotic use in humans. It is important to cite both the data and the gaps in the data that limit a science-driven conclusion regarding the human health effects of antibiotic use in animals. Few projections are made in this report on human health consequences, largely because such projections require the further use of extrapolations and assumptions, still might not answer the question, and could be used out of context. The report makes recommendations that should facilitate the collection and correlation of relevant data that can be accessed by all stakeholders to formulate decision-making policies based on good science and relevant statistics.

THE ANTIBIOTIC ISSUE

Antibiotics are used in food animals for treatment or prevention of disease and for increased production performance or increased efficiency of use of feed consumed by the animal for growth, product output, or modifying the nutrient composition of an animal product. Many times the drugs that improve the health of animals also enhance their growth and production performance because an animal can reduce that portion of the nutrition requirement associated with fighting subclinical diseases and bolstering health defense processes, thereby enhancing the portion of nutrients available for growth and production. Furthermore, there are uses for antibiotics to increase the growth response of animals that are apparently not related to their mechanism of action as drugs that can kill pathogens.

The idea that medical discoveries will defeat whatever threat is posed to animals and humans by infectious pathogens and microorganisms is often taken for granted. Decisions on courses of action are made to obtain outcomes that are beneficial to public health, but the perceived benefits of some decisions often are obscure and in conflict with the priorities of others. The present report stems from concerns—expressed by professionals in human and animal health care, producers of food animals, and segments of the general population—regarding the beneficial and detrimental effects of using antibiotics in food-animal production. The consumables obtained from food-producing animals anchor much of the base of human protein requirements and the needs for other macro- and micronutrients in the United States and many parts of the developed world (NRC 1988). At the heart of the issue are opposing views on the appropriateness of antibiotic drug use in food-animal production. Legitimate questions about the practice are being raised by all sides. Concerns cover a wide spectrum, ranging from the concern that antibiotic use is too permissive to the concern that food production is in jeopardy if drug use in food animals is restricted. Many of the questions regarding this issue are not new, they have been raised before, and they remain largely unanswerable because of the difficulties associated with valid data collection, experimental designs that are nearly impossible to control, and the continuum of microbial adaptation that forces scientists to try to stay apace rather than address future needs.

A Possible Scenario

A dairy farmer has worked for years breeding cattle to achieve the best genetics he can to obtain high-quality milk. A prize calf of the farmer is sick with a bacterial infection and is not responding to any of the traditional treatment strategies of the veterinarian. Elsewhere, a man's immune system is weakened during treatment for a rare form of cancer. His susceptibility to infections is high. Unfortunately, the man has contracted a bacterial infection that must be controlled by antibiotics. The infection is initially unresponsive to "traditional" antibiotics; however, through culture and sensitivity testing, a new-generation antibiotic is found that will ensure the man's longevity. For the farmer, such resources might not be readily available to save the calf, and questions arise as to whether all appropriate measures were taken to prevent the transmission of the organism to other animals on the farm or to the farmer himself.

Questions regarding the appropriateness of antibiotic use in food-animal production and the risks and benefits to human health cannot and will not be answered soon. The issue might be too complex for experimental and epidemiological investigators to generate unbiased study results. Furthermore, some aspects of the research are so expensive that asking who should fund them is a valid question in itself. The data needed to address the issue are sparse, although more aggressive measures for reporting, tracking, and characterizing infections are being used. The lack of appropriate data and the extrapolation of poorly validated data sometimes allow illogical conclusions to be drawn, resulting in fears and demands for regulation that are not founded on scientific information.

The Emergence of Antibiotics in Our Lives

Throughout human history, people have sought remedies for their own ills and those of their animals. Largely through trial and error, and with no knowledge of the biological and biochemical processes at work, people developed herbal and folk remedies that used plants, plant extracts, and fermented food or beverages to relieve their ailments (Florey 1945; Brumfitt and Hamilton-Miller 1988). For example, one German folk treatment was to use the *schaum* or foam from the top of the fermenting vat of sauerkraut, as a drink to relieve pulmonary ailments. Most likely, what was consumed was a broth of penicillin, from the growth of penicillium mold that was effective against an organism causing bacterial pneumonia. The revelation that many diseases were transmitted by bacteria and microorganisms provided an observable explanation for many forms of disease. Serendipity and observation of biological phenomena provided early clues that the presence of some microorganisms prevented the presence or growth of others (Florey 1945; Fleming 1950).

The middle decades of the twentieth century were an exciting time in human and animal medicine because of the scientific processes and new technologies applied to antibiotics and the increased appreciation for their mechanisms of action. Not long after the introduction and widespread use of antibiotics such as penicillin, the realization came that these drugs might not be effective in all situations forever. The term "resistant" came into use to describe classes of bacteria against which an antibiotic was used effectively for some time but became ineffective. Derivatives of classic antibiotics, developed by chemists, provided a quick short-term solution to the resistance problem. Subsequently, bacteria were shown to adapt to these drug-related selection pressures and acquire resistance to multiple classes of drugs.

Researchers in human medicine were not alone in their efforts to exploit the biochemical properties of antibiotics, and the veterinary community soon realized the benefits of using antibiotics to treat diseases in animals. From the 1940s through the 1950s, several reports in the peer-reviewed scientific literature clearly showed that the growth and productivity of animals intended for food were improved with the continuous use of antibiotics. The first true antibiotic with reported efficacy was streptomycin, followed soon after with tetracycline, chlortetracycline, penicillin, and bacitracin (CAST 1981). With the improved health and productivity of farm animals, intensive production practices were developed that allowed food-animal producers to operate more efficiently, as animals were raised more and more frequently in protected, albeit confined, quarters the year around. However, the added intensity and confinement have been partnered with the greater use of low concentrations of antibiotics to prevent or limit disease (CAST 1981; Roura et al. 1992) because of the somewhat higher incidences of naturally occurring diseases, such as respiratory infections in calves and chickens, and because of immune challenge in general. Research on the benefits of antibiotic use in animal feeds, as a disease prevention measure, demonstrated that the effects of these drugs were greater and more apparent in herds with few or no disease control measures (as reviewed by Zimmerman 1986). The higher incidences were not viewed as a problem, however, because continuous, low-concentration antibiotic use was found to maintain or restore the health of animals. As such, the economics of food-animal production depended on antibiotic and antimicrobial drug use in common animal production practices that facilitated the affordable, plentiful supply of meat and eggs, providing the quality, nutrition, and safety that consumers desired.

Less than a decade after the first antibiotics were approved by the FDA for use in livestock (feed applications for enhanced production), concerns arose about the effects of this practice on human health. Initially, concern focused on the issues of antibiotic residues (the drugs themselves or metabolized degradation products of parent drugs) in the food supply and the potential for human pathogens to acquire the antibiotic resistance of animal pathogens. Subsequently, the focus shifted from residues to concerns for human health—specifically to the resistance to antibiotics developed by bacteria that were exposed to the drug in the animal, and survived.

Concern for the consequences of antibiotic resistance in animal agriculture on human health stems not only from what is known about the relationship but also from fear about what is not known. Given some limited facts, authoritative opinions, and some projections on possible—although not necessarily probable—biological events, scenarios can be quickly woven to paint a bleak picture of the future. Consumer interest in this sensationalism was reflected in the summary of popular literature coverage on the topic of antibiotic resistance between 1950 and 1994 in the Office of Technology Assessment (OTA) review of antibiotic resistance (OTA 1995). The OTA report correctly pointed out how synthesized scenarios (in which one is led from the initial use of an antibiotic on the farm, through the development of a resistant *Escherichia coli*, to the development of drug-resistant *Salmonella* by coliform plasmid transfer, to the farmer dying of drug-resistant salmonellosis) are questionably founded in reality.

A comparison of the number of human disease cases confirmed as acquired from animals harboring infectious pathogens and the number of disease cases acquired in hospitals, hints that hospital care poses a greater risk to human health than does the use of antibiotics in food animals. OTA (1995) summarized data from the Centers for Disease Control and Prevention (CDC) supporting the observation that "1 out of 20 patients (2 million per year) acquire infection in the hospital . . . [at a cost of] \$4.5 billion a year in terms of extra treatment. . . . [The infections] directly cause 19,000 deaths . . . and [are] the eleventh leading cause of death in the U.S. population." The number of drug-resistant, hospital-acquired bacterial infections increased close to 300 percent during the 1980s, even with CDC's development and distribution of guidelines for antibiotic use in hospitals and human medicine by the CDC (OTA 1995).

The number of cases of drug resistance in food animals receiving antibiotics is probably much greater than the number of humans developing drug-resistant bacterial disease, but there are fundamental differences in the way that the statistics should be interpreted. Although the use of antibiotics in food animals can cause resistance emergence, not all instances of resistance are clinically significant, not all involve resistance in pathogens, and not all cause actual illnesses. In contrast, because the occurrence of infection in hospitals is often considered life-threatening, the risk to human health of hospital-acquired infections might be thought of as a greater risk. Certainly, the development of hospital-acquired vancomycin resistance in pathogens is a major human health concern largely devoid of input from agricultural sources in the United States (Bingen et al. 1991; Frieden et al. 1993).

Food-Animal Antibiotic Resistance and Human Health

Direct literature citations relevant to instances of transferred antibiotic resistance from animals to humans and development of clinical disease are relatively few, but they do exist. In addition, state and federal public health statistics on food-borne diseases provide useful information to make justified inferences about human health issues related to antibiotic resistance. Some criticisms have implied that public health department conclusions and recommendations on animal drug use are too conservative and that estimates of the effects on public health are unnecessarily high (AHI 1998). However, compiling these data and forming conclusions regarding effects on human health are significant parts of CDC's mission.

Human diseases caused by *Campylobacter* and *Salmonella* serve as a useful example for integrating many of the overlapping issues of animal antibiotic use and human health risk. Most frequently, people become ill after consuming food tainted with these organisms, which originate largely in food animals (ERS 1996b). The statistical databases for both diseases suggest that only a portion of the actual disease occurrences are reported, making the numbers used to state some aspects of risk erroneously low. ERS published a report on the medical and productivity losses associated with bacterial food-borne diseases (ERS 1996b) in which CDC statistics were collected for reported cases and projected unreported cases of salmonellosis and campylobacteriosis. Together, there are an estimated 6.5 million (upper end of the estimate) annual cases of disease occurring from *Salmonella* and *Campylobacter* infections in the United States. Of these, 93 to 95 percent recover fully and require no hospital or physician visit. Five to six percent visit a physician and recover fully. Two percent of the *Salmonella* cases and 0.6 percent of the *Campylobacter* cases require hospitalization. Of these cases, 94 to 95 percent recover fully; 2 to 6 percent die. The occurrence of death is presumed to be associated most frequently with invasive disease that becomes systemic and, to a smaller extent, is further associated with the failure of antibiotic treatment.

A "modern" strain of *Salmonella*, DT-104, is resistant to multiple classes of antibiotics (Glynn et al. 1998). The death rate cited previously is largely affected by how treatable an infection with either of these bacteria is and the success in treatment is dictated by the susceptibility and relative resistance of the bacteria to the antibiotics used. *Salmonella* DT-104 and *Campylobacter jejuni* are becoming increasingly important to human health risk from antibiotic use in animals because with each additional occurrence of resistance to yet another class of antibiotics, the treatment of that infection becomes more difficult and the death rate, and thus, the risk to human health, becomes greater.

These "special" pathogens (e.g., *Salmonella* DT-104) are important. They are among the bacteria that could cause great harm to humans as zoonotic pathogens because of the potential for widespread dissemination and difficulty in controlling infections that become invasive and septic. In the larger setting of the food-animal antibiotic issue, however, the view of several researchers is important in keeping the magnitude of the health threat in perspective. Shah et al. (1993) used in-patient and out-patient hospital infection data as well as in-patient hospital location data to assess some of the relationships between antibiotic health risks to humans. Based on their data collection (incidence of life-threatening and difficult-to-treat infections and the patterns of bacteria and drug-resistant bacteria isolated) they concluded, "if use of antibiotics in the veterinary field [were] to lead to development of (ultimately untreatable) infections caused by multi-resistant bacteria in man, we should be encountering multi-resistant isolates with a higher frequency in community acquired infections than in nosocomial (hospital-acquired) infections." The authors did caution, however, that because some difficult-to-treat pathogens can arise from the use of antibiotics in food animals (albeit at a much lower incidence than for hospital-acquired infections), there is no room for complacency in the use of these drugs in animals, and "close monitoring of antimicrobial susceptibility is warranted."

Human health is intrinsically linked to the health of food-producing animal populations. Factors that affect animal health also will affect human health. That link sometimes leads to conflicting concerns from different segments of the population. The public is concerned about the risks of drug use, residues, and microbial contamination of its food supply, but it also is concerned that the animals produced to supply the food are raised in healthful and humane conditions. The medical community is concerned about the threat of growing antibiotic resistance of human pathogens and about the contribution of antibiotic use in food-animal production to the emergence of resistance in human pathogens. Resistance problems are not solely a concern of the medical community. Animal producers and the veterinarians are concerned that resistance in bacteria in farm animals is interfering with the effectiveness of drugs. They also worry about an impending shortage of effective alternatives for use at therapeutic and subtherapeutic concentrations.

What is the fundamental issue that brought about the commission of the present study? Furthermore, how can the positions of proponents and opponents of large-scale use of antibiotics in food-animal-production practices be summarized? Each question is based on conflicting perceptions: (1) Antibiotic use in animal agriculture is too great, too unregulated, and there is too little accountability—all of which perhaps contributes unnecessarily to a threat to human health. (2) Choices of antibiotics for use in agriculture to ensure animal health and productivity are too few. (3) The process of federal approval to use a drug for a specific purpose in animal agriculture is too rigorous, arbitrary, expensive, and lengthy—all of which impedes the development of new drugs.

Antibiotics are the class of veterinary drugs most widely used in agriculture. However, the veterinary and animal production industries are concerned about the relative lack of approved drugs for use in food-producing animals across the entire spectrum of drugs compared with those for human therapeutic use. On the basis of interpretation of objective data and scientific expertise in the various fields, the committee presents recommendations in this report to improve harmony, understanding, and cooperation among all stakeholders.

The magnitude of drug use in the food-animal industry in the United States is large. The animal populations of various commodity producers are estimated at greater than 100 million beef cattle, 10 million dairy cattle, 10 million sheep, 60 million hogs, and 8 billion poultry. In 1995, those animals supplied 74 billion pounds of meat and poultry, 74 billion eggs, and 156 billion pounds of milk (ERS 1996a). Those commodities contributed more than $87 billion to the nation's economy. To support the industries, 18 million pounds of antibiotics were used in major species in 1985; 90 percent of that was used for subtherapeutic dose applications (IOM 1989). In 1991, approximately 76 million pounds of antibiotics were used for treatment of disease in humans and animals (therapeutic, growth promotion, disease prevention); approximately 25 percent of that was used for food-animal production (treatment, disease prevention, growth promotion) (Carneval, R. 1997. Animal Health Institute, Alexandria, personal communication).

Forty-five years after the initial approval of antibiotic-medicated feeds for livestock to improve overall health and increase productivity, the uses and applications for antibiotics are still growing in animal production facilities in the United States. Some new antibiotics have been developed and incorporated into animal use (for example, ceftiofur, efrotomycin, and a fluoroquinolone), and others have been removed (nitrofurans). Regardless, 60 to 80 percent of all livestock and poultry will receive antibiotics in feed or water or by systemic injection at some time during their production lifespan (IOM 1989). This practice is by choice of the producer (usually driven by economic incentive) where growth promotion is concerned, and by necessity with veterinary input where illness threatens animal well-being and management practices or human well-being. The practice is a strong indication that the economic and management benefits for the producer outweigh the cost of procurement and use.

Concern over the public health consequences of animal antibiotic use, however, also grows steadily among practitioners of human medicine. The public perceives a risk to its health, but in general the perception is diffuse. Specific populations with health problems are more focused on the potential repercussions of antibiotic use in food animals. Risk is certainly greater among persons with immunodeficiency diseases (human immunodeficiency virus positive), patients who receive antineoplastic immunosuppression for cancer therapy, and among a large number of persons with diseases of the endocrine system that reduce natural immunity to infection (Telzak et al. 1991). Individuals who have direct contact with the food animals and the production environment also are identified at higher risk simply because of their increased contact with animals, carcasses, and excrement, for example. As determined by Wall et al. (1994) and Holmberg et al. (1984b), persons who came into contact with domestic or farm animals—especially ill animals—had more infections with the same organisms that affected animals. In fact, pathogen transfer from animals to humans and then from one human to another also can occur, as happened in an infant nursery outbreak in

1980 (Lyons et al. 1980). Therefore, an emerging question is whether immunocompromised individuals with higher risk for exposure to food-animal microorganisms (such as farm families), pathogenic or not, constitute a sensitive population that should be monitored more closely for the emergence of antibiotic resistance from animals?

Since the inception of this report, there have been important changes in perceptions and priorities of federal agencies regarding animal antibiotic use. Those changes are reviewed, and the current focus of several of the federal agencies with responsibility for human or animal health and food safety is described. It appears that some steps are being taken to obtain data to better assess the risks associated with antibiotic use. A prominent part of the process is consideration of active partnering of many agencies and industries to use reduced resources more efficiently for solving problems.

There are risks associated with using antibiotics in animal production as well as not using them. The relationship between risks is dynamic, and the risks dealt with in this report could change, especially as more information is gathered. Through partnership and communication among stakeholders, the effect of the changing of risks inherent in the use of antibiotics can be identified and intervention strategies can be formulated before a true crisis develops.

2

Food-Animal Production Practices and Drug Use

OVERVIEW

Food-animal production has intensified over the past 50 years. The number of livestock and poultry farms in the United States has decreased, but the density of animals on those farms has increased substantially. Production also has become more efficient; a greater quantity of commodities is produced by fewer animals. The increase in efficiency results from several factors, including preventive medicine, genetic selection, and improved nutrition and management. Veterinary medical care in food animals consists of the use of: (1) vaccines and prophylactic medication to prevent or minimize infection; (2) antibiotics and parasiticides to treat active infection or prevent disease onset in situations that induce high susceptibility; and (3) antibiotic drugs and hormones for production enhancement, growth promotion, and improved feed efficiency. This chapter provides a historical description of the major food-animal industries, the challenges faced by each that influence drug use today, and the types of drugs in use and the trends associated with food-animal production. It might appear that some of the data presented are unbalanced with regard to the quantity of information presented and the inferences made regarding health statistics and antibiotic drug use. The imbalance largely reflects the availability of data from quality-assurance programs and feeding and production records.

The structure of the major food-animal industries varies considerably, and this variation has an important influence on accountability (the recorded instances of use, duration, procurement records, containment, security, and appropriateness of use) for use of drugs and the ease of implementing quality-assurance programs within individual industries. The structure of the industries also affects the ease of identifying the source of a problem (whether it is a pathogenic microorganism, a drug residue, or an antibiotic-resistant bacteria) and the ease with which consumer preferences flow back through the system to stimulate changes in the genetics and breeding of stock to produce the desired product.

In all of the animal industries, antibiotic drugs are used for three primary reasons: (1) therapeutically, for treating existing disease conditions; (2) prophylactically, at subtherapeutic concentrations[1] ; and (3) subtherapeutically for production enhancement (increased growth rate and efficiency of feed use). Therapeutic use generally occurs after diagnosis of a disease condition, and treatment is governed by the drug's label instructions or in accordance with extra-label instructions provided by a veterinarian in the context of a valid and current veterinarian–client–patient relationship (VCPR). Subtherapeutic doses are used when pathogens are known to be present in the environment or when animals encounter a high-stress situation and are more susceptible to pathogens. Subtherapeutic doses are smaller than those required to treat established infections. They might also use compounds developed exclusively as production enhancers that have no therapeutic purpose. Although the U.S. Food and Drug Administration (FDA) defines subtherapeutic concentration as <200 g/t of feed, there is a wide range of concentrations below that for which different antibiotics are formulated into feeds and fed to different species.

As summarized in Cromwell (1991), there are three mechanisms of action through which antibiotics appear to enhance growth and production. The first involves direct biochemical events that are affected by antibiotics: nitrogen excretion, efficiency of phosphorylation reactions in cells, and direct effects on protein synthesis. The second involves direct effects on metabolism, including the effects of antibiotics on the generation of essential vitamins and cofactors by intestinal microbes and the way that antibiotics affect the population of microbes that make these nutrients. In addition, the feeding of antibiotics is associated with decreases in gut mass, increased intestinal absorption of nutrients, and energy sparing. This results in a reduction in the nutrient cost for maintenance, so that a larger portion of consumed nutrients can be used for growth and production, thereby improving the efficiency of nutrient use for productive functions. The third proposed mechanism of action is eliminating subclinical populations of pathogenic microorganisms. The elimination of this route of metabolic drain allows more efficient use of nutrients for production.

The goal of an efficient livestock operation is to maintain animals that are free of disease or injury, that gain weight well if they are intended for market, or that stay in optimal condition if they are kept as breeding stock. The producer

---

[1]Antibiotics are used in food animals therapeutically to treat disease and sub-therapeutically (at <200 g/t of feed) to increase production performance, to increase efficiency in the use of feed for growth or output, and to modify the nutrient composition of an animal product.

relies on many methods of disease prevention and treatment. The worst case is having diseased and injured animals deprived of therapeutic treatment. Such a situation results in needless pain and suffering and, in far too many cases, in death. Leaving sickness or injury untreated is the most expensive alternative for the owner and is certainly the least humane for the animal.

The strategies for raising food animals are pertinent to the larger issue of human health effects from drug use in food animals. The intensiveness of farm production in this country has increased because of the advantages inherent in the use of drugs that prevent or control infection and promote growth in animals. Strong incentives for the use of these drugs exist to assure the public that only healthy animals enter the food chain and to maintain the profitability of the industry.

A significant limit to animal production efficiency is any form of disease stress that animals might encounter in their production lives. Traditional growth promoters, such as the steroidal and nonsteroidal estrogenic agents, are less effective when used, because even low-grade disease affects general metabolism. For this reason, pharmacological strategies to prevent or treat animal diseases are used, and the drugs of choice for bacterial infections are antibiotics. Adequate use of antibiotics is necessary for several reasons. Improvements in feed efficiency reduce environmental pollution, for example, through reduced nitrogen and phosphorus losses in animal waste products. Illness in herds and flocks decreases production and nutritional use efficiency (Elsasser et al. 1995, 1997). Klasing and co-workers (1987) suggested that the antigenic challenge of the immune system in animals fighting off disease stress and illness causes repartitioning of nutrients away from growth and production to support the mechanisms that participate in restoring homeostasis and health. Repartitioning of nutrients is a process in which hormone and immune cytokines direct one type of cell to not take up and use a given nutrient and to spare the availability of that nutrient while facilitating other cells (e.g., immune function cells) in increasing their metabolism and uptake of nutrients (Elsasser et al. 1995).

THE POULTRY INDUSTRY

Originating in the 1700s, the U.S. poultry industry grew in size and genetic diversity as chickens were brought to North America on ships from Europe and Asia. In the 1870s, farmers began to select breeding stock, emphasizing specific traits pertaining to meat and egg production. Bugos (1992) outlined the evolution of the broiler and egg-layer industries and the breeding that propelled rapid advances in each. In 1928, before modern breeding began for broilers, the average broiler required 112 days and 22 kg of feed to reach a 1.7-kg market weight. By 1990, broilers required 42 days and less than 4 kg of feed to reach a market weight of 2.0 kg. Laying hens produced an average of 93 eggs per year in 1930, 174 eggs per year in 1950, and 252 eggs per year in 1993. Immediately after

World War II, the broiler industry was concentrated in the northeastern and the midwestern states. However, by 1991, 54 percent of broilers were produced in just four states: Arkansas (16 percent), Georgia (15 percent), Alabama (14 percent), and North Carolina (9 percent) (Knutson 1993). Broiler production in the United States increased from 1.6 billion birds in 1960 to 7.0 billion birds in 1994, a number that corresponds to 13.6 billion kg (30 billion lb) of meat with a value of $10 billion (FSIS 1994b). Annual per capita consumption of poultry meat (chicken and turkey) was projected to be 43 kg (94 lb) in 1995. Similarly, egg production in the United States has grown from 59 million eggs produced in 1950 to 70 million eggs produced in 1994, with average consumption projected to be 240 eggs per capita in 1995. Selective breeding has propelled the poultry industry and allowed the breeders to become relatively independent; at the same time, broiler, layer, and turkey industries have become integrated (Rogers 1993).

An Integrated Industry

Integration is defined as the unified control of several successive (vertical) or similar (horizontal) economic, especially industrial, processes formerly carried out independently. When that definition is applied to the various animal industries, it is notable that the poultry industry is vertically integrated with the exception of the primary breeders who produce the parent strains for commercial production. The swine industry is progressing rapidly toward complete vertical integration. The dairy industry, by its very nature, involves some degree of vertical integration, and the beef and sheep industries remain largely unintegrated. Some effort has been made, starting with the processors, to integrate beef cattle production, but in general the various segments of these industries continue to operate independently.

In vertical integration, the integrator (the poultry company) buys the breeder's eggs that become the parent stock of the broilers and delivers the hatched broiler chicks to others who are under contract to grow the birds, usually in floor pens with 10,000 to 20,000 birds per pen (Lasley 1983). Turkeys are bred and managed similarly to broilers, except that pens of 5,000 to 10,000 birds are more common (Lasley et al. 1983). The integrator maintains ownership of the birds, and supplies the feed and medication to the grower. Integrators also own their feed mills (to control costs and customize feed) where the grain can be purchased in bulk at cost savings to the grower–producer. In addition, integrators own the slaughter and processing facilities, and they generally market the finished product.

Poultry diets, which constitute 68 percent of total production costs, consist of corn and soybean-meal mixtures with vitamins and minerals, and typically include two or three medications (North 1984). Starter, grower, finisher, and layer diets are designed to meet the needs of the birds in each phase of development.

Medications and vaccinations make up 2.16 percent of the total production costs (Agrimetrics Associates 1994).

History and Trends in Drug Use

The growth-enhancing effect of antibiotics was first demonstrated for poultry. Various nutritional studies in chicks showed that antibiotic-fermentation products influenced the growth of chicks (Moore et al. 1946; Stokstad et al. 1949). By 1951, the addition of growth-promoting antibiotics to feed had become standard practice (CAST 1981). The history of antibiotics, growth-promotion compounds, arsenical compounds, and coccidiostats has been reviewed (NAS 1969; Fagerberg and Quarles 1979; CAST 1981; IOM 1989). An earlier review of poultry experiments showed an important advantage in the use of low concentrations of various antibiotics (NAS 1969) that was evident in the superior growth of birds that received antibiotics. The majority of drug use in poultry management practice today is prophylactic, with the bulk of medications encompassing application of antiprotozoal compounds and antibiotic growth promoters.

The poultry production system serves as an interface between animal and human health and affects the environment, so it is important to describe drug use in the context of the overall system as well as to define what process controls are in place to address the safety and quality of the products. In terms of the overall system, intensive management and confinement operations minimize some kinds of infection and facilitate control of others. For example, *Salmonella gallinarum* and *Salmonella pullorum*, which are spread congenitally through the fertilized egg, are controlled by using breeding birds that test negative. Tuberculosis has been virtually eliminated by culling from the flock birds that test positive.

Calnek et al. (1991) assembled a comprehensive treatise on diseases of poultry. Vaccination of day-old chickens controls some viral infections, such as Newcastle and Marek's diseases. Turkeys are routinely vaccinated against Newcastle (5 days of age) and hemorrhagic enteritis (2 to 3 weeks of age), and sometimes against erysipelas, *Bordetella avium,* cholera, and influenza, depending on local experience. Antibacterials and other chemicals are frequently used for controlling other infections such as coccidia, worms, fungi, ectoparasites, and several bacterial infections.

In practice, broiler producers almost always include a coccidiostat (Table 2–1) in grower rations, as well as an arsenical, and an antibiotic (Table 2–2) for improved feed efficiency and body weight gains and for reduced morbidity and mortality. Control of coccidiosis is imperative with modern management systems for broilers and turkeys. Table 2–1 lists 20 coccidiostats labeled for use in broilers (Shepard et al. 1992), 11 of which also may be used in turkeys; only 2 are approved for layer chickens. The ionophores dominate the coccidiostats, but evolution of resistant coccidia has led many broiler producers to alternate

TABLE 2–1   Coccidiostats Approved for Use in Broilers (B), Turkeys (T), and Layers (L)

Sulfonamides	Ionophores	Others
Sulfachloropyrazine (B)	Lasalocid (B)	Amprolium (B, T)
Sulfamethazine (B, T)	Maduramycin (B)	Arsanilate (B, T, L)
Sulfadimethoxine (B, T)	Monensin (B, T)	Buquinolate (B, L)
Sulfamyxin (B, T)	Narasin (B, T)	Clopidol (B, T)
Sulfanitran (B)	Salinomycin (B, T)	Dequinate (B)
Sulfaquinoxaline (B, T)		Nequinate (B)
		Nicarbazin (B)
		Robenidine (B)
		Zoalene (B, T)

Source: Compiled from FDA Approved Animal Drug List (Green Book), 1998a, and Feed Additive Compendium, 1997.

TABLE 2–2   Major Claims of Antibiotics Approved for Use in Chickens and Turkeys

Compound	Growth and Feed Efficiency	Various Infections
Bambermycin	yes	no
Bacitracin[a]	yes	yes
Chlortetracycline	yes	yes
Erythromycin[a]	no	yes
Gentamycin	no	yes
Neomycin	no	yes
Novobiocin	no	yes
Oleandomycin	yes	yes
Oxytetracycline[a]	no	yes
Penicillin	yes	yes
Roxarsone	yes	yes
Spectinomycin	yes	yes
Streptomycin	no	yes
Tetracycline	no	yes
Tylosin[a]	yes	yes
Virginiamycin	yes	yes
Fluoroquinolones	no	yes

[a]Also labeled for use in layer chickens.
Source: Compiled from FDA Approved Animal Drug List (Green Book), 1998a, and Feed Additive Compendium, 1997.

coccidostats in "shuttle" programs. Several turkey farms now use a coccidiosis vaccine with good results.

All of the antibiotics listed in Table 2–2 are marketed over the counter. Several of these antibacterials are labeled for use against some other specific infections, but some viral infections still periodically devastate the industry. For example, in extreme cases of avian influenza, houses can be depopulated and sanitized to eradicate the virus. *Mycoplasma galisepticum* and *Mycoplasma synovia* were ubiquitous and required prophylaxis in broilers, for example, with tylosin or oxytetracycline. On the other hand, mycoplasmas have been controlled in most turkey flocks by using breeders that test negative. According to Shepard et al. (1992), 16 antibiotics are approved for use in broilers or turkeys (Table 2–2), but only 4 of these may be used in layers. In addition, 2 arsenicals are approved for control of blackhead, 4 compounds are available for worms, and 1 fungicide is approved for broilers.

There are three categories of antiprotozoal drugs: ionophores, sulfonamides, and other chemical compounds. They are routinely administered through feed. Some ionophores are not well absorbed across the intestinal wall or are not sufficiently toxic to dictate a withdrawal period and so they can legally be used until slaughter. (Withdrawal is the period required by law between the final administration of a drug and the time when the animal can be harvested for food. The withdrawal period allows drug residue concentrations to fall in the tissue or milk of treated animals to those considered nonthreatening to human health.) Chemical coccidiostats (e.g., amprolium, roxarsone) are most often used in broiler starter diets and traditionally have been followed by ionophores. Most chemical coccidiostats require withdrawal periods.

Antiprotozoal drugs used to combat *Histomonas* infections in turkeys and pheasants are similar to the organic arsenical compounds used in broiler chickens. Nitrarsone (4-nitrophenyl arsenic acid) is the only compound approved to prevent histomoniasis and the subsequent sequella produced by the protozoa in combination with some bacteria. Two other compounds previously approved for this purpose, ipronidazole and furazolidone, were recently removed from the market. Furazolidone is a member of the nitrofuran family of compounds, which were removed from the market by the FDA's Center for Veterinary Medicine because of their carcinogenic potential; however, similar compounds are still in use in human medicine today.

The integration of the poultry industry facilitates tracing a potential residue in meat or eggs to its origin. The integrator companies have much to gain by avoiding altogether any hint of problems, such as drug residues in poultry foods. This constitutes a powerful motivation to control drug and chemical use.

Routes of Drug Administration

Feed

Several diet formulations are typically fed to poultry from hatching to market. Prestarter and starter diets are fed to broilers for up to 19 days after hatching. These diets might contain up to three drug components: (1) a prophylactic coccidiostat, (2) a growth-promoter antibiotic, and (3) an organic arsenical compound that has both growth promoter and coccidiostat activity. A battery of grower diets are fed for the next 8 to 12 days to maintain the metabolic requirements of these fast-growing birds, and withdrawal diets of one or two types are fed in the remaining days before market. Thus, the diets used in each phase are progressively reduced in drug use and cost. To comply with FDA-mandated drug-withdrawal periods, organic arsenical compounds are not used in withdrawal diets.

Most poultry operations routinely monitor withdrawal feed to ensure compliance, for several reasons. First and foremost, monitoring reduces any potential risk that drug residues will remain in tissues, and second, the difference in cost between withdrawal diets and grower diets is substantial. The cost differences might exceed $20/t; if grower feed were fed in place of withdrawal feed, the cost of gain would increase. The industry has adopted what is known as a "two-bin system" for most broiler houses. This system places two bulk tanks at each grower's house and eliminates mixing of withdrawal feed with other types. Further monitoring by tissue analyses is done before slaughter. Fat and other samples are tested for residues of pesticides, herbicides, and heavy metals.

One-Day-of-Age Injection

Two drugs are currently approved (ceftiofur sodium and gentamicin sulfate) for one-day-of-age injection of chicks. Neither drug is absorbed gastrointestinally. Both have been used to protect the poult or chick from injection-site abscesses after vaccination for Marek's disease. Because mass incubation and hatching techniques create significant challenges with aerosols of various genera of *Enterobacteriaceae*, one-day-of-age injections can be used to improve early viability.

Water Medication

Sick poultry are generally medicated through drinking-water systems. Systemic or intestinal medication can be given that way, and the industry has learned how to achieve and maintain therapeutic concentrations of drugs by studying the actual water use for each class of poultry, and accounting for the age of the birds and the environmental temperature. Although the actual overall water-soluble systemic use of drugs in poultry is declining, a recently approved therapeutic-concentration fluoroquinolone antibiotic may now be administered to poultry via drinking water. Summaries of drug use in poultry from 1989 to 1994 are presented in Tables 2–3, 2–4, and 2–5. The amount of antibiotics administered to poultry, especially the amount administered in medicated feeds, declined for the following reasons:

• use of preventive medicine, including implementation of biosecurity procedures, vaccination, genetic selection, and eradication of various pathogens, resulting in specific-pathogen-free stocks;
• reduction in the number of available efficacious compounds for treating respiratory diseases caused by *Escherichia coli* and *Pasteurella multocida*, and for treating other infections such as those caused by *Staphylococcus aureus*;
• efforts to control cost, including improving environmental conditions and culling unhealthy birds;
• concentration and focus on residue avoidance; and
• innovation on the part of manufacturers of vaccines and biological agents to rapidly meet the demands of industry when exotic diseases occur.

These reasons notwithstanding, there is cause for concern in the poultry industry. In recent years only one new systemic antibiotic, a fluoroquinolone, has been approved for treatment of diseases caused in poultry by *E. coli*. The use of that antibiotic is being criticized because its effectiveness as a last line of defense in human antibiotic therapy might be undermined by further FDA approval and use in animals. The removal of the nitrofurans from the market further complicated the situation. When exotic or variant respiratory viruses emerge in an area, septicemic *E. coli* infections cause excessive mortality if no treatment is initiated. In the past, vaccine strategies were developed and implemented to prevent the spread of the newly emerged virus and to decrease the stresses on poultry that facilitate opportunistic secondary bacterial infection such as occurs with *E. coli*.

TABLE 2–3   Cost of Drug and Vaccine Use in Broilers from 1989 to 1994

Treatment	1989	1990	1991	1992	1993	1994
Vaccine (¢/broiler)	0.14	0.15	0.14	0.14	0.13	0.14
Direct medication (¢/broiler)	0.09	0.09	0.07	0.06	0.05	0.06
Feed medication (¢/broiler)	0.58	0.68	0.60	0.56	0.56	0.52
Total (¢/broiler)	0.81	0.92	0.81	0.76	0.74	0.72
Diseased or condemned (%)	1.01	0.96	0.80	0.85	0.67	0.81

Source: Agrimetrics Associates, Inc., 1994.

TABLE 2–4 Turkey Medication and Vaccine Cost Analysis

Treatment	1st Half 1989	1990	1991	1992	1993	1994
Confined hens						
Feed medication ($/t of feed)	2.91	2.93	3.14	3.09	3.171	3.22
Feed conversion (lb feed/lb weight gain)	2.401	2.400	2.380	2.448	2.471	2.397
Field medication						
and vaccine ($/lb)	0.0038	0.0032	0.0035	0.0034	0.0031	0.0035
Feed medication ($/lb)	0.0035	0.0035	0.0037	0.0038	0.0039	0.0039
Confined toms						
Feed medication ($/t of feed)	2.62	2.85	1.64	3.17	3.21	3.03
Feed conversion (lb feed/lb weight gain)	2.686	2.660	2.582	2.579	2.583	2.667
Field medication						
and vaccine ($/lb)	0.0043	0.0039	0.0035	0.0036	0.0034	0.0035
Feed medication ($/lb)	0.0035	0.0038	0.0021	0.0041	0.0041	0.0040

Source: Agrimetrics Associates, Inc., 1994.

TABLE 2–5 Cost of Medication and Vaccination Used for Turkeys and Broilers in the United States

Target Use	Total Live Cost (¢/lb live weight)	Medication[a]		Vaccination[b]	
		Cost (¢/lb live weight)	Percentage of Total Live Cost	Cost (¢/lb live weight)	Percentage of Total Live Cost
Hen turkey	32	0.165	0.52	0.083	0.26
Tom turkey	26	0.231	0.64	0.116	0.32
Broiler	—[c]	0.060	0.22	0.140	0.50

[a]Water-soluble medication only, excluding feed-grade drugs.
[b]Vaccines and vaccine stabilizers.
[c]Total live cost for chicken amounts to 28 ¢/lb live weight.
Source: Agrimetrics Associates, Inc., 1994.

Growth Promotion

The poultry industry no longer uses low concentrations of tetracyclines, penicillin, or tylosin for growth promotion. Arsenical compounds are still used as partial coccidiostats and growth promoters. The primary reason for the use of nonsystemic growth promoters is for specific activity against clostridial species. The current practices of drug use for growth promotion in poultry are (1) use of low concentrations, 1 to 50 g/t; (2) routine use; (3) use of minimally or nonabsorbed drugs; (4) use of antibiotics having activity against Gram-positive organisms; and (5) use of nontherapeutic drugs. These drugs include bacitracins, bambermycins, lincomycin, and virginiamycin. All four of these drugs are classified by FDA as category I drugs, requiring no withdrawal period (Feed Additive Compendium 1995).

Disease Control

The three most serious bacterial diseases in poultry are caused by *Salmonella*, *E. coli*, and *Clostridium*. All have human health implications and highlight the need for safe and effective drugs to control these pathogens in birds as well as for the development of vaccination strategies to prevent clinical infection by pathogens (Cooper et al. 1994).

Salmonella Control

Salmonella infections are a persistent worldwide problem (Houston 1985). The total economic impact of human nontyphoid, foodborne salmonellosis in the United States is estimated to range from $0.6 billion to $3.5 billion annually (ERS 1996b). Efforts to control the spread of *Salmonella* do not have the same momentum in the United States as in Europe. One reason is that more cases of human salmonellosis are reported in Europe than in the United States. About 3 cases per 100,000 population occur in the United States, and at last report, 262 cases per 100,000 occur in Germany. The reasons for the difference are not the subject of this report, but some can be related to food-handling differences and the strains of *Salmonella* that have emerged to infect the human population.

Salmonella control in poultry is a growing concern today, principally because better detection and screening methods are establishing the magnitude of the problem. Also, recent increases in the virulence and in the pathogenicity of many *Salmonella* strains make infections with these bacteria more difficult to control. Official USDA statistics have documented a *Salmonella*-positive broiler carcass percentage rate between 35 and 75. The rate of positives varies by year within the same geographic region and the same processing plant. One major poultry integrator studied 328,000 cultures of *Salmonella* from one processing plant in North Carolina over a 17-year period. The results suggest that cumulative annual rainfall is positively correlated with the incidence of the carcasses, testing positive for *Salmonella* (Colwell and Brooks 1994). The results are supported by the work of Opara et al. (1992) who studied water activity of the litter. On dirt-floor broiler housing, higher water activity of the litter correlates positively with a higher incidence of Salmonella contamination. With careful processing techniques and chlorine rinses, some broiler integrators can achieve as low as a 6 to 8 percent positive incidence of *Salmonella*. In addition, data have been gathered by several large poultry integrators to show that Salmonella-positive flocks are more expensive to raise (Bender and Mallinson 1991).

Escherichia coli Control

E. coli infection in poultry is among the most costly diseases to challenge the industry. The majority of American poultry isolates of *E. coli* are resistant to most if not all of the U.S.-approved poultry chemotherapeutic agents (Raemdonck et al. 1992). The same is true of isolates from Morocco (Filali et al. 1988). Turkeys are equally affected with *Pasteurella multocida* (Walser and Davis 1975) and *E. coli* (Glisson, J. R. 1995. University of Georgia, Athens, personal communication). It has been estimated that 2 to 4 percent of all turkey production losses are due to *E. coli* (Miles and Barnes 1995). Competitive exclusion products (cultures of live mixed populations of normal gut flora that competitively outgrow some undesirable bacteria and, therefore, aid in controlling enteric pathogens) appear to control *E. coli* pathotypes found in poultry (Weinack et al. 1981; Soerjadi et al. 1981). However, they do not inhibit the nonpathogenic commensal *E. coli* present in normal gut flora.

Clostridium Control

Clostridia frequently overgrow normal intestinal flora after infections with the coccidiosis parasite, *Eimeria*. Clostridial infections produce toxins that kill poultry at minimal doses. Coccidiostats are routinely used as prophylactic medication to prevent clinical diseases. Competitive exclusion products appear to control *Clostridium* if the coccidia control is reasonable (Dekich, M. A. 1995. Perdue Farms, Inc., personal communication). *Clostridium* species resistant to bacitracins are emerging in several areas in the United States. Twenty-six isolates of *Clostridium perfringens* were made from poultry in necrotic enteritis outbreaks, and the minimal inhibitory concentration (the concentration of an antibiotic that arrest the growth of a particular organism) was determined for bacitracins, lincomycin, virginiamycin, and penicillin. Preliminary data collected by Cummings et al. (1995) were interpreted by those authors to suggest a trend of increasing resistance to bacitracins and lincomycin in the *Clostridium perfringens* isolates. Most isolates showed sensitivity only to virginiamycin and penicillin. Probiotic organisms such as *Lactobacillus* spp. are efficacious under specific conditions. Those conditions include monocultured birds challenged with *Clostridium perfringens* (Fukata et al. 1991).

In the future, much of the effort to control pathogens in food animals, including poultry, will depend on the increased use of vaccination programs. Advances in molecular biology will permit specific pathogen antigens to be cloned and synthesized, facilitating their use in vaccines to stimulate the animal's own natural defense mechanisms.

THE SWINE INDUSTRY

In 1900, approximately 90 percent of U.S. farms maintained hogs. That percentage fell to 25 percent in 1969 (Hayenga et al. 1985). More than 3 million farms had hogs in 1950, but fewer than 250,000 had hogs in 1992 (NPPC 1994), and fewer than 100,000 are expected by the year 2000 (Hurt et al. 1992). However, the total number of hogs slaughtered in the United States has remained relatively constant, fluctuating between 1950 and 1992 from a low of 70 million (1975) to a high of 97 million (1980). Fewer farms are producing about the same number and total weight of hogs to meet consumer demands of 8 billion kg (17 billion lb) of total pork, or 31 kg (68 lb) of pork per capita, annually.

Substitution of capital for labor was the major force that led to fewer, larger, and more specialized farms. From the standpoint of economics, larger swine farms run more efficiently than do smaller units. Farms with 10,000 hogs enjoy nearly one-third greater efficiency than do those with 3,000 (Hurt et al. 1992).

Eight major breeds contribute to the U.S. hog herd, but marketed hogs are the result of crossbreeding in an effort to capture the best traits from each breed and some heterosis as well (Fredeen and Harmon 1983; NPPC 1994). Heterosis is the beneficial result of animal crosses in breeding to increase disease resistance, growth characteristics, and other physical qualities. Multinational companies offer genetically consistent hogs that produce more lean pork on less feed. Consumer preferences are relayed effectively through the pork processors to the producers on specialized farms, which now produce nearly identical animals delivered to slaughter. Slaughter facilities are now located near the hog farms and have started to move regionally from their traditional location in the Midwest to the Southeast. Iowa is still ranked first in swine production (approximately 25 percent of the market); North Carolina is now ranked second (13 percent) (ERS 1996a).

Marketing of hogs is changing from open markets, where farmers sell hogs to the highest bidder and where the quality of the hog has little effect on price, to contracts by which processors pay farmers a fee plus performance incentives to feed hogs to market weight (Barkema and Cook 1993). To achieve even greater control, a few processors raise and feed their own hogs in a vertically integrated production system similar to that for broiler chickens. These structural changes now in progress in the pork industry have profound implications. The processor will be more sensitive than is a more distant producer to the potential ramifications of drug residues in pork, and tracing a residue to its origin will be facilitated by contracts and integration. Lifetime identification of food animals was recommended previously to facilitate tracing contaminations to their origins (NRC 1985).

Although some farrowings (the process of birthing piglets) are still in small houses on pastures, about 80 percent are in confinement (FSIS 1992) to better manage the environment, and the vast majority are in farrowing crates to optimize survival of the piglets. Commonly, after farrowings the farrowing house is emptied, pressure cleaned with hot water, and disinfected to minimize subsequent infections and optimize productivity. Pigs are weaned at 3 to 5 weeks of age to maximize the number of piglets born per sow per year. Research continues on ways to reduce the age at weaning to as little as 5 to 6 days to control more effectively several of the major infectious diseases of sows and piglets (Dial et al. 1992). Such control involves antibiotic medication of the sows before farrowing and the piglets until after weaning.

In the various management systems, weaned pigs might be moved to a nursery, a grower, or a feeder–finisher facility. Although more than three-fourths of the hogs are produced on "farrowtofinish" farms (FSIS 1992), some producers sell feeder pigs at 8 to 9 weeks of age (about 23 kg [50 lb] of body weight) for finishing on other specialized farms. Market hogs weigh about 114 kg (250 lb) at 4.5 to 6.5 months of age (NPPC 1994).

Disease Control and Use of Drugs and Chemicals

Pork producers and herd veterinarians view human food safety as an integral part of total herd health programs. Producers pay strict attention to the health of their herds, taking precautions and using a variety of management practices to protect herd health. Individual herd health programs are developed in close consultation with veterinarians.

Antibiotic drugs are used in pork production for disease prevention, treatment of disease, and growth promotion. The management system in place for individual swine production operations will determine the antibiotic used and the quantity.

In the extensive management of hogs until after World War II, common diseases, such as erysipelas and cholera, were controlled by vaccinations, slaughter, or treatment of individual hogs (Fredeen and Harmon 1983). Epidemics of the common infectious diseases were kept in check by stocking with low-density population. However, in the intensive management of common diseases today hogs usually are given subtherapeutic concentrations of antibiotic drugs in feed. Shepard et al. (1992) listed 29 antibiotic drugs approved by FDA (21 antibiotics and 8 chemotherapeutics).

Thus, in addition to antibiotics, antiparasitics are another major category

TABLE 2–6   Major Claims of Antibiotics Approved
for Use in Hogs

Compound	Growth and Feed Efficiency	Various Infections
Amoxicillin[a,b]	no	yes
Ampicillin[a,b]	no	yes
Apramycin	no	yes
Arsenilic acid	yes	yes
Bacitracin	yes	yes
Bambermycins	yes	no
Chlortetracycline	yes	yes
Efrotomycin	yes	no
Erythromycin	no	yes
Gentamycin	no	yes
Lincomycin	no	yes
Neomycin	no	yes
Oleandomycin	yes	no
Oxytetracycline	no	yes
Penicillin	yes	no
Spectinomycin	no	yes
Streptomycin	no	yes
Tetracycline	no	yes
Tiamulin	yes	yes
Tylosin	yes	yes
Virginiamycin	yes	no

[a]Only in combination with chlortetracycline and penicillin.
[b]Available by prescription only.
Source: Compiled from FDA Approved Animal Drug List (Green
Book), 1998a, and Feed Additive Compendium, 1997.

of drugs for hogs.   Nine chemical entities are approved in the United States
(Shepard et al. 1992), several marketed by more than one company and in forms
suitable for use in feed or by injection.   They are recommended routinely for
breeding animals, when new animals are introduced into a herd, and when weaned
animals enter the feedlot.   Controlling helminths is the principal objective, but
insects also must be controlled.   In general, although parasites can severely
restrict productivity in hogs, several bacterial and viral infections are more cata-
clysmic (see Tables 2–6 and 2–7).

Growth and Metabolic Performance

Hog performance (growth rate and feed efficiency [pounds of feed consumed for a gain of 1 pound in carcass or body weight]) is improved with the use
of subtherapeutic concentrations of any of 12 antibiotic drugs with claims for

TABLE 2–7   Major Claims of Chemotherapeutics
Approved for Use in Hogs

Compound	Growth and Feed Efficiency	Various Infections
Arsanilate sodium	no	yes
Arsanilic acid	yes	yes
Carbadox	yes	yes
Roxarsone	no	yes
Sulfaethoxypyridazine[a,b]	no	yes
Sulfachlorpyidazine	no	yes
Sulfamethazine	no	yes
Sulfathiazole[a]	no	yes

[a]Only in combination with chlortetracyline and penicillin.
[b]Available by prescription only.
Source: Compiled from FDA Approved Animal Drug List (Green
Book), 1998a, and Feed Additive Compendium, 1997.

increased rate of gain or improved feed conversion. An important result of subtherapeutic use is reduced morbidity and mortality in growing pigs (Cromwell 1991). In breeding animals, feed-additive antibiotic drugs improve farrowing rate, litter size, birth weight, and pigs weaned per litter; and they reduce the incidence of mastitis (bacterial infection of the mammary gland), metritis, and agalactia. It is not surprising, therefore, that antibiotic drugs are used in about 90 percent of starter feeds, in 75 percent of grower feeds, in more than 50 percent of finisher feeds, and in at least 20 percent of sow feeds (Cromwell 1991). Although antibiotic resistance emerges in herds medicated continuously (Tribble 1991), the procedure does not seem to diminish the enhanced productivity effects (Cromwell 1991).

In swine production today, producers vaccinate piglets for some or all of the following diseases or microbes: erysipelas (46 percent), atrophic rhinitis (42 percent), *Pasteurella* pneumonia (28 percent), *Haemophilus* pleuropneumonia (13 percent), *Streptococcus* infections (12 percent), *E. coli* scours, and *C. perfringens* infections (FSIS 1993a). The piglets are castrated by the age of weaning (90 percent), given iron supplements and have tails docked (80 percent), treated for worms (48 percent), treated for mange and lice (40 percent), and given antibiotic injections (33 percent). Among sows and gilts, 60 to 70 percent are vaccinated for leptospirosis, parvovirus, and erysipelas; 50 percent for *E. coli* scours; 33 percent for atrophic rhinitis; and more than 20 percent for transmissible gastroenteritis, *C. perfringens* infections, and pseudorabies (FSIS 1992). Eighty-five percent of sows and gilts are wormed, and 72 percent are treated for mange and lice.

THE DAIRY INDUSTRY

Milk cows were brought to the United States in the 1600s. The dairy industry has changed considerably since then. In 1910, more than 20 million cows
were maintained on 5 million farms, averaging 4 cows per farm. In 1993, a total
of 9.6 million dairy cows were on 159,450 farms (FSIS 1994b). Yet production
of dairy products has increased substantially. Milk production increased from 61
million kg (135 million lb) in 1984 to 70 million kg (154 million lb) in 1994,
while the total number of milk cows decreased by approximately 1.2 million.
Milk production increased from 5,598 kg (12,316 lb) per cow in 1983 to 7,478 kg
(16,451 lb) per cow in 1995 (ERS 1996a).

Consumers drink an average of 104.5 kg (230 lb) of milk and eat approximately 12 kg (26 lb) of cheese, 7.3 kg (16 lb) of ice cream, and 2.3 kg (5 lb) of
butter per capita annually. Providing consumers with milk, cheese, ice cream,
and other dairy products involves collaboration among several specialized sub-
units, including the dairy farm, state health department, milk hauler, processing
plant, and distributor.

Dairy farms are partially vertically integrated in that the dairy producer
controls the genetic selection of breeding stock, breeds the animals, raises the
young stock, manages the producing animals, and sells the raw product. The
processors and distributors are generally independent of the producer, although
some large processors are producer-owned cooperatives. Animal health is closely
associated with milk production and the profits subsequently generated. Therefore, it is important that dairy farmers in conjunction with herd veterinarians
practice sound management and health programs to maintain optimal herd health.
As with the other food-animal species, prevention is the key to the control of
diseases in dairy cattle; however, maintaining a healthy herd is also highly dependent on therapeutic drug use to treat such diseases as laminitis, anaplasmosis,
pinkeye, coccidiosis, foot rot, metritis, respiratory infections, dystocia, enteritis,
and, of course, mastitis.

According to a 1991–1992 survey (FSIS 1993b), 90 percent of dairy calves
are removed from their dams within 24 hours, and essentially all heifer calves are
given colostrum from the first milking to provide maternal antibodies and thus
passive immunity. Most calves are housed individually in hutches or in pens in a
barn and are fed milk until 6 to 8 weeks of age. After weaning, calves are usually
raised in groups, dehorned, have extra teats removed, and are identified, usually
with ear tags. Severe diarrhea (scours, 53 percent) and respiratory infections (21
percent) are the major causes of death before weaning, and between weaning and
calving (11 percent and 31 percent, respectively). These two health problems
together caused the death of 1.2 percent of all heifers—more than half of the total
mortality losses (FSIS 1993b; APHIS 1993).

TABLE 2–8 Intramammary Antibiotics Approved for Dairy Cattle

Compound	Rx[a]	OTC[b]	Lactating Cows	Dry Cows
Amoxicillin	yes	no	yes	no
Cephapirin	no	yes	yes	yes
Cloxacillin	yes	no	yes	yes
Erythromycin	no	yes	yes	yes
Hetacillin	yes	no	yes	no
Novobiocin[c]	yes	yes	yes	yes
Oxytetracycline	no	yes	yes	yes
Pirlimycin	yes	no	yes	yes
Penicillin	no	yes	yes	yes
Penicillin/Novobiocin	no	yes	yes	yes
Penicillin/Streptomycin[d]	yes	yes	yes	yes

[a]Rx = Available by prescription.
[b]OTC = Available over the counter.
[c]OTC for dry cows and Rx for lactating cows.
[d]OTC for low doses and Rx for high doses.
Source: Adapted from FDA Approved Animal Drug List (Green Book), 1998a, and Feed Additive Compendium, 1997.

Disease Control and Prophylactic Treatments

Most dairy producers vaccinate heifers for diseases such as leptospirosis (81 percent), infectious bovine rhinotracheitis (IBR, 90 percent), bovine viral diarrhea (BVD, 87 percent), parainfluenza type 3 (PI3, 85 percent), bovine respiratory syncytial virus (BRSV, 66 percent), and brucellosis (65 percent). In addition, 54 percent are given coccidiostats in their feed and 60 percent are wormed. Dairy farmers also vaccinate more than 30 percent of nonlactating cows for leptospirosis, IBR, BVD, and PI3; and 22 percent for BRSV. Parasiticides are used extensively, mostly in heifers for control of coccidia and nematodes.

Therapeutic Treatment of Disease

Although vaccinations are a major means of controlling viral and bacterial infections in dairy herds, diarrhea and respiratory disease are the most common illnesses among calves and heifers. Therapeutic use of drugs is called for in the treatment of such reproductive problems as retained placentas and metritis. Among the diseases afflicting dairy cattle, mastitis is recognized as the most costly. In fact, intramammary infection (Table 2–8) is the most costly disease to U.S. animal agriculture. In Table 2–9, health costs for dairy animals are divided by functional category (Shook 1989). The mammary-gland category is the largest, accounting for approximately half of the total health costs for the dairy cow.

TABLE 2–9   Distribution of Health Costs ($) per Cow by Functional Category[a]

Category	Labor[b]	Expense[b]	Total[b,c]	Expense (Least-Squares Solution)[d]
Mammary	48.3	23.76	30.20	17.80
Reproductive	17.3	8.93	11.24	11.75
Locomotive	32.2	1.08	5.37	3.74
Digestive	3.7	1.13	1.62	0.40
Respiratory	1.8	1.16	1.40	0.51
Other	13.6	5.83	7.64	3.38
Total	116.9	41.89	57.47	37.58

[a]Compiled by Shook (1989).
[b]From Hansen et al. (1979).
[c]Total includes expense plus labor at $8.00/hour.
[d] From Shanker et al. (1982).

More than 80 percent of dairy farmers used veterinarians to treat sick animals and supply drugs relating back to a high level of accountability for drug use in the dairy industry. However, a substantial number of farmers also obtained drugs elsewhere. In most rural agricultural regions of the nation, many FDA-approved drugs are available over the counter at feed supply, milk plant cooperative, or general farm supply stores. In the dairy industry, as well as in all other food-animal industries, the availability and use of antibiotics make it more difficult to produce accurate statistical documentation of drug use and disease incidence.

Questions have been raised about the appropriateness of over-the-counter drug availability. However, with the dairy industry as an example, most dairy farmers are very good at recognizing commonly-encountered illnesses in their cows and calves, and they opt for the convenience of treating the animals as the need arises. This is rather successful for the dairy industry because of the active residue surveillance program and the penalties associated with drug use violations (discussed in detail in subsequent chapters). As a result, difficulties in tracking and predicting the emergence of drug resistance are increased.

Mastitis was found to be second only to milk yield in explaining variance in profit (Andrus and McGilliard 1975). Annual losses due to mastitis shown in Table 2–10 average $184 per cow (DeGraves and Fetrow 1993). Thus, with a current cow population of approximately 9.6 million, the annual cost of this disease to the dairy industry approaches $2 billion. This figure is approximately 11 percent of the total value of farm milk sales.

Organisms present in milk from mastitic cows pose little threat to human health. The bacteria that commonly cause bovine mastitis seldom cause disease in humans. Some strains of *Staphylococcus aureus*, a common cause of mastitis,

TABLE 2–10   Estimated Annual Losses Caused by Mastitis[a]

Source of Loss	Loss per Cow ($)	Percentage of Total Loss
Reduced production	121.00	66.0
Discarded milk	10.45	5.7
Early cow replacement cost	41.73	22.6
Reduced cow sale value	1.14	0.1
Treatment	7.36	4.1
Veterinary services	2.72	1.5
Total loss	184.40	100.0

[a]Assumptions: One-third of cows infected in an average of 1.5 quarters; milk loss 856 lb per infected quarter; milk price $12.07/100 lb of milk.
Source: Dairy Field Day, Coastal Plain Experiment Station, Tifton, Georgia, June 1994.

can produce enterotoxins that cause nausea, vomiting, abdominal cramps, and diarrhea when ingested. However, if milk is cooled properly, pasteurized, and handled correctly thereafter, the danger of toxin formation is remote.

An important public health concern is the potential for antibiotics used in mastitis treatment to remain as residues in milk or meat. Careful use of antibiotics (avoidance of products not approved for use in dairy cattle, use of proper dosages, and compliance with withdrawal times specified on product labels) is intended to minimize the potential for antibiotic residues to carry over into meat and milk. Given the potential for drug residues in dairy products, the industry is seeking alternatives to antibiotic use in herd health programs.

Antibiotic Drug Use

A comprehensive program of mastitis control has been adopted for reducing the incidence of intramammary infections in dairy cows. The key is prevention of the disease, and prevention is best accomplished by improving milking hygiene and decreasing exposure to pathogens between milkings. However, new infections still occur and must be eliminated to reduce the overall incidence of mastitis in the dairy herd.

Established infections caused by major udder pathogens can be eliminated by spontaneous recovery, culling of chronically infected cows, treatment during lactation, and treatment at time of drying off (Philpot and Nickerson 1992). Spontaneous recovery occurs when the infected cow is cured of an intramammary infection without medical intervention; however, that phenomenon takes place at most in 20 percent of established infections. The majority of spontaneous recoveries occur in mammary gland quarters with mild or recent cases of mastitis and only rarely in quarters with well-established or chronic infections. Culling is often used as a last resort to eliminate chronic infections from herds that are unresponsive to therapy. Consideration should be given to culling those cows whose continued presence in the herd constitutes a reservoir of infection that might ultimately spread to uninfected cows.

Obviously, spontaneous recovery and culling have serious limitations in terms of usefulness for eliminating established infections. Drug therapy remains the principal alternative for eliminating existing infections in a herd. During lactation, treatment is efficacious against some mastitis-causing bacteria and poor against others. Most preparations have been designed with little or no attention to the natural defense mechanisms operating within the udder. In addition, several host factors might influence or be influenced by antibiotic therapy. Thus, because of treatment failures, new strategies are needed to improve cure rates for existing mastitis and to reduce the incidence of new infections.

Production Enhancers

The potential to exploit hormone-dependent mechanisms to increase the production of milk has been understood for several decades. Some 50 years ago, research showed increased growth rates in rats injected with a crude pituitary extract. Later it was discovered that the extract, which contains a protein hormone called somatotropin, also affects lactation, and research with lactating cows ensued. Before the 1980s, progress was slow in bovine somatotropin (bST) research because the availability of bST was restricted to that which could be extracted from pituitary glands of slaughtered animals, limiting studies to a few cows and short time frames (OTA 1991).

In the late 1970s, new research showed that the physiological basis for more efficient milk production in genetically superior cows was the better use of absorbed nutrients. Scientists recognized the need for new concepts regarding nutrient regulation in animals. More recent work demonstrated that somatotropin exerts key control over nutrient use. When administered exogenously, either pituitry-derived or the recombinant DNA-derived analog markedly improves milk production efficiency in lactating cows. In the last decade, the refinement in production technology and development of easily used delivery technologies (i.e., long acting hormone delivery implants) has established an important role for somatotropin in the dairy industry. Today recombinant DNA-derived somatotropin is approved by FDA for use in dairy cattle to boost milk production.

THE BEEF INDUSTRY

Although cattle were brought to America in the 1620s, the practice of animal husbandry was not widespread (Thompson 1942) by current standards. By the time interest in improved cattle evolved in America, stockmen could import breeds that emerged in Europe after Robert Bakewell (1725–1795) demonstrated the improvement in cattle through controlled breeding (Thompson 1942). From that period until after World War II, pure breeds were the focus of beef breeding. Crossbreeding, originally developed for adapting types of cattle for the Gulf Coast region, currently provides heterosis and genetic variation, which are needed for optimal performance in various environments. New European breeds were introduced in the 1960s, and consumer demand for less fat caused breeders to change from small-framed, early-maturing cattle to larger cattle having less fat deposition at market weight. Consumption of beef declined slightly from 48 kg (106 lb.) per capita in 1984 to 42 kg (93 lb.) in 1994. More than 10.5 billion kg (23 billion lb) of beef was produced in the United States in 1994.

The number of cattle fluctuated from 63 million to 100 million between 1925 and 1994 (FSIS 1994c). Breeding-cow herds vary greatly in size. About half have 10 to 99 cows, but 12 percent have more than 500 and 10 percent have fewer than 10 cows (FSIS 1993a). Nearly 75 percent of beef calves are born between February and May. More than 80 percent of the farms have mixed-bred cows; only 4 percent have purebreds exclusively.

At 2 to 4 months of age, calves typically are sorted by sex (bulls destined to be steers are castrated and dehorned) and tagged for identification. In 1992, on average, calves were weaned at about 7 months, when they weighed about 227 kg (500 lb) (FSIS 1993a). Ideally, for about 45 days after weaning (a period called backgrounding), calves should be fed a high-protein, high-energy concentrate and given access to high-quality hay and pasture to optimize their transition to the next phase. Following this period, calves might be fed on pasture or range similar to that for the breeding herd. More typically, they are shipped (often hundreds of miles) to stock farms, where they are fed for growth (not finishing) for up to 1 year on small grain pastures or corn or sorghum stubble (Boykin et al. 1980).

Feeding cattle in western and midwestern feedlots became much more common with the availability of inexpensive grains during the 1960s. Forty years ago, nearly all cattle were fed on small farms, mostly in the north-central region of the country. Today, feedlots are concentrated in the western corn belt, the eastern Great Plains, and the High Plains of Texas. Most feedlot cattle are purchased at auction or through order buyers (VanArsdall and Nelson 1983).

Until the 1960s, most cattle were moved large distances to slaughter plants near major population centers (Koch and Algeo 1983). More recently, meat packers have moved closer to where cattle are fed, providing advantages in labor, waste management, transportation, and efficiency. Most cattle are purchased by meat packers directly from feedlots. Packers distribute more than 95 percent of the beef in boxes directly to retail stores and fast-food chains (Knutson 1993).

Vertical integration, which typifies the broiler industry and is increasing in the hog industry, has not made much progress in the beef industry. Given the relatively disjointed structure of the beef industry, animals can be traced from the slaughter plants to the feeder and sometimes to the stock farm, but only rarely to the farm of origin.

Disease Prevention

To safeguard against disease emergence during periods of stress, calves are given vaccinations against respiratory (for *Clostridium* and respiratory-disease complex) and gastrointestinal (primarily viral) diseases, and they are treated for worms and ectoparasites. After shipping, on entry into the feedlot, cattle are typically vaccinated again for *Clostridium* and respiratory-disease complex, further treated for worms and ectoparasites, and given a steroid-type implant for growth promotion. For 28 to 65 days they also are given a prophylactic combination of tetracycline and sulfamethazine to prevent disease during the initial stressful period accompanying feedlot entry. Other antibiotic drugs are fed throughout the finishing period, including ionophores to improve feed efficiency and growth rate and tylosin to prevent liver abscesses (Koch and Algeo 1983).

The following measures can be taken to prevent diseases in beef cattle:

• use of adequate and balanced nutrition, which is essential for optimal immune functioning in animals;

• elimination or reduction of the population of vectors, for example, the face fly, which transfers pinkeye; the mosquito, which transmits anaplasmosis; and the culicoid, which transmits bluetongue;

• good pasture management, such as weed control, rotational grazing, adequate fertilizing, fresh water, and fenced-out muddy areas to help control disease infestations and prevent stress, which might leave animals, especially newborns, weak and more susceptible to disease; and

• keeping the facilities and environment as clean as possible. Any invasive procedure, such as that requiring an esophageal tube or a syringe, should be done with clean hands and clean equipment to avoid human transmission of disease.

Trends in Drug Use

Anabolic compounds are widely used to promote weight gain and feed efficiency in cattle. Most are derivatives of reproductive steroid hormones (estrogen, progesterone, or testosterone) and generally work by interacting with specific steroid hormone receptors (Hancock et al. 1991). Residue data indicate a wide safety margin for human health in the use of those drugs in cattle (Henricks et al. 1983). Some data indicate that increases in estrogen residues from implanting steers are no greater than are those found in heifers at some stages of the natural estrus cycle (Henricks et al. 1983).

Some of the most devastating cattle diseases, such as foot-and-mouth disease, brucellosis, and tuberculosis, have been controlled through national eradication and surveillance programs. Others, such as clostridial infections, are controlled by vaccination. Respiratory diseases are managed by mass vaccinations and treatment of affected individuals. Such diseases as diarrhea are managed by treatment of individual calves.

Because the largest potential for creating drug residues in beef tissues arises from treatment of cattle in feedlots, feedlot operators emphasize control of infectious diseases at the time cattle enter the lot, 2 to 4 months before slaughter (the duration of this period depending mostly on the price of grain and on market prices for finished cattle). Various feed additives (Tables 2–11 and 2–12) and implant treatments are approved for use throughout the feeding period. Eight feed-additive antibiotics are labeled for improved growth or feed efficiency. Shepard et al. (1992) also list 11 antibiotics with no claims for growth or feed efficiency, 18 parasiticides and 6 sulfonamides for cattle, and 3 estrus synchronizers for beef cattle and dairy heifers. The parasiticides include 11 wormers, 2 coccidiostats, 4 ectoparasiticides, and 1 endectocide. Additionally, insecticides and insecticidal ear tags for beef cattle are approved by EPA.

Therapeutic Drug Use

Therapeutic use of drugs in cattle is often necessary. Most commonly drugs are administered for enteric and respiratory diseases in calves and feeder cattle, and for reproductive infections in breeding herds. Although therapy is more expensive than preventing disease and injury through the use of healthful conditions and vaccination, it is necessary when these measures fail. The costs incurred are for:

* medication;
* visits by the veterinarian;
* additional time required to move infected animals to and from the treatment area;
* segregation of infected animals, which might involve separate feeding, watering, shelter, and observation;
* weight loss;
* reduced value of chronic cases that never return to their original condition; and
* death.

Feeding low concentrations of antibiotics to cattle with the intention of increasing the dose as signs of disease occur is different from subtherapeutic feeding to increase weight gain. The method of administration is through feed rather than injection, but the intention is therapeutic. Cattle are sometimes fed low concentrations of antibiotics during particularly stressful times when they are most apt to get sick—for example, at weaning or after being shipped a long distance. That regimen might be used for 2 or 3 weeks. Data from the former National Cattleman's Association (1995) suggest that penicillins are not used for growth promotion in cattle and that the use of tetracyclines is in sharp decline as

TABLE 2–11   Major Claims for Systemic Antimicrobials Approved for Use in Beef and Dairy Cattle

Compounds	Respiratory Infections	Diarrhea	Mastitis	Other Infections	Growth and Feed Efficiency
Antibiotics					
Amoxicillin[a,b]	yes	yes	no	yes	no
Ampicillin[a,b]	yes	no	no	yes	yes
Bacitracin	no	no	no	yes	yes
Ceftiofur[a,b]	yes	no	no	no	no
Chlortetracycline[b]	no	no	no	yes	yes
Dihydrosteptomycin[b]	no	no	no	yes	yes
Erythromycin[b]	yes	no	no	yes	no
Furamazone	no	yes	no	no	no
Gentimycin	no	no	no	yes	no
Lasalocid[a]	no	no	no	no	yes
Monensin[c]	no	no	no	no	yes
Neomycin[b]	no	no	no	yes	no
Oxytetracycline (oral)[b]	no	no	no	no	yes
Oxytetracycline (injection)[b]	yes	yes	no	yes	no
Penicillin[b]	yes	no	no	yes	no
Streptomycin	yes	yes	no	yes	no
Tetracycline	yes	yes	no	no	no
Tilmicosin[a]	yes	no	no	no	no
Tylosin[d]	no	no	no	yes	no
Sulfonamides					
Sulfabromomethazine	yes	yes	yes	yes	no
Sulfachloropyridazine	no	yes	no	no	no
Sulfadimethoxine[b]	yes	no	no	no	no
Sulfaethoxypyridazine[a]	yes	yes	yes	yes	no
Sulfamethazine	yes	yes	yes	yes	no
Sulfamethoxine	yes	no	no	no	no

[a]Available by prescription only.
[b]Approved for lactating cattle.
[c]For beef and pastured cattle.
[d]Preventive liver abscesses claim only.
Source: Compiled from FDA Approved Animal Drug List (Green Book), 1998a, and Feed Additive Compendium, 1997.

TABLE 2–12   Steroid Products Labeled for Improved Growth and/or Feed Efficiency in Cattle

Compound	Steers	Heifers
Estradiol	yes	yes
Estradiol/Progesterone	yes	no
Estradiol/Testosterone	no	yes
Estradiol/Trenbolone	yes	no
Melengestrol	no	yes
Trenbolone	yes	yes
Zeranol	yes	yes

Source: Compiled from FDA Approved Animal Drug List (Green Book), 1998a, and Feed Additive Compendium, 1997.

a result of the suggestion to limit the use of these drugs pending results of research on human health.

Vaccinations

Like dairy cattle, beef cattle are vaccinated against brucellosis, leptospirosis, clostridial infections, and a bovine respiratory complex of diseases, which usually include IBR and PI3. Many outbreaks of disease in herds can be prevented on farms with good vaccination programs.

THE VEAL INDUSTRY

After World War II the number of calves, mostly cull males from dairy breeds, marketed for veal rose to more than 13 million (Knutson 1993), which at that time was similar to the number of dairy cattle. Most of these calves were "bob" veal, which were only a few days old and weighing about 100 pounds. The number of veal calves fell continuously from 1945 to about 1.4 million in 1992.

The veal calf industry as it exists today originated in the late 1960s. For veal, up to 0.9 million cull dairy bull calves are purchased at less than 1 week of age, mostly at auction (Wilson 1993). Typically, a veal farmer can receive more than 100 calves, originating from about 50 farms, to start a cycle. Throughout its 16- to 18-week feeding period, the veal calf is housed individually in a stall and maintained as a preruminant by feeding commercially available milkbased liquid diets. The starter usually contains an antibiotic (e.g., oxytetracycline). Typically, beginning at 4 to 6 weeks of age, the starter is gradually replaced with a liquid grower diet with less protein and limited iron and containing no antibiotic. The calves are slaughtered at 400 to 500 lb body weight. Iron is limited to create pale muscle, but without anemia, because red blood cells have a higher priority for limited iron. The price paid for the calf is reduced proportionately to the intensity of red color in the muscle.

Veal calves encounter the same diseases as do other calves, particularly enteric and respiratory infections. FDA recently created a new policy for drug usage. Out of concern for veal animal well-being and for the industry, FDA now permits the use of some drugs already approved for beef or dairy cattle when they are used in veal calves under a valid veterinarian–client–patient relationship (VCPR) to ensure safe drug use and optimize animal health. Wilson (1993) listed 8 antibiotics, 2 sulfonamides, and 2 anthelmintics, which were used extralabel in veal calves under valid VCPRs.

Since 1991, 3 drugs have been labeled for veal calves: amoxicillin (respiratory infections), ampicillin (enteric infections), and decoquinate (coccidiosis). To assist in labeling new drugs for use in veal calves, USDA recently classified veal as a minor-use species, making research on calves eligible for funds in the IR4 program for new-drug approval.

THE SHEEP INDUSTRY

The number of sheep worldwide has risen almost continuously. In the United States, however, after a peak of about 56 million in 1942 (Parker and Pope 1983), the stock declined to about 10 million in 1985 (the lowest since records were begun in 1867), and remained relatively constant thereafter. Sheep now account for less than 1 percent of the U.S. red-meat consumption (Knutson 1993). Most marketed sheep derive from one or more of eight major breeds. Numbers of sheep in the smaller breeds have declined, while the larger breeds increased, reflecting demand for larger carcasses. Texas (20 percent), California (9 percent), Wyoming (9 percent), Colorado (7 percent), South Dakota (6 percent) and Montana (5 percent) account for 56 percent of the U.S. sheep flock (Knutson 1993).

Typically, in the western states, federal ranges have provided half of the feed for commercial sheep (Parker and Pope 1983). In that region, most ewes lamb in the spring on open range under the care of herders. Others are housed and fed feeds stored for the winter, and are lambed in sheds to optimize lamb survival. Grazing begins in the spring at the lower elevations and follows the receding snow toward higher elevations as spring and summer progress. Some slaughter lambs come directly from these ranges, more when forage is better, but most range lambs are sold or contracted to feedlots for finishing. Some feedlots have a capacity for more than 30,000 lambs.

Sheep are managed much more intensively in most of the rest of the country (Parker and Pope 1983). For example, in the north-central states, lambs often are weaned at 4 to 6 weeks of age and moved directly to dry lot feeding. This reduces the need for high-quality forage, minimizes worm infections and predation, and

TABLE 2–13   Major Claims of Antibacterials
Approved for Use in Sheep

Compound	Growth and Feed Efficiency	Various Infections
Chlortetracycline	yes	yes
Erythromycin	no	yes
Neomycin	no	yes
Oxytetracycline	no	yes
Penicillin	no	yes
Penicillin/Streptomycin	no	yes

Source: Compiled from FDA Approved Animal Drug List (Green
Book), 1998a, and Feed Additive Compendium, 1997.

increases the number of lambs marketed at seasonally high prices. Although this
system requires more grain feeding, grains are readily available and can be the
most economical source of energy in the region. The system also permits the
farmer to maintain about 50 percent more ewes and to optimize the proportion of
ewes that breed to lamb at 12 to 14 months of age. The most intensive management achieves 3-lamb crops with up to 6 lambs every 2 years; more than double
the current national average. This system includes estrus synchronization, the
use of gonadotropins to optimize twinning, hand mating or artificial insemination, pregnancy diagnosis, induced parturition, and artificial rearing of lambs,
especially when ewes are not good mothers (Newton 1982; North 1984). However, most of the appropriate hormones required for this kind of management are
not approved for use in sheep.

Kimberling (1988) outlined the diseases of sheep, most caused by bacteria,
viruses, and parasites. Vaccines are available to prevent several infections, such
as vibriosis, enzootic abortion, epididymitis, enterotoxemia (*Clostridium
perfringens*), and bluetongue. Although antibacterials are helpful for treating
lambs with enteritis, enterotoxemia, or colibacillosis, they are critical to control
respiratory diseases, including shipping fever. Six antibiotics are approved for
use in sheep (Shepard et al. 1992, [Table 2–13]). There are no sulfonamides
labeled for sheep, although they apparently have been used (Parker and Pope
1983).

Parasites, both internal and external, can be devastating to sheep. In two
model programs in the United States, the screwworm has been controlled by
release of sterile flies, and mange mites have been eradicated by mandatory
dipping of sheep before interstate movements (Parker and Pope 1983; Kimberling
1988). Four compounds are labeled to control worms in sheep, and at least one
anthelmintic treatment is critical for pastured lambs. Lambs entering a feedlot
typically are given an anthelmintic, a broad spectrum antibiotic, and an implant

of zeranol. One antibacterial has claims for improved feed efficiency and growth rate, in sharp contrast to the numbers approved for cattle (Table 2–8), hogs (Tables 2–6 and 2–7), and broiler chickens (Table 2–2). Sheep are known to respond like cattle, with improved growth and feed efficiency, when given various steroids, but only zeranol is approved for sheep. Similarly, like cattle, sheep respond with improved feed efficiency when given ionophores, but none is approved with this claim for sheep. Lasalocid, an ionophore, which is approved for enhanced growth and feed efficiency in cattle, has a claim only for the control of coccidiosis in "confined" sheep.

Sheep numbers could increase as management strategies for this industry shift from an extensive, range-based program to intensive management systems, with an attendant increase in the need for some kinds of drugs and chemicals. The examples are feed-additive antibiotics, products for growth promotion, and steroid implants approved for cattle. At this time, however, the sheep industry is too small to justify the investments required to develop many drug products, particularly those that would be used only for sheep.

MINOR SPECIES

Goats are the most important of the minor food animals. The minor species suffer from most of the same kinds of diseases that are found among major species. Goats, for example, have the same variety of enteric, respiratory, nematode, and ectoparasite infections as do sheep and cattle. However, only 6 drug products are labeled for goats (Shepard et al. 1992): 2 for coccidiosis, 2 wormers, and 2 antibiotics (Table 2–14). Potential profit from such products usually is too small to recover the costs of developing them, often even when the active ingredient is already marketed for major species. This shortage of drugs to manage disease is even more vexing for the other minor species. In fact, there are no drugs labeled for use in species such as bison, geese, and squab.

Undoubtedly, the lack of drugs, the discouraging marketing opportunities, and the limited research and information assistance from the government all contribute to contain growth of the minor-species industries. For producers, the only access to many drugs is through extra-label use of products developed for other species with the aid of a valid VCPR. FDA allows this kind of use for some drugs to promote animal well-being and because the industries probably could not exist even in their current form without some of the key drugs.

THE AQUACULTURE INDUSTRY

Aquaculture in the United States is growing rapidly. This industry is now considered an important supplier of food products for U.S. consumers. Inventories of food-size catfish in 1995 were estimated at 202 million fish, up 7 percent in 1994; tilapia production increased to 6.8 million kg (15 million lb) in 1994 and

TABLE 2–14   Major Claims for Drugs Approved for Use in Minor Species

Species	Compound	Claims
Reindeer	Ivermectin	Grubs
Duck	Chlortetracycline	Growth, feed efficiency, various infections
	Novobiocin	Various infections
Goat	Decoquinate	Coccidiosis
	Monensin	Coccidiosis
	Neomycin	Enteritis
	Penicillin/	
	streptomycin	Various infections
	Phenothiazine	Worms
	Thiabendazole	Worms
Pheasant	Amprolium	Coccidiosis
	Bacitracin	Growth, feed efficiency, various infections
	Penicillin	Growth, feed efficiency
	Thiabendazole	Worms
Quail	Bacitracin	Growth, feed efficiency, various infections
	Monensin	Coccidiosis
	Penicillin	Growth, feed efficiency
Rabbits	Penicillin/	
	streptomycin	Various infections
	Sulfaquinoxaline	Coccidiosis

Source: Compiled from FDA Approved Animal Drug List (Green Book), 1998a, and Feed Additive Compendium, 1997.

continues to rise; and salmon production was approximately 11.8 million kg (26 million lb) in 1993 and remained the same in 1994.   In 1995, farmer sales of catfish to processing plants were approximately 20.9 million kg (460 million lb), up 6 percent from 1994.   U.S. oyster growers have not been able to increase production sufficiently to meet increasing demands for exports to Asia, Japan, Taiwan, and Canada.   Total sales of trout rose 13 percent in 1995, an increase attributed to higher sales of food-size fish, which rose 6 percent to $60.8 million. Exports of oysters reached $6.9 million in 1994, up more than 180 percent from exports in 1991.   Because of the near collapse in the stocks of cod, halibut, and several other species, the U.S. and Canadian governments have imposed severe harvesting cutbacks in the Georges Bank fishing area of the northern Atlantic.   As a result, both countries have placed increased priority on cultivation of these species.

As with other food-animal industries, aquaculture is becoming a more concentrated industry of fewer but much larger farms. The vast majority of fish-
farming enterprises in the United States where medications might be used are
pond-like or tank structures, rather than open-water habitats, such as oceans and
lakes. In contrast, some countries like Norway utilize natural structures, such as
the fjords for salmon farming, and there are concerns about the wastes collecting
in fjord bottoms. In the United States, approximately 158,800 acres of ponds
were devoted to catfish production in 1995, but the number of farms decreased.
Tilapia production in the United States has focused on the live-fish market,
because import requirements and high costs restrict live-fish import. This market
continues to expand, however, and production of tilapia in tank systems for
processed products is likely to grow.

Aquaculture encompasses production of various sizes and types of fish.
Brood fish are kept to produce the fertilized eggs that go to hatcheries. Food-size
fish include (1) small fish, weighing 0.34 to 0.7 kg (0.75 to 1.5 lb); (2) medium
fish, weighing 0.7 to 1.4 kg (1.5 to 3 lb); and (3) large fish, weighing more than
1.4 kg (3 lb). Large stocker fish weigh from 82 to 341 kg (180 to 750 lb) per
1,000 fish, and small stocker fish weigh from 27 kg to 82 kg (60 to 180 lb) per
1,000 fish. Fingerlings or fry fish weigh 27 kg (60 lb) per 1,000 fish.

The use of antibiotics and drugs in the fish industry is complicated because
of the need to administer the compounds, for the most part, directly into the water
in which the fish swim. The safety of aquatic food products, the integrity of the
environment, the safety of target animals, and the safety of persons who administer various compounds are important issues that have an effect on drug use in the
aquaculture industry. As with other food-animal industries, industry-developed
and industry-directed aquaculture quality-assurance programs are preferred to
monitor compounds that come into contact with food fish.

Compounds commonly used in the aquaculture industry that might be considered a potential threat to food safety and consumer health include animal drugs
and veterinary biologics, pesticides, disinfectants, and water-treatment compounds. New animal drugs that are added to aquaculture feed are subject to FDA
approval and must be specifically approved for use in aquaculture feed. These
drugs must be mixed in feed at concentrations that are specified in FDA medi-
cated-feed regulations.

Water treatments used in aquaculture include chemicals that are applied
directly to water for control of algae or water-borne parasites. The selection of
the federal agency that will have jurisdiction over a particular chemical depends
on the intended use of the product in the water. Chemical residues in fish can
occur from improper use or application of water treatments to improve fish health
or improper use of products to control weeds or water quality.

New animal drugs approved by FDA for use in the aquaculture industry
appear in Table 2–15. There are several unapproved compounds of low regula-

TABLE 2–15   FDA-Approved New Drugs for Use in Aquaculture

Drug	Active Ingredient	Indication	Species
Finquel, MS-222	Tricaine methanesulfonate	Sedation/anesthesia	Fish (*Ictaluridae, Salmonidae, Esocidae, Percidae*), other aquatic poikilotherms
Formalin-F; Paracid-F; Parasite-S	Formalin	Control protozoa and monogenetic trematodes (*Icthyopthirius, Chilodonella, Costia, Scyphidia, Epistylis, Trichodina* spp. and *Cleidodiscus, Gyrodactylus, Dactylogyrus* spp.)	Salmonids, catfish, largemouth bass, bluegill
		Control fungi of the family *Saprolegniaceae*	Salmodi and esocid eggs
Parasite-S	Formalin	Control protozoan parasites (*Bodo* spp., *Epistylis* spp., and *Zoothamnium* spp.)	Panaeid shrimp
Romet-30	Sulfadimethoxine and ormetoprim	Control furunculosis (*Aeromonas salmonicida*)	Salmonids
		Control enteric septicemia (*Edwardsiella ictaluri*)	Catfish
Terramycin	Oxytetracycline monoalkyl tri- methyl ammonium	Mark skeletal tissue	Pacific salmon
		Control ulcer disease, furunculosis, bacterial hemorrhagic septicemia, and pseudomonas disease (*Hemophilus piscium, Aeromonas salmonicida, Aeromonoas liquefaciens, Pseudomonas*)	Salmonids
		Control bacterial hemorrhagic septicemia and pseudomonas disease	Catfish
		Control gaffkemia (*Aerococcus viridans*)	Lobster

Source: Adapted from Drugs Approved for Use in Aquaculture, Center for Veterinary Medicine, U.S. Food and Drug Administration, Revised June, 1995; http://www.fda.gov:80/cvm/fda/infores/other/aqua/appendixa.html

tory priority to FDA. FDA's enforcement position on the use of these substances is not one of approval or affirmation of their safety.

QUALITY-ASSURANCE PROGRAMS AND ANIMAL HEALTH MAINTENANCE

Animal health products must be handled and administered properly if producers are to maintain public trust and be competitive in U.S. and world markets. Important objectives to producers are reducing the risk of drug residues in food products, and, ultimately, eliminating irresponsible drug use, so that public perceptions of poor drug management are changed with the result that consumer confidence increases.

Food-animal producers know that the profitability of the production facility is directly linked to not only the quality and efficiency of animal management but also to the perceptions of the public regarding the industry and the overall appeal of the product. Stresses on animals must be managed and minimized, so that the animal can achieve its genetic potential for growth and productive metabolism rather than expend energy fighting disease. Quality-assurance programs in the food-animal industry focus on helping producers supply products that are as free as possible of microbiological hazards, and drug and chemical residues. The consumer is presented with products obtained from animals that received proper care.

All major livestock-producer groups have initiated quality-assurance programs to address their responsibilities in producing safe, wholesome products. Among such groups are the National Pork Producers Council (NPPC), the National Cattlemen's Beef Association, the National Milk Producers Federation, the American Sheep Industry Association, the American Veal Association, the National Broiler Council, the National Turkey Federation, the United Egg Producers, the Catfish Farmers of America, the National Aquaculture Association, and the U.S. Trout Farmers Association.

The following sections describe the quality-assurance programs initiated by the National Broiler Council, the National Turkey Federation, NPPC, the National Cattlemen's Beef Association, and the National Milk Producers Federation.

Poultry Quality-Assurance Programs

In the United States, with the help of various public and private institutions and the implementation of the National Poultry Improvement Plan (NPIP) of 1935 and the National Turkey Improvement Plan of 1943, the poultry industry has been able either to eradicate or to minimize disease exposure. That undertaking has improved profitability and expanded the industry.

The eradication of various diseases caused by *Mycoplasma gallisepticum*, *Mycoplasma synoviae*, *Mycoplasma meleagridis*, *Salmonella pullorum*, and *Sal-*

monella gallinarum; velogenic Newcastle disease; and highly pathogenic avian influenza could not have been accomplished without the NPIP system.

The goal of the National Turkey Federation's Chemical Residue Avoidance Program is to ensure that the tissue of turkeys produced and slaughtered in the United States will not contain any chemical residues and will meet or exceed all tolerance and action levels for known harmful residues as established by the federal regulatory agencies (the U.S. Environmental Protection Agency, FDA, and the USDA Food Safety and Inspection Service [FSIS]).

The National Broiler Council's recommended Good Manufacturing Practices address every quality-control point in the production and processing of broiler chickens to enhance product quality and consumer protection. The procedures are drawn from quality-control programs throughout the broiler industry, from the scientific literature, and from existing regulatory documents. In production, recommended practices include:

- maintaining proper facility standards,
- providing growers with pesticide information,
- including pesticide-use statements in grower contracts, and
- enforcing biosecurity programs.

Regarding animal health care, the following practices are recommended:

- ensuring that pharmaceutical laws and regulations are followed (only FDA-approved pharmaceuticals and regimens are to be used), and
- enforcing company standards for pharmaceutical use.

In breeder operations, standards are to be maintained for feeds and animal health. In addition, procedures to control poultry-borne and egg-borne pathogens and diseases should be a routine part of breeder-monitoring programs. Hatchery recommendations address sanitation and microbiological controls, which continue through the growing period, transport, slaughter, and processing. Testing for microbiological quality, pesticide and chemical residues in feed ingredients is recommended for feed preparation during the growing period. Maintaining records of feed distribution and pharmaceutical inventories, and ensuring that FDA regulations are adhered to, are important aspects of good poultry management practice.

Pork Quality-Assurance Programs

In June 1989, NPPC introduced a management education program called the Pork Quality Assurance (PQA) program. It was designed to help producers avoid violative drug residues, improve management practices, reduce production costs, and increase awareness of food safety concerns. The PQA program emphasizes good management practices in the handling and use of animal health products and encourages producers to review their herds' health programs annually.

The program provides information covering the following topics:

- food safety and the pork industry,
- products used today,
- routes of administration,
- on-farm feed preparation,
- minimum withdrawal times,
- current regulatory system, and
- on-farm testing.

The PQA program (NPPC 1997) was developed by NPPC to institute safety, uniformity, and consistency in the production of pork. The program refers to three achievement levels in the quality-assurance certification process. Levels I and II are self-instructional and self-paced reading from a booklet obtainable from NPPC. All producers are encouraged to learn and implement the 10 "good production practices" defined in the booklet. Producers can achieve Level III through a professional consultation, which takes them step-by-step through the design of a herd health program. For producers this 10-step program is developed around the appropriate uses of medications and the need for accountability. The plan results in an understanding of the need for the oversight of the veterinarian and in written accounts of animal-by-animal drug use. Level III of the PQA program applies principles from the Hazard Analysis and Critical Control Points (HACCP) to the production of pork. The HACCP involves determining where problems could develop and establishing procedures to monitor those problems. To complete Level III, a producer must annually perform the following 10 critical control points:

1) Establish an efficient and effective herd health-management plan.
2) Establish a valid veterinarian, client, and patient relationship.
3) Store all drugs correctly.
4) Use only FDA-approved over-the-counter or prescription drugs with professional assistance.
5) Administer all injectable drugs and oral medications properly.
6) Follow label instructions for use of feed additives.
7) Maintain proper treatment records and adequate identification of all treated animals.
8) Use drug-residue tests when appropriate.
9) Implement employee and family awareness of proper drug use.
10) Complete quality-assurance checklist annually.

In the implementation of the PQA program, extensive cooperation has been received from veterinarians, packers, media, agriculture teachers, FDA, FSIS, extension personnel, feed manufacturers, and pharmaceutical companies.

Producer response to the PQA program has been favorable. As of July 1, 1995, approximately 32,000 pork producers who provide 63 percent of the market hogs in the United States were enrolled in the program. Thirty percent of U.S. pork is from producers who have completed the program and an even larger percentage comes from producers who have implemented some aspects of the program.

According to the 1993 nationwide monitoring program administered by FSIS, violative residues for sulfamethazine and antibiotics in market hogs have decreased (FSIS 1993c). The violation rate for sulfamethazine has continued to remain low in recent years. FSIS has congratulated NPPC for its work in reducing the violation rate and has encouraged the NPPC membership to continue to follow the recommendations in the PQA program to avoid illegal residues. To continue reducing violative drug residue rates and reach the industry goal of no violative residues, NPPC urges all producers to enroll in and complete the PQA program.

In addition to its Compliance Policy Guides directed toward use of animal health products by veterinarians, FDA has issued a Compliance Policy Guide on Proper Drug Use and Residue Avoidance by NonVeterinarians. The objective of this guide is to ensure proper use of animal health products in food-producing animals when administered by producers. The guide describes the records FDA inspectors would ask to see when doing on-farm investigations after a violative drug residue has been discovered. The guide addresses identification of treated animals; maintenance of treatment records; storage, labeling, and accounting of medications; use of prescription products only through a valid VCPR; and education of employees and family members. The PQA program provides a means for producers to comply with the FDA guide.

Dairy Quality-Assurance Programs

To ensure that only the highest quality dairy foods and residue-free products reach the consumer, two important documents have been developed. The first was the Grade A Pasteurized Milk Ordinance, also known as the FDA PMO (FDA 1995b). The premise of the original PMO, developed in 1924, was that effective public-health control of milk-borne diseases required the application of sanitation measures through the production, handling, pasteurization, and distribution of milk and milk products.

The second document was the Milk and Dairy Beef Residue Prevention Protocol (Boeckman and Carlson 1995), which addresses the need to market residue-free milk and dairy beef. That 10-point plan for the Milk and Dairy Beef Quality Assurance Program was developed by the National Milk Producers Federation and the American Veterinary Medical Association (AVMA). Both organizations emphasized that the plan would require cooperation and communication between dairy farmers and veterinarians, so that the industry could remain active in preventing drug residues in milk and beef. In the plan's guidelines, the producer is viewed as providing a safe product, and the consumer as benefiting by drinking uncontaminated milk. The 10-point plan has been adopted as part of the PMO by individual states, and it is mandatory for all producers after one contaminated load of milk is detected.

An extremely important aspect of quality-assurance programs is the estab-lishment of a valid VCPR. This relationship ensures that farm animals receiving antibiotics will be withheld from the food chain until drug concentrations are below those permitted by FDA. Both the producer and the veterinarian must work closely with quality-assurance program coordinators and extension person-nel to ensure that the drug-avoidance programs are followed.

The 10-point quality assurance plan deals specifically with the drug-residue issue and for milk and dairy beef production includes:

1) Practicing healthy-herd management. Investments in disease prevention are more cost-effective than is disease treatment. Some examples include proper milking management versus treatment of clinical mastitis, good hoof care and trimming versus treatment of foot infections, calving cows in a sanitary location versus treatment of uterine infection, and proper vaccination versus treatment. Producers are encouraged to practice herd health management by consulting with licensed veterinarians and other related professionals.

2) Establishing a valid VCPR. AVMA (1998) defines a VCPR as follows:

> An appropriate veterinarian/client/patient relationship is characterized by these attributes: (1) [t]he veterinarian has assumed the responsibility for making med-ical judgments regarding the health of the animal(s) and the need for medical treatment, and the client (owner or other caretaker) has agreed to follow the instructions of the veterinarian; and when (2) [t]here is sufficient knowledge of the animal(s) by the veterinarian to initiate at least a general or preliminary diagnosis of the medical condition of the animal(s). This means that the veter-inarian has recently seen and is personally acquainted with the keeping and care of the animal(s) by virtue of an examination of the animal(s) and/or by medical-ly appropriate and timely visits to the premises where the animal(s) are kept; and when (3) [t]he veterinarian is readily available, or has arranged for emer-gency coverage, for follow-up in the event of adverse reactions or failure of the treatment regimen. (Pp. 49–50)

A valid VCPR is mandatory if drugs are to be used for reasons different from those stated on the label; this is called an extra-label use. Dairy farmers need the benefit of a valid VCPR to make sure they are following the veterinarian's instructions properly.

3) Using only FDA-approved over-the-counter or prescription drugs with a veterinarian's guidance.

FDA-approved drugs have been tested extensively to show that they perform consistently according to the manufacturer's claims and that they cause no harm to the animal when administered according to the label. As a result, dairy farmers will reduce the risk of violative drug residues in the milk and meat of animals receiving drugs and protect their market by supplying safe and wholesome milk and meat.

FDA-approved over-the-counter drugs are those that can be purchased anywhere without a veterinarian's prescription or supervision. Drugs are labeled for over-the-counter sale when instructions that are adequate for a layperson can be printed on the label, including the package insert.

4) Ensuring that all drugs have labels that comply with state or federal labeling requirements. Because dairy farmers are ultimately responsible for any drug residues, they should be careful to follow drug label instructions. They should not be concerned about the accuracy of a label, because the manufacturer must meet all the requirements to get the drug approved, and veterinarians are responsible for all labels of drugs they prescribe for their clients' animals.

5) Storing all drugs correctly. All medications for cattle must be properly stored, so that they will not come into contact with milk or the milking equipment. Topical antiseptics, wound dressings, vaccines, and other biological products and vitamins or mineral products are generally exempt from labeling and storage requirements. However, some states might have specific storage regulations.

6) Administering all drugs properly and identifying all treated animals. The best way for dairy farmers to avoid problems associated with this critical control point is simply to follow the drug's label and package insert, and to identify each animal that receives the drug at the time it is administered. Immediate identification of the animal will greatly reduce the risk of putting adulterated or contaminated milk into a tank or sending an animal with tissue residues to slaughter.

7) Maintaining and using proper treatment records on all treated animals. Dairy farmers must identify treated animals with a paint stick, leg bands, hock markers, neck strap, numbered ear tags, or other marking devices. Proper identification is crucial for keeping violative drug residues out of milk and meat. Equally important is maintaining a record of all treated animals. The records should be accessible to everyone who works with the animals. The records need to be used to ensure that cull cows, dairy beef, steers, or calves whose markings have worn off are not sold before the withholding time has expired. The records also should be permanent, so the veterinarian can refer to them to prescribe effective therapy and to serve as protection in case of a regulatory follow-up.

8) Using drug-residue screening tests. New technology has made it possible to conduct milk, urine, and blood tests that are easy to use on the farm. Many of these tests are as sensitive as those done at milk or slaughter plants. On-farm testing gives dairy farmers an additional way to avoid violative drug residues in

meat and milk. The key is to match the drug administered with the correct drug test at the desired level of sensitivity.

9) Implementing employee and family awareness of proper drug use to avoid marketing adulterated products. Many cases of adulterated meat or milk occur because one person treats the animals and someone else takes care of the milking or decides to sell the animals. If different individuals are carrying out those tasks, it is important that the critical control points of the quality-assurance program be explained to everyone involved with the animals.

10) Performing the 10-point Milk and Dairy Beef Residue Prevention Protocol annually. Producers need to go through these 10 points with their veterinarians at least once a year. Conditions on the farm change; new employees are hired and different drugs are used because of a change in herd health. In addition, new drugs or screening tests come onto the market. These factors make it worthwhile for producers to review the plan with their veterinarians and farm staff a minimum of once each year.

Voluntary implementation of the 10-point plan has met with varied success. Even highlighting the incentive of reduced costs associated with a herd health program and the reduced need for drugs has not been completely effective. The Implementation and Communication Subcommittee of the Drug Residue Committee (Buntain et al. 1993) reviewed the quality-assurance initiatives and suggested that insurance companies sponsor premium reductions or price breaks on liability insurance for voluntary participants. Another suggestion was for milk processors and cooperatives to include plan participation in their requirements for quality bonuses. The cooperatives and processors could then use the information as a marketing advantage and advertise that a high percentage of their producers participated in the residue-prevention program. Another possible incentive mentioned was to have voluntary implementation of the 10-point plan defer the penalty of a first violation under the PMO. Suggestion was also made for veterinarians to go through the 10-point plan at no charge to producers who implement the plan voluntarily.

Although the incentive of reduced costs associated with a sound herd health program has not enticed a majority of producers to adopt the 10-point plan voluntarily, it still should be a major focus of preventive herd health management. The resulting decrease in disease and increase in production also would lead to a decrease in finding violative drug residues. Residue avoidance would be best served by encouraging and emphasizing the need for on-farm treatment records. The use of treatment records as a source of residue information for withholding milk and meat from the market is obvious. Establishing drug use patterns from treatment records on each farm also would provide a basis for discussing changes in or alternatives to current drug use. This information could provide opportunities for educating producers about better management alternatives in certain stages of the production cycle.

Continuing-education programs on current and changing regulations are necessary for inspector, veterinarian, and producer groups. A centralized task force, perhaps encompassing extension personnel, would be helpful in gathering and reviewing the educational, labeling, and form material available, and distributing the most up-to-date information to producers. Along with details on changing regulations, information needs to be made available on sources such as Food Animal Residual Avoidance Databank (FARAD) project for determining withholding times of extra-label drugs, on drugs prohibited from use in food animals, on the liability associated with drug labeling and signing the 10-point plan, and on the definition of a valid VCPR. The relationship and importance of FARAD to drug use policy in the United States is further detailed in Chapter 3.

Beef Quality-Assurance Program

In 1996, the beef industry initiated the Beef Quality Assurance (BQA) program, a voluntary initiative designed by producers for producers (NCBA 1997). Because of the tremendous diversity across the United States in the beef cattle industry, the BQA program is implemented state by state. Although the National Cattlemen's Beef Association provides technical support and national leadership to beef cattle producers, the administration and implementation of the BQA program are carried out by state cattle affiliates and state beef councils, with the assistance of practicing veterinarians.

The BQA program is designed to educate and train beef cattle owners, their employees, and their veterinarians on the day-to-day management practices that influence the safety, wholesomeness, and quality of beef. Subjects emphasized through producer and veterinarian seminars, workshops, and chute-side demonstrations are (1) the importance of proper and safe animal drug use; (2) adherence to product label withdrawal periods; and (3) record-keeping relative to animal product use, drug inventories, and animal treatment regimens. The program teaches testing procedures for sampling and analyzing feed and feed ingredients for potential chemical and pesticide residues at the farm or feedlot. Through the BQA program, residue drug violations for feedlot cattle essentially have been reduced to zero, as reported by the USDA Residue Monitoring Program (FSIS 1994b).

In the past few years, the BQA program has launched an aggressive effort designed to eliminate injection site tissue damage resulting from intramuscular administration of animal health products. Educational efforts regarding injection site awareness have resulted in a significant reduction in tissue quality defects. The success of these efforts demonstrates the ability of the BQA program to create an effective and responsive network of cattlemen and veterinarians.

The BQA initiative is structured to reach all segments of beef cattle production, including cow and calf, stocker, backgrounding, and feedlot operations. To date, 42 states sponsor aggressive BQA programs. These states produce more than 98 percent of the feedlot cattle and account for more than 95 percent of the cow and calf producers in the United States.

More recently, the state BQA programs have implemented producer BQA certification programs. The certification procedure requires a specified amount of structured quality-assurance training and the verification of quality-assurance practices implemented in the actual operation. It is expected that the momentum for quality-assurance certification will increase throughout the industry.

Finally, the BQA program is prepared to launch a major quality-assurance initiative for cull dairy and beef cows. Violative drug residues in cull dairy and beef cows remain a major concern for the industry.

The industry's BQA program is an effective producer network for addressing product safety concerns now and in the future. However, on-farm food safety interventions must develop around sound science if these efforts are to be effective and further enhance the safety of beef and beef products.

SUMMARY OF FINDINGS

Across all major species of animals used in food production, the development of intensive production practices has changed the way animals are exposed to pathogens in their environment. All species, including fish, derive some benefit from the use of antibiotics to treat active infections, prevent disease outbreaks, or modify their internal environment for faster growth with the use of less feed. Because animals typically are raised in close proximity to one another, the emergence of disease in one animal can result in the rapid infection of many more in a short time, underscoring the need to use subtherapeutic concentrations of antibiotics. Animal producers must adhere to strict guidelines on antibiotic use to ensure that drug residues are not carried over into the human food chain. As such, medication is halted before slaughter to curb the inappropriate introduction of drugs and their residues into the human food chain. Opportunities exist with the use of HAACP quality-assurance programs to modify production and animal-handling strategies, to minimize the incidence and management of disease, and to control the misuse of drugs and pharmaceuticals that could allow drug residues to enter the food chain or for disease pathogens to pose a risk to human health.

3

Benefits and Risks to Human Health

OVERVIEW

The public has long-standing concerns over potentially harmful drug residues in foods. Many consumers fear that neither the facts regarding the consequences of drug use in food animals are being made available nor are enough animal-derived foods available—or affordable—that allow them to select safe products. The possibility that chemical additives, drugs and their metabolites (drug residues) could cause allergic reactions or disease is not taken lightly by the public or by health care professionals (ERS 1996a). Similarly, the threat of human disease posed by microbial contamination is well documented and increasingly acknowledged and publicized (IOM 1998).

The threat of antibiotic resistance is most commonly associated with the emergence of resistance outbreaks in hospital settings and with improper human applications of antibiotic therapy (CDC 1994; IOM 1998). The cause-and-effect relationship between therapeutic administration of antibiotics and resistance is more readily ascertained—and statistically quantifiable—in hospitals than it is in animal production sites, processing and packaging plants, and transport depots common in animal agriculture. It has been difficult to track and document the link between antibiotic use in farm animals, the development of antibiotic resistance, and disease transference to humans. However, the reporting of such data is increasing with the development of larger and more accessible databases, refined culture and detection methods, and the overall heightened awareness and concern for this potential source of disease. The statistics are more apparent for zoonotic transfer of overt pathogens that cause specific diseases that must be reported to state or federal health agencies (Lyme disease, rabies, salmonellosis).

The data are increasing (and referenced later in this report) on the transfer of pathogens from farm animals to humans where issues of antibiotic resistance patterns in the invading organism are more frequently tracked. Many of these data come from case studies that followed reported infection and disease in higher risk groups, such as farmworkers (where epidemiological tracking has identified the source). Increased data collection on antibiotic resistance patterns is occurring largely as a result of implementation of newer technologies (developed within the past 5 to 10 years) on a broader, more affordable, and "user friendly" scale and format. In addition, databases on disease occurrence in particular food-animal species are increasing at a rapid rate.

In large part, the appearance of increasing health problems in food animals does not reflect an increase in incidence. Rather, it indicates an increase in documentation of what was probably there all along. The new data arise because of increased vigilance among producers and veterinarians who want to identify problems and provide treatments quickly to maintain productivity. Many of the successes in this effort are the direct result of voluntary implementation of quality-assurance programs and accountability procedures that are expanding throughout the food-animal industry.

The operating premises can be summarized as follows:

• Antibiotic resistance is a documented major health threat around the world that has been given high priority by many health agencies (WHO 1997; IOM 1998).

• Inappropriate or irresponsible uses of drugs in humans and animals in subtherapeutic and therapeutic regimens contribute to the development of drug resistance (IOM 1998).

• There are opportunities in the microbial environment for interconnected ecosystems to allow exchange of DNA, promoting the spread of resistance from one genus to another. The combination of increased bacterial virulence and increased drug resistance creates a potential for increased risk of morbidity and mortality for animals and humans that some have extrapolated to a catastrophic potential. "Catastrophic" and "crisis" are words often applied to this issue, and they evoke emotional, sensational, and oftentimes inflammatory reactions that tend to distract the focus from the goal of factual assessment and hypothesis testing.

• Human exposure to pathogens from animal-derived foods has been documented and can result in human disease. The relationship between those diseases and the emergence of antibiotic-resistant disease is less clear, less frequently tracked, and constitutes an area in which there is a fundamental dearth of valid data. Between the farm and the table, the large number of places and opportunities for bacteria to be introduced into the human food chain is an important factor in the emergence of food-related illness. Irresponsible actions by individuals both before and after harvest of the food (improper storage, poor home sanitary practices, improper cooking techniques) undermine the effort to control microbial proliferation through responsible regulatory compliance, surveillance, and quality assurance. However, sterile packaging and irradiation could substantively alter (eliminate) the capability for even drug-resistant organisms to proliferate in foods prior to cooking and decrease the assessed risk to humans.

• Increased international trade, reduced barriers to transport, increased efficiency in processing and delivery, and higher consumption approach or, in some cases, exceed the capacity of current surveillance mechanisms. It is virtually impossible to prevent infectious agents in food from reaching consumers, and efforts toward this end need to be strengthened.

• The federally established standards and allowable tolerance levels for many drugs and residues are not zero, and detection of residues should not be equated with adulteration. No assurances can prevent ignorant action, accidents, or breaching of ethical standards in the use of animals that result in animal-derived foods, being adulterated with drug residues. Sophisticated methods for monitoring residues can be used to remove tainted products from the food chain, but every carcass cannot be monitored.

PREVENTION

Bacteria are a natural part of the body's internal and external ecology and environment. Some bacteria are beneficial, most are benign, and their presence is kept in balance through the functions of the immune system, naturally produced antibacterial peptides in skin and epithelial tissues, and microbial populations normally competing with "foreign" bacteria within a stable internal environment. Bacterial infections in any animal, including humans, fall into two categories: subclinical and occult; clinical and overt. Animals and humans can have low levels of pathogens that do not cause detectable disease or illness. A stable internal environment is critical for maintaining health. If environmental, nutritional, or behavioral stresses impinge on an animal or human population, the imbalance in the internal environment (altered adrenal and glucocorticoid hormone concentrations, altered cytokine concentrations, metabolic acidosis, and ruminal disturbances) can trigger the proliferation of bacterial populations that become harmful by spreading infection or release of endotoxins and exotoxins.

Antibiotics are used to treat infections, but maintaining the animal's internal environment (the gastrointestinal tract and absorptive processes) is another use in animal production. This involves giving antibiotics for longer periods of time and at concentrations lower than those administered for therapeutic treatment (Fagerberg and Quarles 1979).

Antibiotics can be applied in three ways. In one, a single antibiotic is administered at subtherapeutic concentrations for an extended period to maintain the normal population of gastrointestinal microorganisms and prevent emergence of any that could be pathogenic. The second is the use of rotating classes of multiple antibiotics at low, subtherapeutic concentrations. Again, the aim is to eliminate the development of opportunistic bacteria that could emerge as pathogenic or be passed from one animal to another. This strategy is used when animals are transported from one location to another, where the surroundings and feeding methods are different and the animals are reared with more-intensive management practices. The potential for antibiotic-resistant populations of organisms to develop still persists. Therefore, a third application strategy, involving a gradient subtherapeutic regimen, is introduced. Antibiotic concentrations are gradually increased, so that the effective dose for bactericidal action is greater, at least in theory, than a concentration of antibiotic to which microorganisms might have resistance. This strategy is effective because both the efficacy of a drug in controlling disease and the development of resistance are dose dependent. The benefits to animals and humans associated with overall therapeutic antibiotic use in food animals outweigh the risks of use because the development and spread of pathogenic organisms are held in check (CAST 1981).

TREATMENT

In assessing the risk–benefit ratio of antibiotic use in food-producing animals, the nature of the applications for which antibiotics are either prescribed or administered must be known. The exercise of ranking risks and benefits to animals and humans of antibiotic use in food animals might change dramatically according to who assesses the risk and how the availability of related facts strengthens or weakens hypotheses derived from conceptual possibilities. A significant threat to humans exists in the form of zoonotic transmission of diseases. Zoonotic infection results from an animal pathogen that is transmitted directly to humans causing a similar infection. Examples of potentially life-threatening zoonotic infections are tuberculosis, leptospirosis, toxoplasmosis, brucellosis, salmonellosis (DT-104), hemorrhagic *Escherichia coli* O157:H7 (colisepti-cemia), and rabies, to name a few. Treatment is the first response when microbial disease is diagnosed in any animal. For a clinically infected animal, the choices are to treat it with therapeutic concentrations of antibiotics for a defined course of administration or not to treat it at all. If the animal is not treated, the organisms can spread throughout the environment to infect other animals and humans and possibly to decrease the animal's productive lifetime (Fagerberg and Quarles 1979).

If the animal is treated, there is a small chance that some microorganisms could become resistant to the class of antibiotics administered. In some cases, the bacteria developing resistance might, in fact, not even be the species causing the disease (CAST 1981). The risk in antibiotic use in food animals (that is, giving antibiotics to cure or prevent disease) is seen by some as a human health benefit, because treating a sick animal directly maintains the health of other animals and humans (Carneval, R. 1997. Animal Health Institute, Alexandria, VA, personal communication). Some risk is involved in the practice of giving antibiotics to animals, but the ranking of risks and benefits cannot be accomplished easily because of the lack of validated data and controlled studies.

BENEFITS OF ANTIBIOTIC USE

Antibiotics are used in food-animal production for the primary benefit of (1) the health and welfare of the animal (Gustafson 1986; Ziv 1986), (2) carcass quality and overall efficiency of growth and production (Langlois et al. 1986; Mackinnon 1993), (3) economics (CAST 1981; Walton 1986), and (4) human public health. The benefit to human health in the proper use of antibiotics in food animals is related to the ability of these drugs to combat infectious bacteria that can be transferred to humans through direct contact with the sick animal, through consumption of food contaminated with pathogens, or through proliferation in the environment. The advantages of antibiotic use in animals are related to the prevention of overt bacterial disease and improvement in animal performance through reducing the physiological costs of limiting growth that are incurred in the process of fighting low-level and overt disease (Hays 1986; Espinasse 1993). Those limitations need to be minimized to permit better nutrient use, enhanced growth rate, and feed efficiency (Elsasser et al. 1995, 1997; Beisel 1988; Roura et al. 1992; see earlier discussion in Chapter 2). However, because of the controversy surrounding the development of antibiotic drug resistance in animal and human populations, and because of the consequences for human health and clinical practices, use of antibiotic drugs in food-producing animals has been questioned by the Food and Drug Administration (FDA), policy makers, health care professionals, and consumer organizations, among others, and has been studied regularly since the 1960s (see IOM 1989; OTA 1995) as directed by several federal agencies. Some groups have argued for a substantial reduction in the use of antibiotic drugs in food-animal production. Others contend that microbial contamination of animal-food products would increase without the use of these drugs. The following summaries of data and studies suggest that antibiotic use in farm animals is largely beneficial:

• Antibiotic treatment of humans who have enteritis caused by *Salmonella* is generally contraindicated. General intestinal enteritis usually is self-limiting and resolves relatively quickly; a greater risk is associated with the development of resistant *Salmonella* in individuals who have used oral antibiotics within a month of *Salmonella* exposure (Riley et al. 1984). Systemic, invasive *Salmonella* requires antibiotic intervention, and the newly emerging multidrug-resistant strain of *Salmonella*, DT-104, could pose an even more significant threat to human health because of the increasing number of treatment failures encountered as isolates emerge for which treatment options are limited (Wall et al. 1994; Wall et al. 1995).

Treatment of *Salmonella* infection is widely used in veterinary medicine, particularly for swine. As several investigators (DeGeeter et al. 1976; Gutzmann et al. 1976; Wilcock and Olander 1978; Jacks et al. 1981; Schwartz 1991) reported that vigorous antibacterial therapy (in combination with supportive therapy) early in the course of septicemic salmonellosis significantly reduces the magnitude and the duration of shedding of organisms. These investigators pointed out that if such septicemic cases were not treated, shedding of the organisms would increase, and *Salmonella* isolations from carcasses (from apparently healthy animals) would increase. The significance of this would be apparent in the greater risk for *Salmonella* to enter the food chain at slaughter and even more directly contaminate the hog environment, fostering the persistence of the problem.

• Drug therapy is effective in controlling and reducing the spread of a number of zoonotic infections, including leptospirosis in cattle. In one clinical case, proper treatment of that disease eliminated shedding of the organism. Without drug therapy, however, *Leptospira* can contaminate the environment, including milk and water, to create a health risk for humans (Jackson 1993). Similar reduction in the shedding of pathogens with drug treatment has been shown for *Campylobacter fetus* (Kotula and Stern 1984; Wokatsch and Bockemuhl 1988; Jackson 1993). Other major food-borne bacterial pathogens that cause significant human health problems associated with contamination of meat products are *Streptococcus suis*, *E. coli*, especially O157:H7, *Salmonella* spp., *Enterococcus* spp., and *Yersinia* (Clifton-Hadley 1983; Walton 1985; Tauxe et al. 1987; IOM 1992; CDC 1994). Proper treatment of infections from those pathogens at clinical presentation can reduce or eliminate the spread of infectious agents. "In the absence of evidence to the contrary," Mackinnon (1993) inferred that use of antibiotic drugs in pigs could reduce the transmission of some of these zoonotic diseases.

• From an economic standpoint, the therapeutic use of antibiotics to combat active infection in individual animals and herds is unquestioned. The economic benefit of subtherapeutic antibiotic use is more often debated—especially by those not aligned with the animal production industries. However, the overall economic benefit is made possible because of a 1 to 15 percent increase in feed efficiency and performance (growth rate, egg production) over similar animals that do not receive antibiotics (see earlier discussion in Chapter 2). The magnitude of the production response to low concentrations of antibiotics is influenced by animal age, diet, stress, duration of drug usage, and general cleanliness of pens, and stocking rates (Fagerberg and Quarles 1979). One could argue that this occurs only because of the impetus to intensify production practices, but this is the way that food-animal production is accomplished, and the economic benefit is apparent for these systems (CAST 1981).

Inspection at slaughter results in rejection of a proportion of carcasses—most commonly for abscesses, arthritis, pneumonia and pleurisy, peritonitis, and fever (including septicemia). Survey results on 1.3 million pigs slaughtered at abattoirs in the United Kingdom (Hill and Jones 1984a,b) indicated that 262,149 kg of meat and 273,080 kg of liver, heart, and lungs were rejected, contributing to millions of dollars lost in the production of the animals and an inability to recoup the investment input. The greater problem was that the pigs that went to market were not visually different from any other pigs that were slaughtered and that had passed inspection. The investigators concluded that many of the rejections were associated with localized lesions and further suggested that this valuable data resource (slaughter rejection data) was substantively underused in the identification of cost-effective practices to enhance animal health.

The effects of antibiotic drug use in many species are associated with a generalized decrease in health problems in the animals in which they are used (CAST 1981). For example, in the summary prepared for the Council for Agricultural Science and Technology report on antibiotics in animal feeds (CAST 1981), the use of chlortetracycline, oxytetracycline, erythromycin, tylosin, and bacitracin in cattle was associated with a significant reduction in the incidence of liver abscesses. Additional data demonstrate that the decrease in weight gain in abscessed cattle was lower than it was in nonabscessed cattle. All of these subclinical issues add to the expense of raising food-producing animals, and the use of the drugs is associated with improvements in animal health and in economic productivity (CAST 1981). In addition, Mackinnon (1993) summarized data from 12 swine-finishing farms where, throughout the year, a veterinary preventive medicine scheme was implemented to curb the effects of infection on production characteristics and carcass rejections. The introduction of veterinary advice coupled with selective use of medication to eradicate pneumonia and swine dysentary led to a progressive decline throughout the year in offal losses and carcass rejections and decreased carcass rejection variation (Table 3–1).

• Among other pathogenic microorganisms cited as food-borne hazards, *Erysipelothrix rhusiopathiae* (in swine and turkeys) and *Listeria monocytogenes* (in sheep and cattle) also cause clinical disease in animals that might be treated successfully with antibiotics.

• Human health concerns associated with antibiotic use often focus on the more nebulous connections between subtherapeutic use in animals and their consequences, but therapeutic uses also present a set of risk concerns. An assessment of some aspects of the economic consequences of partial or total restriction in subtherapeutic drug use appears in Chapter 7.

POSSIBLE HAZARDS OF ANTIBIOTIC USE

Scientific literature can be cited to support the opinion that antibiotics used in food-animal industries are fundamentally benign to human health (Frappaolo

TABLE 3–1   The Effect of Implementation of a Veterinary Preventive-Medicine Scheme on Offal and Carcass Rejections from 12 Finishing Farms

Survey Date	Total Offal Losses[a] ± SD[b]	Carcass Rejections[c] ± SD
April 1988	9.4 ± 5.0	306 ± 267
September 1988	8.1 ± 6.9	303 ± 287
March 1989	6.4 ± 5.0	219 ± 139
November 1989	5.0 ± 3.1	216 ± 77

[a]Value of rejected lung, heart, liver, and intestines, pence.
[b]SD = standard deviation.
[c]Weight (g) of meat and bone rejected per pig slaughtered.
Source: Mackinnon 1993.

1986; Van den Bogaard 1993). However, the Institute of Medicine (IOM 1989) and the Office of Technology Assessment (OTA 1995) reported on circumstantial evidence linking subtherapeutic use of antibiotic drugs in farm animals to potential human health hazards. The committee members who prepared those reports suggested that caution be used in extrapolating conclusions too generally given the paucity of data on the reviewed issue.

Antibiotic Resistance as a Human Health Risk

Many bacterial species multiply rapidly enough to double their numbers every 20 minutes. With even the simplest bacterial genome, the replication processes are imperfect and, statistically, chromosomal mutations and genetic DNA alterations develop that result in the expression of altered biochemical makeup of some feature of the affected bacterium. The ability for bacterial populations to adapt to changes in their environment and survive otherwise inhospitable conditions often results from the development of favorable mutations that allow for the coding of specific proteins or processes that are not affected by the impinging condition. For example, a hypothetical case can be constructed to suggest how easily an invading bacteria could proliferate to cause disease (Cooper 1991). Suppose a favorable alteration in a bacterial phenotype (the physical expression of the genetic coded information) occurs with the unlikely frequency of 1 in 1 billion. Assume that the average time for bacterial replication is 20 minutes. If an infection were initiated with 1,000 organisms, a first mutational event might occur in one organism after only 7 to 14 hours. Once that occurred, the relative proliferative capacity of the bacteria would allow it to attain significant numbers within 24 to 48 hours, given the longer replicating time in vivo in contrast to in vitro, or in a healthy animal in contrast to one whose immune system is overwhelmed. These events are fundamentally random, and the proliferating numbers are a function of statistics and probability. Therefore, the task of assessing the actual biological consequences is extremely difficult.

Bacterial populations respond to imposed environmental conditions and pressures by adapting and proliferating to become versions of the original populations that are better able to survive in new conditions. The new offspring are strains, and the term applied to the developed ability of the strain to fend off the survival threat is *resistance*. The factors that allow the resistant organisms to proliferate in the prevailing conditions are *selection pressures*.

The interaction of the animal's biological host defenses, coupled with the action of antibiotics, even when those antibiotics are used at subtherapeutic concentrations, is often overlooked. It often is either forgotten or dismissed because of the difficulty of assessing in vivo responses compared with the simplicity, cost, and turn-around time of in vitro antimicrobial experiments. The sensitivity of the organism to selection pressure is complex. There are clearer boundaries in vitro to define the effectiveness of antibiotics to achieve killing and conversely to suggest the degree to which a bacterium is sensitive to a given drug. Very low drug concentrations might be ineffective in vitro in incapacitating the growth of a given bacterial population, and high concentrations might be required to be effective. However, as a caveat, the concentration of antibiotic that kills an organism in vitro might not affect the organism's survival in vivo. Certainly, the ability of the animal's immune system to interact with a chemotherapeutic agent to clear and eliminate invading organisms must be considered. There are clear data from biomedical research to suggest that the natural host defenses against invading bacteria are increased with the use of antibiotics. Furthermore, several studies illustrate the fact that the use of subtherapeutic concentrations of antibiotics increases specific immunological responses of the host to the invading bacteria (Easmon and Desmond 1982; Veringa and Verhoef 1985; Hand et al. 1989). Although many of these effects are reported for phagocytosis and opsonization of bacteria, the story is far from clear. Other data suggest that some antibiotics, such as the cephalosporins (Gillissen 1982), increase immunoglobulin production but decrease lymphocyte blastogenic capability (Chaperon 1982); still others, such as the rifamycins (Bassi and Bolzoni 1982) affect immunosuppression.

The drug concentrations that can kill a given microbial species also might be toxic to humans or animals. For example, chloramphenicol is highly effective against many pathogenic microorganisms. Although well tolerated in domestic animals, this antibiotic in humans results in the non-dose-related development of aplastic anemia. As a result, chloramphenicol has been banned from use under any circumstance in food-producing animals because of possible residue carryover (Merck Veterinary Manual 1986).

The emergence of resistance in a bacterial population does not automatically signal the emergence of a pathological disease corollary. Similarly, in animal production, the emergence of resistance does not necessarily confer inefficacy on subtherapeutic antibiotic use. However, several cases of human illness from antibiotic-resistant pathogens that originated in antibiotic-treated livestock have occurred (IOM 1989). Likewise, there is a report in the literature of a *Salmonella* infection of a mother and nursery infants that was associated with the mother handling sick calves that had recently arrived on the farm from several locations. The resistance patterns of the bacteria (chloramphenicol, sulfa-methoxazole, and tetracycline) were unique, but the calves presumably were infected before coming to the farm and without direct administration of those antibiotics (Lyons et al. 1980).

Recent studies on plasmid transfer between bacteria have suggested that resistance factors can be linked with genes that code for enhanced virulence (the capability to cause disease). Consequently, the potential for animal-to-human transfer in this fashion exists. The risk is greater than zero, but basically incalculable, and the threat is perceived to be significant (WHO 1997; IOM 1998). The use of *perceived* here is stressed. The threat might be real, and case studies have shown that the passage of resistant organisms from animals to humans can occur and be perpetuated and amplified through food (Spika et al. 1987).

The question remains, How likely is that to happen? The answer is not available and can be addressed only with the development of the proper database and effective risk analysis. The database should be generated jointly by regulatory agencies; animal, pharmaceutical, and health-care industries; and academic basic and clinical science departments. It must be open to all concerned parties.

Antibiotic Resistance Trends

A 1994 *Science* editorial, "The Biological Warfare of the Future," described the issue of antibiotic resistance as "a menace of major proportions to the health of the world" (Koshland 1994). Most of the issue in which the editorial appeared was devoted to a discussion of the problems in antibiotic resistance. With current funding restricting the development of new agents (Culotta 1994) and with a paucity of promising new antibiotic drugs for veterinary and human use occurring at a time of emerging multidrug-resistance problems, the health and well-being of the U.S. and European human populations are seriously threatened (Kingman 1994). Microbial resistance to antibiotics is a global issue that amounts to what some health professionals consider a crisis (Kunin 1983 and 1993; Levy 1992; Burke and Levy 1985; Neu 1992; Cohen 1993). This is reflected in the stand taken by the World Health Organization (WHO) in its world health report statement (WHO 1998). Kunin (1993) outlined the response of many multinational groups and their efforts to control the problem, particularly in human use and applications. Many of those efforts involve increased education and broadened awareness of the proper and improper use of these powerful drugs, largely based on documentation of disease in hospitals and health care facilities. Concerns about the agricultural use of antibiotics were raised because of the large amount of the drugs used and the potential for disease to occur in humans—

despite the low rate of documented cases. Witte (1998) reemphasized the human clinical stand on the use of antibiotics in agriculture as a health risk to humans, citing specific examples of avoparcin-related, vancomycin-resistant enterococci disease transfer from animals to humans and the speculation about the relationship between *satA-gene*-mediated streptogramines-resistance development and the use of virginiamycin in food animals. The concern is that the unwarranted use of antibiotics "can lead to unexpected consequences that limit medical choices."

A full discussion of the problem of worldwide multidrug resistance is beyond the scope of this report, but in an era of crisis, defining the contributing factors is of paramount importance in designing solutions. There is a great deal of disagreement over who or what is responsible for the spread of antibiotic resistance. Clearly, much evidence suggests that most of clinically important resistant pathogens in humans result from inappropriate uses of antibiotics in human medicine (IOM 1989 and 1998; Amabile-Cuevas 1993; Hickey and Nelson 1997). There are some data that support the idea that antibiotic resistance in agriculture can result from the use of antibiotics in subtherapeutic and therapeutic regimens in the food-animal industry (for example, Berghash et al. 1983; Kobland et al. 1987). The challenge is to determine the extent to which resistant microbes of animal origin affect human health. The challenge addresses the interconnectedness of the respective ecosystems and might not be resolved with current clinical data. If resistance to a drug develops but the microorganism is not a pathogen, is there a propensity for human disease? Similarly, although possible in laboratory settings, the passage of resistance plasmids from clinically benign to pathogenic bacteria might be clinically irrelevant. However, the answer to this concern is incomplete because of very limited data on passage frequency outside the laboratory.

The issue of antibiotic resistance in bacteria from animals is relevant to human health (Dupont and Steele 1987). A component of the concern could arise from the relationship of humans and the farm animal environment (Haapapuro et al. 1997). Levy (1992) voiced concerns regarding antibiotic use in farm animals and the consequences of resistance in humans from environmental exposure to animal manure:

> For example, the amount of feces excreted by a cow per day is 100 times more than that of a human each day. If an animal is given an antibiotic, the fecal bacteria that survive the antibiotic treatment are resistant to it. Hence, via their excrement, animals are contributing a large amount of resistant bacteria to the natural environment, much [more] than are people. (P. 140)

Clearly, the use of antibiotics in food animals has been associated with the development of human antibiotic resistance. The development of resistant microbes with antibiotic use is regarded as a fundamental underlying assumption of antimicrobial chemotherapy. The increase in resistance with the assumptions of antimicrobial chemotherapy and use in agriculture was cited in the report from a Rockefeller University workshop on antibiotic resistance as a threat to human health because of the increased propensity for this practice to set up conditions favorable to the selection of resistant bacteria (Tomasz 1994). In that report, however, the conclusion regarding agricultural use of antibiotics as a threat to human health was derived from a single previous review of the issue (Dupont and Steele 1987). The report failed to critically assess data that would take the conclusion to the next logical step—a substantive review of the actual development of disease (incidence, severity) directly related to antibiotic resistance in bacteria of food animals, and not to the mere potential for this to occur.

Threlfall (1992) reviewed the issue of drug resistance and antibiotic use with regard to selection of food-borne pathogens. He concluded that the prophylactic and therapeutic use of such antibiotics contributed substantially to the emergence of multidrug-resistant strains. He cited many examples of the emergence of such organisms from poultry, dairy calves, and pigs that he believed resulted in human disease. Conversely, Shah et al. (1993) reviewed the major pathogens involved in antibiotic-resistant human infections and their resistance patterns, compared them with the organisms and resistance patterns isolated from animals, and concluded that the veterinary pool has not contributed substantially to the overall profile of clinically significant antibiotic-resistant infection in humans. Wiedmann (1993) summarized the monitoring and origin of resistant organisms in humans and suggested that development of resistance could not be generalized but had to be discussed on the basis of specific drugs, bacterial species, or locations. Although he stated that the use of antibiotics in food-animal production had minimal consequences for the treatment of human infections in hospitals, those conclusions must be viewed from the perspective that the effects were minimal because there were alternative antibiotics that could be used to treat the infections.

All of these studies reached valid conclusions based on the interpretation of their data; however, none fully accounted for the issues of interconnectivity between species, genera of bacteria, or human and animal ecosystems. There are studies that critically examine the extent or mechanisms by which microbes pass from animal to human populations. Some microorganism transfers between animals and humans are clinically significant and result in invasive infections. There is no doubt that the passage of antibiotic-resistant bacteria from animals to humans occurs and that it can result from direct contact with animals or their manure (as might occur with workers on the farm [Holmberg et al. 1984b; Bates et al. 1994; Haapapuro et al. 1997]), through indirect exposure to food contaminated with animal-derived bacteria (Witte and Klare 1995), or from person-to-person contact after a primary exposure of nonfarm persons (Lyons et al. 1980). The passage of microorganisms from animals to humans probably also occurs without clinically overt disease in humans or animals, or more frequently, with self-limiting disease that is untreated. Clinically relevant diseases also can be misdiagnosed with respect to the source or nature of the infection. Chalker and Blaser (1988) suggested that, for each case of salmonellosis that is confirmed by cultural methods, there are as many as 100 undocumented cases (see also, ERS 1996b). Perhaps more insidious to unraveling the causes and effects of the relationship between animal drug use, resistance emergence, and the potential for human disease are the inherent problems of the tests of antibiotic sensitivity and the interpretation of results (Murray 1994).

The resistance of microorganisms arising from subtherapeutic use of penicillin, tetracyclines, and sulfa drugs in agriculture is suggested by WHO (WHO 1997) to be a high- priority issue. WHO would phase out the use of antibiotics—particularly penicillin, tetracyclines, and others used to treat human diseases—as subtherapeutic-concentration growth promoters in food animals. Arguments persist that even if low-level resistance to antibiotics exists in bacteria from treated food animals, illness resulting from infection by organisms resistant to these drugs could easily be controlled by newer medications available for humans or animals strictly by prescription (AHI 1998). Levy (1998) suggested that even low-level drug resistance is a factor that predisposes bacteria to develop resistance more easily to other antibiotics. For some people, alternative antibiotic therapy might not be viable because of physiological or even economic limitations, and for these individuals some level of assurance and accommodation might need to be in place. Until more accurate data on animal antibiotic use, patterns and rates of resistance transfer to humans, occurrence of actual disease emergence, and mechanisms of resistance are available, actions aimed at regulating antibiotics cannot be implemented through a science-driven, well-validated, justified process.

The consequences of inappropriate use and accountability of antibiotics in human and veterinary medicine and in agriculture are (1) a shortened lifespan of an antibiotic's usefulness, (2) additional complications in surveillance, (3) the ability to predict resistance patterns, and (4) the consequences for human health. Certainly, over-the-counter availability of antibiotics for domestic animals and the absence of professional oversight in many uses contribute to the frustration encountered by regulatory officials for the lack of accountability (Scott 1987) and limit the ability to make a true estimate of the magnitude of resistance problems that threaten human and animal health. Records of sales do not necessarily imply proper use, and there is no centralized repository of records of antibiotic use by animal species. Newer generation antibiotics are available only by prescription and this facilitates control over these drugs. In contrast, ethical issues of illegal and black market drug use in agriculture as well as in human medicine could pose an undocumentable risk.

HUMAN HEALTH RISKS FROM DRUG RESIDUES IN FOODS

The toxicity of drugs is an inherent part of all uses of medication, and there are differences from one animal or human to another, especially in allergic reactions. Residues of drugs or their metabolites in food products from treated food animals are major considerations in the safety of drugs approved for use in food animals. FDA approval of drug dosages, routes of administration, durations of treatment, withdrawal times, and residue tolerances is designed to ensure the safety of foods derived from treated animals.

In the United States today, residues of carcinogenic chemicals or their genotoxic metabolites are rare in meat and meat products. FDA regulations have effectively prevented allergenic, toxic, and carcinogenic animal drug residues from entering the food supply. A review of the medical literature from 1966 to 1994 (National Library of Medicine 1994) yielded no evidence in short- or long-term studies of human cancers traceable to carcinogenic animal drug residues in foods. Chronic toxicity related to drug residues might be manifested by mutagenic, teratogenic, or carcinogenic potential. FDA operates under the 1958 congressional mandate that "no proven carcinogen should be considered suitable for use as a food additive in any amount." Many other countries and international organizations apply the same stipulation to prevent carcinogenic residues in foods (FAO/WHO 1961, 1988). Although FDA approves new animal drugs and permits the continuance of approvals of animal drugs that have potential carcinogenic properties in food animals, it does so under strict guidelines: (1) The compound must be used only at authorized concentrations. (2) The compound must have no demonstrated carcinogenicity in the target animal species. (3) No carcinogenic residues can be detected in the edible animal tissues or products after a suitable drug withdrawal time (FDA 1992). Some drugs, such as diethylstilbestrol, nitroimidazole, internal-use nitrofurans, and quinoxaline di-N-oxides, have not been approved or have been removed from use in food animals because they have demonstrated a carcinogenic and mutagenic potential (nitrofurazone as a topical ointment is permitted).

Maximum residue concentrations for these drugs vary from 0 to 10 ppm. In 1993, FDA proposed a maximum safe concentration of 1 ppm in the total daily diet for noncarcinogens; 2 to 3 ppm would therefore be permitted in meat, assuming meat would constitute only one-third of the daily diet. FDA states this concentration has no adverse effects on intestinal ecology (Kidd 1994).

Some 30 antibiotic drugs are approved by FDA for oral administration in food animals. Several are antiprotozoal coccidiostats and anthelmintics for control of intestinal parasites. The rest are systemic or nonsystemic antibiotics. Systemic antibiotics are absorbed from the intestines in substantial amounts and include tetracycline, penicillin, erythromycin, and lincomycin. Nonsystemic antibiotics are not absorbed or are absorbed in trace amounts. This group includes bacitracins, neomycin, streptomycin, tylosin, oleandomycin, novobiocin, virginiamycin, and the bambermycins. When drugs are supplied to animals in feed or water, only those that are absorbed from the alimentary tract can induce residues in edible animal products.

In 1994, residue-monitoring tests for 9 antibiotics in food animals sampled at slaughter plants were positive at violative concentrations in 0.5 percent of 3,595 cattle; 0.3 percent of 960 sheep and goats; 0.2 percent of 1,298 swine; and 0.3 percent of 2,112 poultry. The most frequently detected antibiotics were tetracycline (27 percent of total), penicillin (27 percent), gentamicin (16 percent), and neomycin (20 percent) (FSIS 1994a).

Residues of drugs used in food animals can enter the human diet directly (as compounds of edible animal tissues and products) or indirectly (from the environment). The possible clinical implications of consuming residues of antibiotics are: toxicity, allergenicity, and infection by drug-resistant disease-causing microorganisms. Drug residues are considered unintentional food additives and thus come under regulatory scrutiny, as do other chemicals added to or entering the food supply. The Food Safety Inspection Service (FSIS) of the U.S. Department of Agriculture (USDA) conducts and coordinates an intensive program of residue screening, detection, and research, and publishes annual summaries of those data (Domestic Residue Data Book, USDA, Washington, D.C.).

Antibiotic Toxicities

Most antibiotic drugs administered in therapeutic and subtherapeutic form to domestic animals also are approved for human use. The drugs have been shown to be relatively safe as based on the therapeutic index of the drug and largely through the historic database that can be used to link adverse responses to residue concentrations. Patterns, distribution, and residue concentrations in food animal tissues vary according to how the drug is administered. Treatment through water or feed avoids the potential complications of high localized concentrations that might accumulate at the site of injection, where intramuscular or subcutaneous routes of administration could be needed or used. Injection sites can pose special concern in regard to residues. Care should be exercised to ensure that the smallest possible amount is left at injection sites. Strict adherence to withdrawal times and suggested withdrawal intervals is critical, and sometimes removal and discarding of the tissue at and surrounding the injection or treatment site is required.

Acute and chronic toxicities have been evaluated and are well documented. In most cases, the amount ingested by an individual who consumes the drugs as tissue residue will be considerably less than that consumed as a primary drug (Wilson 1994). The likelihood of direct toxicity from antibiotics or their metabolites in animal tissues is extremely low, as indicated by the lack of cases documented in the literature (Corry et al. 1983; Black 1984). There is exception in chloramphenicol, a drug that produces toxic aplastic anemia that is not related to dosage. Chloramphenicol has been implicated as the causative agent in several cases of fatal aplastic anemia (in one case, a 73-year-old woman died after receiving chloramphenicol) after its use as an ophthalmic drug at an estimated total dose of only 82 mg (Fraunfelder et al. 1982). In another study, chloramphenicol residues were found in 13 calves of 3,020 tested (Settepani 1984), confirming that the residues can be consumed in human food. That finding led to a ban on the use of chloramphenicol in food animals in the United States.

The responsibility for monitoring food for violations of animal-drug-residue limits is shared by USDA (meat, poultry, and eggs) and FDA (milk and seafood). All standards are set and enforced by FDA. Details of the residue-monitoring program are discussed in Chapter 5.

The nitrofurans, quinoxalinedinoxides, and nitroimidazoles require restrictions as carcinogens, mutagens, or inducers of DNA synthesis, but the inherent hazards of their genotoxicity could be overcome by appropriate use and adherence to conservative withdrawal protocols (Somogyi 1984). For example, a conservative withdrawal period might be increased two- or three-fold from the last drug administration to ensure that any potential residues would have been eliminated. Such use and withdrawal regimens would preserve the value of these drugs in animal infection control. The toxicity of the sulfonamides in thyroid gland stimulation (Swarm et al. 1973) and phenotypically variable detoxification rates in the liver (Peters et al. 1990) require restrictions in food-animal use and continuation of residue monitoring.

Sulfonamides have been used widely at subtherapeutic and therapeutic concentrations in food-animal production, but increasing concern over their carcinogenic and mutagenic potential and their thyroid toxicity has led to decreased use, longer withdrawal times, and tighter residue monitoring. The sulfonamides approved for use in food animals are sulfamethazine, sulfadimethoxine, sulfaquinoxaline, sulfachlorpyridazine, sulfathiazole, sulfacetamide, and sulfanilamide (Compendium of Veterinary Products 1993).

Allergenicity

A literature search of published records and clinical epidemiological testing indicates that allergic reactions in humans from ingesting antibiotic-contaminated foods of animal origin are rare. Most reactions resulted from β-lactam antibiotic residues in milk or meat. The allergic reactions occurred in people exposed to the antibiotic drug residues in the foods. Many of the people went through prior medical treatment and were hypersensitized to a degree that subsequent oral exposure evoked a response (Dayan 1993). Dayan (1993) and Dewdney and Edwards (1984) presented several biochemical and biological reasons that antibiotic residues present in animal-derived foods are considered a relatively small health risk to humans: (1) The molecular weight of the free antibiotics is too low to make them immunogenic by themselves; (2) when complexed to larger molecular weight proteins that would make them immunogenic, the number of immunogenic epitopes per protein molecule is extremely low (less than 0.01 epitopes per protein molecule), which minimizes the ability of such residues to initiate a hypersensitivity reaction; (3) heating as would occur in food preparation further degrades residue epitopes and reduces the potential for allergic response; and (4) sensitizing reactions are more directly related to intramuscular drug administration than to oral administration and the epitope distribution of protein-bound drug is so low as to be relatively insignificant as a potential cause for initiating and sensitizing responses when they are eaten. A summary of those rarely reported allergic reactions follows, with a commentary on conditions resulting in the adverse responses.

Four reports (two from the United States and two from England) of allergic reactions in persons previously sensitized to penicillin were identified between 1958 and 1969, when milk residues of penicillin were more prevalent. Vickers et al. (1958), Zimmerman (1958), Borrie and Barrett (1961), and Wicher et al. (1969) reported patients with dermatitis, urticaria, and subacute eczematous eruptions after drinking milk that contained residues of penicillin. Dewdney et al. (1991) cast doubt on (haptenized) penicillin residues as the causative factor in development of penicillin hypersensitivity. They argued that the immunogenicity, epitope density, and overall concentration were too low to contribute to allergy development. However, they did not point out that oral consumption of penicillin was less sensitizing than was parenteral administration. Questions still exist regarding the ability of parenteral administration to be the sensitizing stimulus and regarding the consumption of penicilloyl residues as a trigger for hypersensitivity reaction.

Other cases of allergic reactions reported between 1972 and 1980 were traced to consumption of penicillin-residue-containing meat. One reaction was to residues in pork, which originated from swine treated with penicillin 3 days before being butchered. Another reaction was to the beef in a frozen dinner, which subsequently was found to contain penicillin residues (Tscheuschner 1972; Schwartz and Sher 1984). Two patients experienced pruritus on the face and fingers, and one suffered an anaphylactic reaction. No deaths occurred.

Relative Risks: Residues versus Microbial Contamination

Microbial contamination of food is a major health problem worldwide. Great difficulty exists in ensuring that foods are free of microbial contamination, and there are many points in the chain of processing, storage, sale, and preparation that provide opportunities for microorganisms to proliferate in food. Initializing contamination events might be innocuous, but under conditions that permit these organisms to proliferate, the build-up of pathogenic bacteria and toxins will contribute significantly to food-borne illness (Altekruse et al. 1997). Surveillance and monitoring of contamination and disease outbreaks associated with microorganism-based food-borne illness is spread across several federal agencies, including FSIS, FDA, and the Centers for Disease Control and Prevention (CDC). There are now 10 organisms identified and tracked by the federal agencies under a collaborative interagency Pathogen Reduction Task Force that produces updated Sentinel Site Study reports. Of these 10 pathogens, FSIS has identified *Campylobacter, Salmonella* and *Shigella* as the 3 most frequently encountered pathogens causing reportable diarrheal disease in humans (FSIS 1997). Surveys of disease incidence data between 1980 and 1994 (Bryan 1980; Bean and Griffin 1990; CDC 1994) demonstrate that, of almost 5,000 food-borne illness outbreaks, fewer than 10 percent were traced and confirmed to have arisen from meat or meat products.

Protection of the public from animal products contaminated with animal-drug residues that could cause human toxic reactions could be considered much more effective than protection from products contaminated with microorganisms. This is because there is little chance of residues entering the food after the point of slaughter and because so much of the opportunity for bacteria to multiply in an animal-derived food occurs long past the time when federal inspectors can monitor contamination and take action. Inspection at food-processing facilities can detect and monitor residues with accuracy, and inspectors can respond to violations quickly. But after a product is beyond the live animal, the risk of microbial contamination and microbial load increase with time. The number of handling steps and the care retailers and consumers use in preserving the integrity of the product affect the potential for bacteria to increase. Human infections and intoxications by food-borne microorganisms originating from infected food animals are commonly from commensal organisms of carrier animals. Prevention and elimination of carrier states in food animals requires an armamentarium of drugs and vaccines, professional decisions on their administration, and measures to ensure the safety of their products for human consumption. Safety of foods from animals that have been given medical treatment requires that the therapy eliminates primary or secondary infectious agents that might remain in carrier and shedder states. Antibiotics are needed for specific application in eliminating carrier states in food animals subclinically infected with agents that are infectious to human consumers.

SUMMARY OF FINDINGS

There appears to be a hierarchy of concerns regarding animal-drug use and human health. Principles of animal microbiology, antibiotic use, and food processing and preparation all relate to human health. Antibiotic resistance is a global problem found in human and animal environments, and is fostered by overuse, inadequate oversight, and inappropriate use in all areas of human and animal medicine. Only a multilateral effort can contain resistance. Inappropriate use of antibiotics must be controlled in all environments. Although resistance will develop in any animal, including humans, in which antibiotics are administered, the resistance itself cannot automatically be linked to a disease state. Current evidence indicates that microbial contamination of food causes many more cases of human illness than are caused by antibiotic-resistant organisms transmitted from animals to humans.

There is no doubt that the passage of antibiotic-resistant bacteria from food animals to humans occurs. It can result from direct contact with animals or manure, from indirect exposure to food contaminated with animal-derived bacteria, from person-to-person contact, and from the use of antibiotics in food animals. A demonstrable link can be found between the use of antibiotics in food animals, development of resistant microorganisms in those animals, and zoonotic spread of pathogens to humans. Although occurrence is historically rare, the data are woefully inadequate to show whether changes in disease rate are occurring. It is difficult to establish whether an increase in resistance detection is the result of increased antibiotic use in food animals or the result of the perpetuation of resistant species in food animals, the environment, or other reservoirs. Thus, a significant limitation is that the real number of incidents of zoonotic antibiotic-resistant passage to humans that resolve in clinical disease might not be well documented or even trackable.

Although therapeutic and subtherapeutic antibiotic treatment might be effective in decreasing a small percentage of the microbial load of food animals at harvest, the greatest proliferation of organisms occurs during inappropriate handling and processing after slaughter. A concern is that available data for critical review are scarce and that the information that is available is used opportunistically to support or refute claims by interested groups. In contrast to microbial contamination of food, drug residues appear to constitute a relatively lower risk as assessed by the available monitoring data.

4

Drug Development, Government Approval, and the Regulatory Process

Today, Americans don't have to worry about safety or effectiveness when they buy [drugs and medical devices] from cough syrups to the latest antibiotics and pacemakers. The Food and Drug Administration has made American drugs and medical devices the envy of the world and in demand all over the world. And we are going to stick with the standards we have, the highest in the world. But strong standards do not mean business as usual.

President Clinton, 1995
National Performance Review

OVERVIEW

The history of federal government involvement in controlling, regulating, and assuring the quality of therapeutic drugs in the United States dates back to the mid-nineteenth century and the congressional enactment of the Drug Importation Act (to stop entry of adulterated foreign drugs into the United States). Subsequent to this, President Lincoln (1862) appointed a scientist to the U.S. Department of Agriculture (USDA) to begin the Bureau of Chemistry, which ultimately would evolve into the modern Food and Drug Administration (FDA). President Theodore Roosevelt signed into law the Pure Food and Drug Act, further defining aspects of adulteration and healthfulness of food and drug preparations. In 1927, an enforcement agency was authorized, the Food, Drug, and Insecticide Administration, which, in 1930, was renamed the Food and Drug Administration. A significant act of Congress was passed in 1938, the Federal Food, Drug, and Cosmetic Act (FDCA), which set standards for safety, efficacy, prevention of adulteration, tolerances, factory inspections, penalties, and seizures associated with drugs, cosmetics, and medical devices. FDA was transferred from USDA to the Federal Security Agency, and a final reorganization in 1968 placed it in the Public Health Service of the U.S. Department of Health and Human Services (DHHS).

The federal structure that oversees animal drug use is complex, extending through the Centers for Disease Control and Prevention (within DHHS), the Center for Veterinary Medicine (CVM, within FDA), the Food Safety and Inspection Service (within USDA), and the U.S. Environmental Protection Agency.

Other organizations, such as the Agricultural Research Service (within USDA), work in support and they generate the necessary research data to answer questions of scientific importance in agriculture and human nutrition.

It is not main charge of this report to review the responsibilities of each federal agency that influences animal drug use, but the principal organization, CVM, is highlighted here because of its work in the approval and monitoring activities that govern animal drug use in the United States. Specific issues of monitoring drug use and drug residues are discussed in Chapter 5.

CVM has the important tasks of protecting society from harmful animal drugs and maintaining public confidence in the drugs that are in use. These objectives are achieved by ensuring that new drugs pass a rigorous approval process. CVM has pledged to be more active in its efforts to increase the availability and diversity of safe and effective animal drugs (CVM 1997b).

Under the larger structure of FDA, CVM regulates the manufacture and distribution of drugs and feed-additive drugs intended for food animals and companion animals. The structure of CVM has evolved to its present state after a series of reorganizations initiated with the change from the Bureau of Veterinary Medicine to CVM in the early 1980s. The current structure reflects the larger drug approval and monitoring process. In essence, the process through which a sponsor (a party interested in developing a drug to market) develops, manufactures, and markets a drug product is divided into two main categories: preapproval and after-market monitoring. The preapproval process is overseen by a section of CVM called the Office of New Animal Drug Evaluation, and the monitoring activities of CVM are overseen by the Office of Surveillance and Compliance. The CVM structure is shown in Figure 4–1.

The regulations that govern all aspects of the drug approval, marketing, and monitoring process are detailed in the Code of Federal Regulations (CFR): Title 21, Parts 500 to 599 govern animal drugs, animal feeds, and associated products; Parts 200 to 299 govern registration, labeling, and good manufacturing practices; good laboratory practice (GLP) regulations are contained in Part 58. The GLP regulations are an essential part of the regulatory process. They contain the standards of uniformity for study conduct, and they influence the uniformity and validity of data needed to sustain the review process. Some aspects of the requirements for environmental assessment are found in Part 25. Updates to these procedures are printed in the weekly editions of the *Federal Register*.

To obtain approval to manufacture and sell a product, developers must contact CVM with an investigational new animal drug (INAD) application and, ultimately, submit a New Animal Drug Application (NADA). Because of the reading and interpretation of the regulations, an animal drug is technically "unsafe" without an approved NADA on file at CVM, and the use or sale of an unsafe compound is illegal. The director of the office of New Animal Drug Evaluation, within CVM, is responsible for evaluating data and information submitted by the sponsor in one of several submission modes to satisfy the require-

Department of Health and Human Services (DHHS)
Food and Drug Administration (FDA)

Center for Veterinary Medicine (CVM)

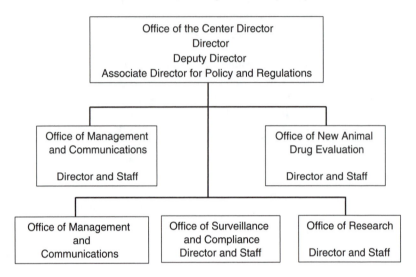

FIGURE 4–1   CVM Organizational Structure.   Source: htpp://www.fda.gov/dvm/fda/ aboutdvm.html; May, 1998.

ments for intended-use effectiveness, animal safety, human drug-residue-consumption safety, environmental impact, manufacturing processes, and NADA completeness.

Armed with preliminary data to justify further processing, a sponsor seeks initial permission from CVM to conduct animal studies. This step constitutes an INAD application and provides CVM with the data and information necessary to evaluate the stated claims of safety and efficacy for the compound with respect to proposed studies. The INAD is critical because it permits unapproved drugs to be transported to sites where they can be used legally in animal evaluation studies and contains the information needed to obtain an investigation withdrawal time and permission to slaughter test animals. FDA is notified when the animals are slaughtered, and the animals must be slaughtered at a federally inspected facility. A USDA inspector is assigned to the facility.[1] Tissues from test animals may not be used for food. The protocol for clinical study or trial dictates that animals be slaughtered after allowing a withdrawal time for drug depletion.

---

[1]For additional information on the INAD and NADA process, see CFR Title 21, Parts 511 and 514; CVM Staff Manual Guides 1240.300, 1240,3030 and 1240.31000; and FDCA, Section 512.

A newly evolving feature of the approval process added flexibility to relationships between CVM and sponsor companies. The levels and timing of dialogue, communication, and the structure of the review are more flexible. CVM is developing new strategies to be more responsive to sponsors' schedules within the approval process by allowing sponsors to establish the nature of the communications and review process through which approval is sought. For example, initial discussions between CVM and the sponsor will establish early in the development and approval process the expectations for data submission (phased review of data and studies at critical development points versus review of the total data package) and field testing.

RESTRUCTURING THE REGULATORY AND APPROVAL PROCESS

One fear in the U.S. animal and drug production industries and allied industries is that agriculture in the United States is in danger of losing its competitive edge to foreign interests because of the unusually long approval process. Drug products often are available in other countries before they are on the market here. However, it is an equally valid fear of regulatory agencies and the medical community that rushing the review process might jeopardize human health by allowing critical information to be overlooked and, thus, potentially introducing new problems to the nation. This is the price paid for ensuring a high level of confidence in the "unadulterated" condition of the food supply—a condition sometimes unattainable in other parts of the world. In recent years, the CVM's practices and procedures for reviewing submissions and approving products have been substantially revised but have maintained the goal of ensuring the human health. Sometimes problems that develop with the use of a given drug do not become apparent until the product has been on the market for a significant period. Oftentimes, neither reviewers, developers, nor manufacturers can determine whether an adverse reaction will develop in animals or humans. Therefore, it is critical that, after a drug has been approved and marketed, additional tracking information is collected on that product to ensure that new problems are detected quickly.

In the recent past, drug sponsors devoted 10 to 11 years in developing and obtaining FDA approval to market a drug. A substantial portion of that time was spent fulfilling CVM requirements and waiting for documents and responses to be evaluated and returned. As a major contribution to the "drug crisis," the federal approval process was considered ill-defined and slow by sponsors and animal producers and added years of additional work and expense to the frustrating experience of seeking approval (AHI 1982, 1992). Of particular concern was the burdensome requirements to continuously revalidate safety and efficacy results for compounds and drug combinations already established for other intended uses and to conduct costly multiple field trials in several locations. In part associated with constituent pressure and in part associated with the Clinton

INAD/NADA Elements

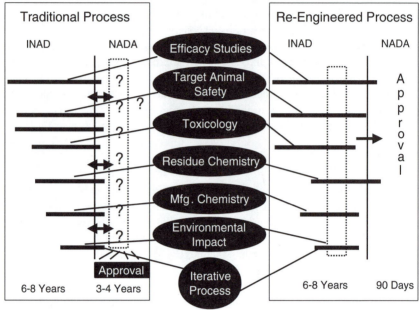

FIGURE 4–2   Comparison of the Traditional and Re-Engineered Approval Processes. Source: Adapted from a statement by Michael A. Friedman, M.D., lead deputy commissioner, FDA, DHHS, before the Subcommittee on Agriculture, Rural Development, and Related Agencies, Committee on Appropriations, U.S. Senate, May 1997.

Administration's larger goal of "reinventing government," CVM initiated newly streamlined processes to decrease some of the cumbersome paperwork that slowed the approval process. The most recent contributions to streamlining are in the areas of drug availability and "extra-label usage," which allows veterinarians to exercise their judgment to recommend uses for drugs beyond those specified on labels or package insert.

A comparison of the old and new approval processes, including schedules, is presented in Figure 4–2. The "traditional" approval process often was cumbersome and unresponsive to sponsors. During a 6 to 8 year period, developers and manufacturers would initiate and conduct the experiments needed to generate the data for efficacy, target animal safety, toxicology, residue chemistry, manufacturing chemistry, and environmental impact. After these data were collected, the sponsor would enter into iterative negotiations with CVM, refining the requirements of data to support the approval. Often, the sponsor would need to undertake additional studies to satisfy the review process, and this added significantly—

up to 4 years (AHI 1993)—to the time required to obtain approval. The new process is considerably more interactive with the sponsor, and it is more dynamic. The new process incorporates the iterative discussion phase early in the data-gathering and study-design phases and gives the sponsor immediate feedback on the requirements sought by the review. In the traditional system, the combined length of time of INAD plus NADA stages was as much as 12 years, with 3 to 4 years in the iterative NADA stage alone. In the re-engineered process, the initial INAD stage is comparable to that in the old process, but the NADA stage is reduced significantly to 90 days.

Dispute settlement in the past often was time-consuming, because there was no formal process, and adversarial attitudes often added needlessly to the time required to reach a decision.

Revisions occurring within CVM are reducing the time a drug application stands in review before approval. During the past few years, the trend has been to shorten of the average time to NADA approval from 47.7 months in 1992 to 39.1 months in 1995 (Figure 4–3). Although FDCA calls for FDA to make a decision on NADA approval within 180 days, even with the improvements in review time, it now takes 6 to 7 times longer than that (AHI 1994). Data were unavailable to determine whether the shortening of time to approval between 1991 and 1995 resulted from the increased efficiency of the review process or from decreased filings. The adoption of the revised policies was phased in beginning 1993 and

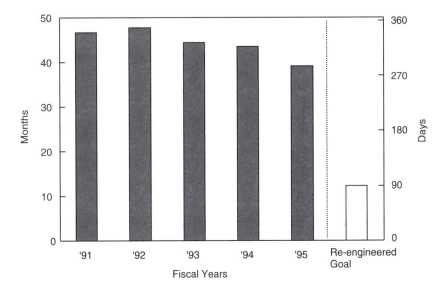

FIGURE 4–3   Effect of Re-Engineering the Approval Process on the Time to Approve New Animal Drug Applications. Source: CVM Summary of NADA Approvals, 1996.

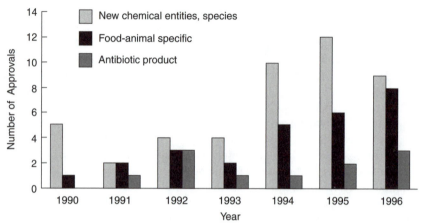

FIGURE 4–4   Trends in Animal Drug Approvals since 1990.   Source: DHHS, FDA, CVM Office of New Animal Drug Evaluation, 1996.

continues. Overall, there is a trend toward increased approval by CVM since 1991, and many of approvals are for new chemical entities or new species uses (Figure 4–4). Still another factor that influences the approval turnaround time is the overall increased quality of sponsor applications.

The aquaculture industry is one area of food-animal production that is truly hampered by a shortage of medications to treat diseases. Most compounds available are not antibiotics in the true sense but rather chemicals with limited specificity that are applied to the water. They include acetic acid, calcium salts, some vitamin preparations, herbals such as whole onion, formalin, oxytetracycline, and sulfa compounds. Treatments with nonapproved materials can be permitted for use by CVM through the filing of a "compassionate INAD," which permits the use of a nonapproved drug when the only recourse would be death or euthanasia. The requirements of the compassionate INAD are that some measure of public safety be demonstrated for the application and that data are derived from the process to support a formal NADA. The compassionate INAD is issued for a specified number of animals and is valid for 1 year with refiling necessary for extension. CVM considers the compassionate INAD a sound measure for offsetting the shortage of approved drugs in aquaculture and in its recommendations for these uses weigh the potential for excessive use against the safety of the intended use.

Important new changes in many aspects of the approval process are aimed at clarifying the expectations of submitting and approving parties alike. Multiple presubmission conferences iron out the details of required documentation of efficacy and safety. New regulations on multiple and repeated field trials are being implemented to eliminate the redundancy of information processing, thus reducing the time and cost to conduct, summarize, and justify such trials by the sponsor and reducing CVM's need to review such documents.

Reforming the Regulatory Process

In addition to the time required for approval, criticisms of the CVM policies also have focused on the cost and time associated with redirecting the use of a drug already approved for other purposes or species and the perception that finding flaws in approval applications is more important than is facilitating the approval process. There also are concerns that some of the requirements for accountability in manufacturing are too stringent and that the tissues used as drug-residue sentinel sites do not adequately reflect the risk of carryover into the food chain. Stringent drug approval requirements and processes that are questionably rooted in scientific data have been blamed for contributing to the shortage of available animal drugs and slow decision making that forces manufacturers to avoid research and development of new antibiotics and applying for approval for use in food animals (AHI 1992, Feedstuffs 1996). Substantial redundancy appears to exist in the CVM regulatory process. Animal-drug approval decisions that address potential human health concerns are handled conservatively, and progress on approving new drugs is hindered. The clash in views between manufacturers and regulators is affected by the lack of rigorous data upon which to base decisions and questions regarding exactly whose responsibility it is to provide data beyond a reasonable set of criteria or concerns. For example, the argument can be made that concern for the consequences of antibiotic use in animals on human health is valid even though few data address that concern. In reviewing the issues presented in commissioned papers and invited workshop presentations, the committee identified 6 points for which control over animal drug approval might be too stringent:

• FDA technical and regulatory requirements for manufacturing animal drugs are nearly identical to those for human drugs.
• Extensive, rigid, and statistically bound efficacy requirements for animal drug applications are equivalent to those for human drug applications; statistically significant dose titration studies for each claim of effectiveness and pharmacokinetics support studies for each species are required.
• Extensive target-animal safety studies are required for each species and claim. All are done under the rigorous GLP regulations. Many of the terms used in the GLP regulations are vague and poorly defined. Acute laboratory studies must be done for the Poison Control Center. It is often necessary to clarify the relationship between regulations and guidelines. In this instance, when a law or act is written, *regulations* are written to clarify and interpret the law. *Guidelines* (as might be presented by CVM) offer ways to meet and satisfy the terms and criteria in the regulations. This does not mean that the only way to meet the

regulations is by way of the guidelines, but they do offer one or more ways to fulfill obligations.

• For food animals, a rigorous, rigid, repetitive, expensive, and time-consuming food-safety research program is required for each species. This requirement alone takes 3 to 6 years and between $5 million and $8 million to complete. The food safety research and development program represents 50 to 70 percent of the research expenditures for a new chemical entity; those funds are committed early in the development procedure. The food safety requirements include extensive toxicological testing to calculate acceptable daily intake of residues of the drug. Then, elaborate metabolism and withdrawal studies are required to determine withdrawal times.

• The environmental concerns for drugs developed for use in companion animals are equivalent to those for drug use in humans; a major concern is in manufacturing. Food-animal use requires an extensive and expensive research package for evaluation of environmental fate. That area continues to grow. A minimum projected cost of $300,000 and 18 months of testing environmental impact are required for the simplest nontoxic compounds.

• A factor of concern in the United States and Europe is the emergence of socioeconomic and political pressure to shape the approval process. These sources of input can be driven by political and special interests and beliefs, generally with little consideration of scientific data.

The implication of the points is that, even with re-engineering, in many cases, there could be significant opportunities to further shorten the approval process. Those opportunities may need to be reviewed.

The Animal Medicinal Drug Use Clarification Act

In 1968, when the congressional animal drug amendments to the FDCA created the Bureau of Veterinary Medicine (changed to CVM in the early 1980s), Congress prescribed an animal drug regulatory system no less strict than that for human drugs. During the ensuing years, new animal drugs were approved on the basis of increasingly stringent safety and efficacy regulations. One important requirement for the safe and efficacious use of an animal drug relates to how and under what circumstances a drug can be used. This information must be contained on package instructions (inserts or directly on the label) and is called labeling. A drug can be used only for the specific purposes stated on the label; any departure from that use is called extra-label use. However, enforcement was minimal, and approved uses and dosages were widely ignored, because they were considered ineffective or inapplicable for animal health needs.

In its policy statement on extra-label drug use, CVM (1984) recognized that strict enforcement of product labeling would be detrimental to livestock producers, veterinarians, the pharmaceutical industry, the consuming public, and the animals themselves. Strict enforcement would result in unnecessary animal pain and suffering, increased animal losses, decreased use of animal drugs, and higher prices for animal products. To practice a high standard of medicine, veterinarians must resort to extra-label drug use when, in their professional judgment, the clinical situation demands it for the well-being of animals.

Extra-label use may be classified in three broad categories: (1) drugs approved for human use that are used in animals, (2) approved animal drugs used in nonapproved species, and (3) approved animal drugs used in the approved species but for a nonlabeled purpose or dosage.

The provisions of the CVM (1984) extra-label drug use policy were as follows:

• A careful diagnosis is made by a veterinarian who has a professional knowledge of the animal's health.
• No other drugs are specifically labeled to treat the condition diagnosed, or the dosages recommended on the labels of available drugs are ineffective.
• Thorough treatment records are kept on the animals, and the treated animals are identified.
• A withdrawal period between drug treatment and marketing of the animals is carefully observed and extended if necessary to ensure that the meat, milk, or eggs are free from illegal residues.

The extra-label drug use policy provided the means for CVM to address public health concerns by taking enforcement action against those who placed animals or public health at risk. This policy made the attending veterinarians responsible for drugs prescribed for or administered to food animals. Professional decisions on withdrawal times from all extra-label drug use were made by attending veterinarians, and the government continued to monitor animal products for violative residues.

The authority granted by CVM for extra-label drug use did not include lay persons. Extra-label use did not extend to medicated feeds and, because of human food safety concerns, some drugs were not allowed to be used in food animals under any circumstances. These include diethylstilbestrol (DES), chloramphenicol, ipronidazole, dimetridazole, and the nitrofurans.

On October 7, 1994, legislation legalizing discretionary extra-label drug use by veterinarians within the framework of a valid veterinarian–client–patient relationship (VCPR) was passed by the 103rd Congress. On October 22, 1994, President Clinton signed the Animal Medicinal Drug Use Clarification Act of 1994 (AMDUCA) into law. FDA published final regulations in the *Federal Register* (21 CFR Part 530) November 7, 1996 (Federal Register 1996). Some of ADMUCA's key provisions are as follows:

- Extra-label use of FDA-approved animal drugs or human drugs is permitted under the following conditions:
    —by the lawful written or oral order of a licensed veterinarian
    —within the context of a VCPR, and
    —in compliance with regulations promulgated by the secretary of Health and Human Services.
- Extra-label use of animal drugs in or on animal feed is not permitted.
- Extra-label use of an animal drug is not permitted if another animal drug contains the same active ingredient, can be administered in the same form and concentration, and lists the intended use in its specifications.
- The secretary of Health and Human Services may prohibit particular uses of an animal drug.
- Use of an animal drug that results in residues, exceeding established safe concentrations is considered an unsafe use.
- The secretary may provide access to the records of veterinarians to ascertain any use or intended use that the secretary has determined might present a risk to the public health.
- The secretary may, after allowing opportunity for public comment, prohibit an extra-label use of an animal drug if it presents a risk to the public health or if an analytical method has not been developed for testing residue concentrations.
- If the secretary finds that an extra-label use of an animal drug might present a risk to the public health, the secretary may establish, either by regulation or order, a safe concentration for residues of that animal drug and require development of a practical analytical method to detect unsafe concentrations of residues.

Even though extra-label drug use has been legalized, it is less than ideal, because a veterinarian's involvement might be peripheral or intermittent and, from an enforcement perspective, difficult to assess. An important question is how to establish "an appropriate withdrawal time" for a compound in a species for which hard data are lacking. One asset to AMDUCA is the Food Animal Residual Avoidance Databank (FARAD), a nationally sponsored project of USDA's Cooperative State Research, Education and Extension Service funded through the Food Safety and Quality national initiative. FARAD developers largely are associated with CVM, and are located in Florida, North Carolina, and California. Each location has separate but overlapping responsibilities. For example, the University of California at Davis is responsible for helping veterinarians establish safe and appropriate withdrawal times for extra-label drug formulations. The University of Florida serves as a repository for information on FDA-approved animal and veterinary products in a database that is readily accessible through the Internet as well as by phone and fax.

Under AMDUCA, a veterinarian who works in a valid VCPR (which involves total accountability for the use of the veterinarian-recommended extra-label product) can access the database or be referred to a professional pharmacologist to obtain information on the use, dose, and suggested withdrawal interval for an extra-label product. A distinction is made between a *withdrawal interval* and a *withdrawal time*. Only FDA can establish a withdrawal time, as the term is used in its legal application. FARAD establishes a conservative withdrawal interval or withdrawal time period, to provide a large margin of safety in eliminating residues from treated animals. In addition, FARAD makes no claims as to the efficacy of the intended treatment and responds only to inquiries from licensed veterinarians with suggestions for withdrawal intervals and periods. The use, dose, and withdrawal specifications listed in FARAD are obtained from several sources, including international compendiums of the same or similar products and formulations that are already approved abroad, and from published literature citations and data extrapolations based on referenceable data that can be used for the specific applications (Craigmill, A. 1998. FARAD, personal communication).

It would be desirable to improve the process of reviewing and approving animal drugs at CVM to enhance the availability of safe and efficacious drugs for use in food animals and companion animals under CVM-established conditions of use. Drug manufacturers and FDA should set boundaries for safe and effective use of drugs in animals as they do in humans. Approvals are needed for the dosage ranges (rather than for specific dosages) found to be minimally effective and maximally nontoxic, and withdrawal times for maximum dosages should be established. Local evaluations and decisions by veterinarians with appropriate training in drug prescription are needed to optimize effectiveness and ensure the safety of animals and consumers. However, if the issue of animal drug availability is not addressed aggressively, the legal extra-label drug use actually could be a deterrent to the animal drug industry in its attempts to discover and develop new pharmaceutical products.

The Animal Drug Availability Act

Given current drug efficacy requirements, relatively few food-animal species and a small number of diseases or production improvement uses are seen by the animal health industry to warrant the risk and capital investment now required for successful drug development. If those drugs or other new drugs are to be made available to a broad range of species, efficacy requirements must be interpreted to maximize rather than limit the potential of a drug for approval.

Clinical trials need not be the sole or predominant measure of a product's effectiveness. The realities of livestock production and drug use are that, in the case of food animals raised in flocks or herds, any drug product will be tested quickly in the marketplace, and those found uneconomical or ineffective will be eliminated. To remedy many of these problems and facilitate the approval of drugs, CVM undertook a major investigation of how it conducted its affairs. The second piece of legislation awaiting final rule is the Animal Drug Availability Act (ADAA), signed by President Clinton in October 1996, which introduced many new ways for the regulatory process to approve animal drugs and medicated feeds more rapidly. ADAA's overall intent is to lessen the burden placed on the animal health industry to follow the approval process while maintaining the protection of the public, summarized as follows:

• ADAA eliminates the strict requirement for field studies (except as requested and justified by CVM) by redefining and broadening the interpretation of what constitutes "substantial evidence" of efficacy. However, CVM still maintains strict requirements for proof of efficacy; where valid alternatives do not exist, the field study is the recommended and required evidence.
• ADAA provides for greater interaction between the sponsor and CVM; studies can be identified that must be conducted to provide needed data.
• ADAA creates a new category of animal drugs: veterinary feed directive drugs.
• ADAA supports flexible labeling to permit a range of recommended and acceptable dosages within a given species.
• ADAA defines *adequate* and *well controlled* more explicitly with regard to the conduct of field trials.

Collectively, the act reflects a significant improvement in partnership and in interactive and constructive discourse between CVM and other interested parties.

HUMAN HEALTH RISK, RESIDUES, AND APPROVAL

Risk depends not only on the nature and severity of a hazard but also on the probability of its occurrence. The probability of an adverse health effect occurring depends on the exposure of consumers to a compound. Thus, exposure assessment has as much of an influence on overall risk characterization as does toxicity assessment. In the extreme, there is no risk from even the most hazardous compound if no one is exposed to it. A more relevant risk assessment approach could be designed by identifying the residue of toxicological concern for a particular compound. The portion of the residue that is still potentially bioactive and bioavailable to the consumer could be identified. An assessment could be performed to determine the exposure of consumers to residues in their diets. The information would then be used to determine the most relevant approach for determining the risk posed by a compound (Mulligan 1995).

This type of assessment would require more expertise and evaluation by CVM and drug sponsors. It would require use of all available scientific information and extensive communication between CVM and sponsors rather than reliance on guidelines that spell out requirements. However, this approach would enable manufacturers to spend time and resources on those tests that would be most beneficial in identifying relevant toxic end points for the consumer and still protect public health (Mulligan 1995). The costs and delays associated with preparing inordinately comprehensive environmental-assessment reports have hampered research and development of new products. A modified, simplified environmental assessment, perhaps based on standard and uniform tests, could be implemented to circumvent an aberrant oversight. The ecological interactions that shape the evolution of pathogens (*Pfisteria*, for example) are only beginning to be understood and could substantively affect decision making in the future for farm animals, drugs, and the environment. By adding to the already escalating costs of drug development and by increasing the quantity of data needed for approval, this area of the approval process might have contributed to industry reluctance for developing new drugs for animal use, and it might have produced a shortage of new drugs to treat diseases with new resistance patterns. The effect of the costs and delays has been seen especially in the development of drugs for minor species and minor-use claims.

Perspectives on Developing Drugs

To better explain the position of animal producers, animal health professionals, and the animal health industry and how availability of drug choices affects their work, it is useful to view the problem in terms of the size of the related industries. As shown in Table 4–1, the sheer number of food animals raised in the United States is staggering. There are approximately 10 million dairy cows and more than 7 billion poultry. Actually, the efficiency of production (remembering that a substantial portion of increased efficiency relates to animal health and animal drug use) serves to hold the numbers of production animals down.

Table 4–2 shows that, as of 1996, the total comparative values of the animal drug industry, encompassing prescription drugs, over-the-counter preparations, and feed efficiency drugs, amounts to $3.2 billion. That is approximately 6 percent of the value of human prescription drugs.

Finally, as seen in Table 4–3, 87 percent of all animal drugs have annual individual product sales of less than $1 million, and only 5 percent of the available compounds generate sales of more than $5 million.

Animal pharmaceutical companies and animal health divisions of large parent corporations are expected to be financially independent and profitable. The number of corporations with animal drug development programs is declining through mergers, sales, or downsizing in relation to profitability and competitiveness. The number of CVM animal drug approvals had declined up to 1991. Some questions have arisen regarding the rate at which new approvals were authorized. In particular, few new drugs were approved for use in production of veal calves, sheep, goats, and fish. Reassessment of human risk by FDA actually resulted in the removal of some animal drugs from use in production, including

TABLE 4–1   Food-Animal Populations in the United States

Species	Population (in thousands)	
	1991	1996
Cattle and calves	96,393	103,819[a]
Beef cows[b]	32,320	35,333[a]
Milk cows[b]	9,966	9,412[a]
Hogs and pigs[c]	54,416[d]	60,190[e]
Sheep and lambs	11,174	8,457
Goats[c, f]	1,900[d]	1,900
Chickens[c]	363,594	384,241[a,e]
Broilers	6,137,150	7,017,540[a,g]
Turkeys[h]	284,910	289,025[a,g]

[a]Preliminary data.
[b]Cows and heifers that have calved.
[c]Data as of December 1 of preceding year.
[d]Data from 1990.
[e]Data from 1995.
[f]Texas only.
[g]Data from 1994.
[h]Poults that hatched less death loss of poults and young turkeys.
Source: USDA Agricultural Statistics 1995–1996.

TABLE 4–2   Comparative Value of FDA-Regulated Industries

Industry	Value ($ Billions)
Human prescription drugs	51.3
Human medical devices	39.4
Cosmetics, toiletries, and fragrances	20.0
Human over-the-counter medications	9.8
Pet food (dog and cat only)	8.5
Animal prescription, over-the-counter drugs, and feed drugs	3.2

Source: AHI 1994.

the nitroimidazoles, nitrofurans, and DES, which have been identified as carcinogens and which, by the Delaney Clause[2] of the FDCA, were prohibited as "additives" to the food supply.

---

[2]The Delaney Clause, which was included in the 1958 Food Additives Amendment to the FDCA, directs that "no additive shall be deemed to be safe if it is found to induce cancer when ingested by man or animal, or if it is found, after tests which are appropriate for the evaluation of the safety of food additives, to induce cancer in man or animal."

TABLE 4–3 Annual Sales of Animal Drugs

Total Sales of Individual Animal Drugs (%)	Total Amount Generated by Individual Animal Drug Sales ($ Millions)
87	1
8	1–5
2	5–10
2	10–25
1	25

Source: AHI 1994, with input from commissioned paper by Dr. John Welser, Pharmacia-Upjohn. Kalamazoo, Michigan.

For the animal production and health industries, the issues regarding antibiotic development, approval, and use are in some ways more complex than are those for human health. The human health industry focuses on approval processes for a single species, even though within that species, drug use applications are further subdivided and classified as to route of administration (because the safety profile differs by local and systemic toxicity as do the pharmacokinetics) and disease (because some are more severe and more risk might need to be tolerated). These drug criteria also are stratified by age, health status, sex of the patient, and so forth. Animal drugs traditionally were approved for each species and each application within a given species, and manufacturers were required to validate the claims of efficacy and safety for each use. For example, drugs for bovine use need separate government approval for applications in milk production, meat production, reproduction, and juvenile uses; poultry drugs are approved separately for laying hens, broilers, and turkeys. The reason for the separate approvals for each use is similar to that for humans: Relative local and systemic toxicities vary with the pharmacokinetics and these are affected by age, health, disease virulence, and sex of the animal. But also separate approvals are needed because, for residue regulatory actions, husbandry practices differ for the uses of drugs and thus the potential to affect human health varies. The redundancy in expected paperwork to substantiate an application submission for government approval and the response time on the part of the authorizing federal agencies were considered by the animal industry to be major impediments to the process and progress of drug development. Historically, the authorizing federal agencies have held firm that the health of the human and animal populations was of paramount importance in the approval process and that the integrity of the process would not be violated. Ultimately, the preservation of human health was the standard by which all drug-related decisions were made.

WORLDWIDE HARMONIZATION OF
THE ANIMAL DRUG APPROVAL PROCESS

Data packages are increasingly comprehensive, and multinational development of products is becoming more common. Harmonization of U.S. and foreign approval standards should be a major goal supported by CVM and the animal drug industry. In reviewing an application for a drug that has already been approved elsewhere, regulatory officials should take advantage of the valuable resources of other countries whenever possible. For example, approval of a product in the United States that has already been registered by the European Economic Community (EEC) should be a straightforward, speedy process. If a product is approved outside of the United States in a country with a comparable approval process, the process in the United States could be expedited.

The areas of human food safety, target-animal efficacy and safety, and environmental fate and worker safety are the major areas of data required in all countries for approval of a veterinary compound. Harmonized review requirements could be envisioned for these data packages. Data would include the following:

• *Human food safety.* This area includes toxicology, metabolism, biological effects, residue profiles, and consumption calculations.
• *Target animal safety and efficacy.* This area includes basic principles and studies on the use of the drug, such as its mechanisms, toxicities, interactions, and limits. These data would be needed to show that the product works and to define the limits. Exact dose forms, local clinical trials, and support use studies would be done for each country.
• *Environmental safety.* This area includes all the basic transformation studies, fate studies, environmental-toxicity studies, and worker safety studies.

Harmonization of testing procedures and standards for the approval of human drugs as part of the International Conference on Harmonization is continuing among the United States, EEC, and Japan. Many of the guidelines generated for human drugs also could be applied to animal drugs. Every effort should be made to harmonize such requirements as toxicity testing of human drugs, animal drugs, and pesticides.

Under the United States and Canada Free Trade Agreement, scientists from CVM and the Canadian Bureau of Veterinary Drugs (BVD) have harmonized human food safety requirements for approval of drugs used in food animals. The United States and Canada are to use a 6-step procedure for human food safety evaluation of new animal drugs. Using these harmonized standards, both countries have agreed on identical tolerances for 37 animal drugs (Brynes and Yong 1993).

Two important lessons can be learned from the efforts of CVM and the

Canadian BVD under the free trade agreement. The first is the importance of involving working scientists in the harmonization efforts. Having scientists who used testing protocols and standards as part of their everyday review work helped to ensure that harmonization was achieved. The scientists were familiar with the background and rationale for each requirement and could easily determine which areas were open to compromise and which were not.

The second and perhaps more important lesson is that harmonized standards do not automatically result in harmonized acceptable residue tolerance levels. Setting standard concentrations is the ultimate goal of most current harmonization efforts. For example, differences between the U.S. and Canadian tolerance levels resulted from different but equally valid conclusions made by different scientists about the same data. Harmonized standards and requirements would not have changed the outcome to any significant degree.

Although harmonizing testing protocols and standards is a worthwhile goal, until countries conduct joint reviews that lead to a single tolerance level, more emphasis must be placed on delineating guidelines for determining the equivalence of different tolerance levels for the same compound. One mechanism is to use dietary exposure estimates to determine the equivalence of tolerance levels, which normally are calculated from the acceptable daily intake (ADI) determined for a compound for human consumption. ADI is the amount of residue of a compound that can be ingested daily over a consumer's lifetime without appreciable health risk. Therefore, ADI can be considered the safety standard for a compound. If use of one country's tolerance level does not result in residues above another's ADI, then the tolerance level should be considered equivalent for purposes of consumer safety, trade, and, perhaps, regulatory decisions (Fitzpatrick et al. 1995). Again, agreement on the definition of terms affects how harmonization processes can proceed. The United States and the EEC have similar requirements for animal drug approval in all of the major data areas, and decisions regarding ADI revolve around a "no observable effect" definition. Japan differs in its approach to evaluating the human food safety aspects of an animal drug. Rather than calculate an ADI for a compound, Japan bases its regulations on a "no-residue" standard. On the basis of the most sensitive analytical method available, no residues of a compound can be found in edible animal products. Essentially, one definition constitutes a form of bioassay where the other is pure analytical chemistry.

The drug review process also could be harmonized by using expert panels to report their recommendations to regulatory groups for action. The panels should be international, so that their findings would be accepted by all regulatory groups as definitive summaries of scientific evidence. The panels would be charged with reviewing documentation by using the harmonized approach described above. The panels would evaluate the data and compile expert summaries. If the panels found the databases satisfactory, they could then recommend approval of drugs.

If the databases were inadequate, the panels would report deficiencies and recommend studies needed for complete evaluation.

Two examples of the panel approach currently exist in the animal drug area. The panels are involved only in the review of human food safety data for an animal drug. The first is the EEC Committee on Veterinary Medicinal Products (CVMP). The initial step in the approval of an animal drug in one EEC country is the calculation of an EEC tolerance level for the compound by the CVMP. The CVMP consists of animal drug regulatory officials from the various EEC nations. The CVMP reviews all available data from toxicology studies and residue metabolism and depletion studies, and establishes a tolerance level for residues of that compound in edible animal products. That tolerance level is then adopted by all EEC countries that approve the compound for use.

A second example of an international panel is the WHO and Food and Agricultural Organization Joint Expert Committee on Food Additives (JECFA), which evaluates human food safety data on selected animal drugs for the Codex Committee on Residues of Veterinary Drugs in Foods (CC/RVDF). JECFA is an ad hoc committee of animal drug experts from the codex committee countries. The committee evaluates toxicological and residue data on priority animal drugs submitted by the CC/RVDF. These animal drugs are already approved in at least one codex member country. JECFA establishes tolerance levels for the animal drugs; those levels are then sent through CC/RVDF for acceptance by other member countries. The United States currently does not accept a codex tolerance level for an animal drug if it differs from the level established here.

The issue of harmonization, however, can not be considered purely in black and white. Sometimes, harmonization of drug regulations is not feasible or practical. Although it is beyond the scope of this report to go into detail, it must be mentioned that some countries have regulations significantly different from those implemented in the United States. In part, the decision could be shaped by socioeconomic factors that make the greater risk in the use of a drug to resolve a rampant health problem more acceptable then the potential risk of the drug's side effects.

SUMMARY OF FINDINGS AND RECOMMENDATIONS

There are several points in the process of drug development and federal approval at which the added cost and time to acquire data and review them impede drug approval. Although historically the development of antibiotics was more-or-less a slow process of trial and error, the evolution of newer biochemical and molecular biological techniques has changed that situation. Newer methods provide tools that allow scientists to predict quickly how chemical modifications of basic parent antibiotic compounds can keep pace with the natural microbial changes that help populations of bacteria to develop resistance. The economics of drug development, however, make antibiotic discovery a matter of industrial priority setting. In the process of discovery and development, antibiotics are more readily prepared for human clinical use than for animal use. The high cost of new drugs makes them impractical for widespread use in agriculture, especially when a potential use is for disease prevention at subtherapeutic concentrations. In addition, in the past, approval of animal drugs in the regulatory process had the added burden of needing to show human food safety as well, thus adding costly and time-consuming projection studies to the food-animal drug development process. Recent developments at CVM, in part facilitated by the 1995 reforms to streamline the federal government, have shifted the regulatory process for animal drug approvals to a more interactive, quicker process. Examples of laws that have added and promise to add increased efficiency to the food-animal drug approval process are AMDUCA and ADAA. Additional considerations limit the availability of some newer antibiotics for animal use, as exemplified by the prohibition on the extra-label use of fluoroquinolone antibiotics for sub-therapeutic uses in food animals.

Veterinarians and animal producers are concerned that the recent increase in emergence of antibiotic-resistant strains of pathogens jeopardizes the future use of the sparse number of available antibiotics. The use of large amounts of antibiotics in food animals has been justified by the suggested benefits to human and animal health (that is, drug use ensures the healthfulness of animal-derived foods). That view might need to be reassessed. A growing concern is that the occurrence of disease and drug-resistant microorganisms in food animals as well as development of multidrug resistance in human pathogens poses a threat to human health. The development of a sound database needs to continue and expand rapidly to assess the relationship between the use of antibiotics in the United States in food-animal production and the impact on human health. The relationship will need to be reassessed continuously, and new procedures will need to evolve, just as microorganisms evolve.

The committee concludes that the pursuit of increased drug development and approval efficiency should be continued in a formalized reiterative process that integrates human and animal health needs with continuously updated data on patterns of antibiotic resistance, efficacy, and usefulness. With sound judgments based on data and emergence projection models, the availability of drugs for human and animal applications can be better coordinated. Decisions to approve or restrict the use of antibiotics must be based on rational and valid data.

Recommendations

The committee recommends that CVM continue procedural reform to expedite the drug approval review process and to broaden its perspective on efficacy and risk assessment to encompass data review on products already approved and used elsewhere in the world. Particular emphasis should be placed on adverse reactions, residue carryover into food, and antibiotic-resistance-emergence patterns. Efforts need to continue to further streamline the iterative INAD period, and, based on the time required for target animal safety trials and efficacy studies, the following are reasonable areas to streamline more:

• *An arbitration procedure should be developed to expedite the regulatory approval process.*

A formal written procedure needs to be established for resolving scientific and regulatory issues between the sponsor and CVM in a timely manner. CVM and the industry could compile a list of experts in the various disciplines willing to serve as consultants to CVM. In the event of an impasse, the consultants would be asked to provide a written opinion on the dispute within a certain period.

• *CVM should eliminate the guideline that all studies be conducted in multiple locations.*

The number and location of the studies should be determined for the specific drug, claim, and species. CVM could save additional resources by placing more emphasis on data from other countries that have previously demonstrated an ability to provide reliable data. The original policy that suggested the need for three locations of study was a CVM guideline and sometimes has been misinterpreted as a requirement.

• *CVM should review the requirement that all studies provide the same quantity of evidence to establish efficacy for supplemental applications as for original applications.*

The quantity of evidence required to establish efficacy should depend on scientific data supporting the relationship between the existing claim and the proposed one. If a supplemental claim is closely related to the one approved, fewer additional studies should be required.

• *More flexibility in CVM's evaluation of manufacturing requirements is needed (Stribling 1992).*

The issue is not whether an animal drug should meet the same standards of safety, effectiveness, potency, quality, and purity as a human drug. The issue is the quantity of the data required to demonstrate that the animal drug meets the standards. In every instance, the amount of data required should be assessed individually with a scientific proposal submitted by the sponsor and the obligation residing with the sponsor to substantiate the case.

• *More realistic estimates of human dietary exposure should be made when residue tolerance levels are developed.*

The requirements for human food safety testing for drug-related residues in meat, milk, and eggs are complex, and demanding toxicological tests of the parent drug and any potentially toxic metabolites, residue identification and quantitation, and method development for quantification of residues in edible animal products are required. In evaluating residues and contaminants, CVM assumes that all residues present in food have the same toxicity as the parent drug based on enterohepatic recirculation and hydrolysis of metabolites to the parent drug. It also assumes that residue is present in a food commodity at its highest permitted daily concentration over the lifetime of the consumer, based on a worst-case scenario. Those assumptions do not account for what the consumer is actually exposed to in the daily diet. Often, the residue remaining in food is no longer bioactive or bioavailable to the consumer. The food commodities in which residue is present might not be part of the daily diet of the consumer, or the residue might not be present in the edible portion of the commodity (Farber 1995).

* *To improve drug availability, worldwide harmonization of requirements for drug development and review should be considered and further enhanced within the federal agencies responsible for ensuring the safety of the food supply.*

Data and criteria for review should be standardized among countries, with final approval remaining with each country. Such harmonization could lead to direct savings in costs of drug development and even greater savings in time and return on investment for the sponsor and the animal producer. The harmonization process needs to be coordinated with drug-resistance-emergence surveys, so that the trends and patterns of antibiotic resistance in other regions of the world— developing countries in particular—can be modeled and structured into the drug development and approval process. Ultimately, increased use of international harmonization agreements will allow FDA to make more efficient use of its resources. Initiating the process of harmonization reform could prove slow and cumbersome, but diligence in this effort should produce a more efficient and responsive collective review and monitoring process. Desirable advances in the regulatory process would be to establish drug use guidelines based on maximum safe regimens for the target food animals, to set drug withdrawal times accordingly, and to develop tests for use on farms to certify the absence of violative residues of toxicologically active drugs or their metabolites.

5
Drug Residues and Microbial Contamination in Food: Monitoring and Enforcement

A principal goal of U.S. food-safety programs is the control of contaminants that might appear in food because of drug use in animals or inadvertent introduction of microorganisms. Drug residue control and microbial-contamination surveillance are accomplished through a rigorous, extensive process of sampling, testing, notification, and enforcement. Tens of thousands of samples are collected and processed annually in routine screening procedures aimed at statistically identifying the occurrence of residues and microorganisms. Three agencies do most of the work to protect the public from residue and microbial hazards: the U.S. Department of Agriculture (USDA), including the Food Safety and Inspection Service (FSIS) and the Agricultural Marketing Service (AMS); the Food and Drug Administration (FDA); and the U.S. Environmental Protection Agency (EPA).

USDA is charged with enforcing the Federal Meat Inspection Act (FMIA), the Poultry Products Inspection Act (PPIA), and the Egg Products Inspection Act (EPIA). Within USDA, FSIS is responsible for the wholesomeness and safety of fresh meat, poultry, and processed meat and poultry products intended for human consumption. It inspects slaughtering and processing establishments and samples and analyzes tissues derived from livestock and poultry at the time of or after slaughter. Inspection and analysis are intended to ensure, among other things, that meat and poultry do not contain residues of drugs, pesticides, or pathogens that cause them to be adulterated as defined in FMIA or PPIA. When residue violations are detected, FSIS notifies FDA, as FDA is authorized to take legal action against violators.

AMS is responsible for the wholesomeness and safety of egg products. It conducts inspections and analyzes samples for chemical residues to ensure compliance with EPIA at plants that process egg products.

FDA enforces the federal Food, Drug, and Cosmetic Act (FDCA). FDA is directly responsible for ensuring the safety of milk and seafood for human consumption and that animal feeds are safe and contain no illegal residues of drugs, pesticides, or other environmental contaminants. FDA also approves drugs used for food-producing animals, establishes tolerance and safe levels for animal drugs and establishes action levels for unavoidable environmental contaminants that might adulterate food. (The section on "Tracking Residues in Food: Regulatory Input" describes tolerance, safe, and action levels.)

EPA is responsible for administering and enforcing the Federal Insecticide, Fungicide, and Rodenticide Act, which regulates the manufacture, sale, and use of pesticides. EPA also is responsible under FDCA for establishing tolerance levels and recommending action levels to FDA and FSIS for residues or pesticides in food. Under the Toxic Substances Control Act, EPA also regulates other chemical substances (such as industrial chemicals) that can adulterate food.

DRUG RESIDUE STANDARDS AND SCREENING

Under the provisions of FDCA, FDA's Center for Veterinary Medicine (CVM) is responsible for ensuring that drugs are safe and effective for use in animals, and that food derived from animals is safe for human consumption. In line with the requirements for approval of a drug, the company developing and sponsoring the animal drug is responsible for furnishing CVM with the scientific information and experimental data showing that the presence of residues from a compound in edible animal products is safe for consumers. The sponsor often must develop and validate analytical methods to extract, purify, and quantify the residues and metabolites of a drug in tissue. Detection and measurement of drug residues are scrutinized by two approaches, assay level and analytical method status (FSIS 1995b). Methods are classified by level as summarized below:

Level I Assay results with highest validation and credibility; considered unequivocal at concentrations of interest; single or combination methods can be used to determine concentration and identity of residue; when used in combination, methods are confirmatory.

Level II Assay results are not unequivocal but accurate and capable of detection at the concentration of interest; sufficiently reliable to be used as a reference method.

Level III Screening methods developed to detect the presence of residue and needed for the high throughput of samples; samples that are positive by Level III methods are analyzed further by Level I or Level II methods.

Practical considerations influence the nature of analyses that FSIS will consider and accept as regulatory methods of residue detection. The criteria for acceptance are the following: (1) the method should take no more than 2 to 4 hours to perform; (2) the instrumentation must be common to all analytical chemistry laboratories; (3) the method must have a minimum proficiency level to detect the residue at the concentrations needed; (4) a quality-assurance program must accompany the method; and (5) the method must have been successfully tested and found reliable for detection of residue at 0, 0.5, 1, and 2 times the levels of published (40 CFR 180; 21 CRF 556) tolerance levels. The method status is further classified according to the source and validation of the method. Examples of method classification status are Official Methods of AOAC INTERNATIONAL, interlaboratory-study-validated methods, *Federal Register* methods, historical official methods, non-validated methods, published methods, and correlated methods.

The confirmatory methods are extremely sensitive and validate the presence of exact residue structures and their concentrations as determined by the mass ion of the molecule, using gas or liquid chromatographic separation and isolation procedures followed by mass spectroscopy. Over the years, the action levels of some drug residues have been lowered because of issues related to "sensitivity of the method," which refers to the accuracy and precision of measuring the lowest concentration of a compound. Over the years, as chemical separation and isolation chemistry methods have advanced, smaller and smaller amounts of compound have been measured. The relative safety of a drug, or its metabolites in edible tissues or milk, is related to the drugs being present in concentrations that have no substantial risk of toxicity or to its being present in such an innocuous form as to be biologically inert. The issues of toxicity become complex and well beyond the scope of this report when the toxic character of the compound arises from the animal's metabolism of the drug and not from the drug itself. The metabolism of some drugs varies according to species, and the toxic character of a compound in one animal species is not necessarily the same as that in humans.

Residue is defined by CVM as any compound or metabolite of a compound that is present in edible tissues from food animals because of the use of a compound in or on animals. Residues can be from the compound itself, its metabolites, or any other substances formed in or on food as a result of the compound's use.

CVM has a rigorous program for establishing the safety of residues present in food-animal tissues. Data are required for toxicity testing, residue and metabolism testing, and development of analytical methods. Toxicity testing is used to establish the maximum safe residue concentration in the edible tissues of the target animal. CVM evaluates toxicity with tests designed to monitor acute, short-term, and chronic toxicity over time. Within the scope of these tests, concentrations of drug residues are determined that affect morbidity and mortality as well as reproductive toxicity, teratology, and carcinogenicity. For monitoring the hundreds of possible compounds that might create residues, FSIS decides where available resources and testing efforts should be assigned, and assesses "relative concerns for those residues most likely to have the greatest impact on public health" (FSIS 1995b). Those decisions are made on the basis of data related to (1) the nature of the FDA or EPA withdrawal period, (2) the rapidity with which the compound is biodegraded to nontoxic products, (3) the absorption and excretion patterns and temporal profiles, and (4) the physical stability of the drug or metabolite in the environment (FSIS 1995b). If the tolerance levels of a compound are not available through FDA or EPA, the pharmacokinetics of absorption, excretion, and tissue distribution can be obtained from the literature. The chronic toxicity of a compound is often given a higher priority than is its acute toxicity simply because the chances of tissues having acutely toxic concentrations are remote. Finally, concern for the presence of residues also should be based on patterns of exposure. For example, for most chemical residues that occur in meat, USDA considers the likelihood of ill effects of one-time or infrequent eating of the meat to be of negligible consequence and risk to the population.

TRACKING DRUG RESIDUES IN FOOD

Investigators can use sophisticated chemical detection methods or drugs labeled with radioactive markers to study the pharmacokinetics, tissue distribution, and metabolism of a drug or test compound and establish the total residue content of the drug present in the edible tissues and in specific test site tissues of treated animals. Typically, muscle, liver, kidney, and fat are analyzed because they are the tissues that are typically eaten in large amounts, tissues that function as storage points for fat-soluble residues, or tissues that metabolize the major portion of the drug in the process of bodily elimination. Drug residue levels in milk and eggs are determined when appropriate. The metabolic profile of the test compound is determined in a sample of each representative edible animal tissue and in animal fluids such as urine or milk, when applicable. Urinary and fecal excretion patterns of the drug are useful in determining the biochemical events that regulate elimination of the drug from the body. For example, biochemical events in liver and kidney increase the aqueous solubility of otherwise poorly water soluble compounds by adding glucuronide or sulfate moieties. Most drugs are either metabolized and broken down to inert forms or metabolically conjugated to anions such as sulfate or glucuronide in the liver or kidney. Another use for the metabolizing and elimination data is to assist in establishing withdrawal times for drugs used in food animals.

The task of tracking drug residues would be considerably more complicated if all important tissues from animals had to be tested for residues. To facilitate inspection and detection of the carcass or product, regulatory agencies have determined that a single tissue site should be targeted for routine residue monitoring. On the basis of pharmacokinetic, drug distribution, and accumulation–depletion data, a target tissue is that tissue from which residues deplete at the slowest rate. In the target tissue, either the parent drug or a metabolite is selected as the marker residue. A tolerance level is then determined for the marker residue. The tolerance level is the concentration of the marker residue in the target tissue when all the residues in every edible tissue are at or below what is considered the safe concentration for that drug. This amount or concentration is derived from an acceptable set of toxicology, metabolism, and residue studies conducted by a drug company that has submitted those data as part of a New Animal Drug Application (NADA). A tolerance level for residues of a drug in the meat, milk, and eggs of food-producing animals is also the amount that is formally established and published at the time of CVM's approval of the drug. The tolerance level is established to facilitate monitoring drug residue entry into the food chain and to further aid in regulating the uses of animal drugs.

Some producers and drug developers are concerned that this conservative measurement practice is counterproductive to the use of many animal drugs, because the drug concentrations measured in marker tissues are irrelevant. The residue concentrations actually consumed in tissues frequently are much lower, and they are eliminated much faster than are those in the marker tissue. Some regulatory pharmacologists believe that the conservative approach is justified because of the possibility that another drug or pathophysiological condition could alter drug metabolism enzymes (for example, cytochrome P 450 complex) and slow the clearance of the drugs from the animal's body.

The maximum residue level (MRL) is not used by the CVM in its regulation of animal drugs. It is used by other countries and by the Codex Alimentarius Commission. In general, the MRL approximates the CVM tolerance level. CVM also uses safe level as a conservative estimate of the residue of a drug in food animals that is considered safe by CVM on the basis of the available safety data. However, it might not be sufficient to set a tolerance level. A safe level is intended to serve as a guide for estimating the safety of residues in meat or milk when no official tolerance level exists. Safe levels are not intended to supplant tolerance levels, and they do not have the same legal status. Generally, safe levels are assigned only when residues appear in meat or milk because of an unapproved use of an animal drug and because a formal tolerance level does not exist. The safe levels for an animal drug are the same for every species of food animal for which the drug is approved.

An action level is a conservative estimate of a residue level of an unavoidable contaminant in food that will not pose a human health risk. CVM initiates regulatory action if a residue found in food is above the action level.

An analytical method for quantifying residues in various tissues and biological fluids and for measuring the concentration of marker compound must be developed for the approval process. This work is done by the drug manufacturers and submitted as part of an NADA. CVM, in conjunction with USDA, submits these analytical methods to independent testing facilities for a systematic battery of tests. The analytical method must be specific, accurate, and repeatable when performed at different laboratories by different personnel. USDA and the FDA review the method and the uniformity of the results developed from the independent testing laboratories to ensure that the assay is based on sound scientific principles and is technically ready for testing. Typically, three USDA and FDA laboratories participate in the trial. If the method passes the trials, it is then submitted to FSIS.

DRUG RESIDUES IN MEAT AND POULTRY

The National Residue Program (NRP), operated by FSIS, is an essential part of the total inspection effort to prevent adulteration of the meat and poultry supply. Under NRP, FSIS monitors, detects, reduces, and controls violative residues of drugs, pesticides, and other potentially hazardous chemicals and contaminants in meat and poultry products. NRP collects samples of livestock and poultry tissues at slaughtering establishments under its inspection authority and from import shipments at ports of entry. The samples are analyzed for the presence of unacceptable residue concentrations of animal drugs that might contaminate meat and other tissues. Most samples for testing are selected either randomly or based on criteria such as incidence of past violations or questionable practices detected on the farm or processing site. Sometimes, informed sources provide information that leads to testing.

To narrow the effort, residue testing in the United States is divided into two major activities: animal population and product sample testing programs (monitoring, exploratory, and surveillance) and violation enforcement. Monitoring provides annual profiles on the occurrence of residue violations in specified animal populations. Compounds are selected on the basis of potential hazard and on the availability of a laboratory method suitable for regulatory monitoring. Information is obtained through a statistically based random selection of samples of normal-appearing tissues from carcasses that have passed visual inspection. Generally, the number of samples provides a 95 percent probability of detecting at least 1 violation when 1 percent of the sampled population is violative.

In addition to profile information, the monitoring program can identify producers marketing animals with violative residues. When such producers subsequently offer animals for slaughter, the animals will be subject to surveillance sampling and testing until compliance is demonstrated. The collected data also indicate incidences and levels of residues; enabling evaluation of residue trends and identification of problems within the industry where educational or other corrective efforts might be needed.

Exploratory projects are conducted for a variety of reasons, but whatever their objective, they have in common the fact that test results normally are not used to take regulatory action or to trigger follow-up surveillance testing. For example, FSIS might conduct a study to develop information on the incidence and concentrations of a trace metal, industrial chemical, or animal drug for which no safe level has been established.

Surveillance is instituted for investigating and controlling the movement of potentially adulterated products. Sampling is biased and is directed at particular carcasses or products in response to information from monitoring programs. In surveillance, the carcasses and organs might be retained until test results are available.

In enforcement testing, specimens are obtained from individual animals or lots based on herd history. Testing is performed to detect individual animals with violative levels of residues. It is emphasized in problem (high-prevalence) populations and used as a tool to prevent residues from entering the food supply.

Through 1996, NRP made use of the Compound Evaluation System (CES) to provide a systematic approach to categorizing compounds with respect to the likelihood of their occurrence in meat and poultry and their potential conse-quences for public health. CES evaluated the risk of residues in meat and poultry on the basis of hazard (adverse effects that might result from a given compound), and exposure (residues and factors affecting concentrations, such as drug use patterns, withdrawal times, and frequency of consumption) (FSIS 1995b).

CES ranked compounds in 24 categories. Compounds of greatest concern were designated A-1—those with a high health hazard potential and high likeli-hood of residue occurrence. Compounds of least concern were designated D-4—those with a negligible health hazard potential and negligible likelihood of resi-due occurrence. The CES coding was an alphanumeric system expressing the two parts of the risk assessment where it is apparent that the detection of a residue would be possible.

Compounds are included in the NRP monitoring plan if they leave a detect-able residue in meat and poultry and have an established tolerance level, action level, or other referenceable regulatory limit. FSIS must have a suitable regula-tory method that has been validated as capable of confirming the identity and quantity of the residue. A compound can be cycled out of the NRP monitoring plan when its residue potential has been evaluated and is no longer of concern. The exposure potential of such compounds is evaluated annually. When infor-mation indicates a possible increase in exposure potential, the compound is re-considered in the plan.

In 1997, FSIS performed monitoring analyses of 7,375 samples of meat and poultry for residues of 12 antibiotics and 7,284 samples for residues of 4 sulfona-mide drugs. The service also monitored 1,056 samples of food animals for ar-senic compounds; 7,409 samples for 27 chlorinated hydrocarbons and organo-phosphates; 1,196 samples for halofuginone; 3,327 for ivermectin; and 4,101 samples for levamisole. In addition, enforcement-testing analyses were per-formed: 219,193 samples for antibiotics; 15,638 samples for sulfonamides; 12 samples for arsenic; 296 samples for chlorinated hydrocarbons and organophosphates; 31 samples for ivermectin; 1 sample for levamisole; and 324 samples for clenbuterol (FSIS 1997). Data on the number of violations identified and violation rates are shown in Table 5–1.

The data in the table suggest that the risk of violative residues entering the food chain is very low. Most measured residues are obtained from tissues (liver, kidney, fat) that are much slower to clear (deplete) residues than is muscle (measurable amounts do not in themselves constitute violative contamination levels). There is a relatively large safety margin in the use of animal drugs when proper withdrawal times and uses are followed. The introduction of more rapid tests (such as FAST, the fast antimicrobial screen test) for antibiotics, which allow more samples to be tested suggests that the actual violation rate could be lower than that estimated given fewer samples.

Greater assurance that the food chain is protected from contamination with drugs, chemicals and other compounds is evolving in the restructuring of new monitoring processes by FSIS (1998) and with a reclassification of health risk ranking of the various monitored drugs. The assessment of risk embraces safety aspects of residues in foods as they might affect the health of populations where the effect is greatest, even though the size of populations could be very small. For example, penicillin is (and was under the old CES system) ranked relatively high (A-1) in the risk assessment. This was not due to any inherent toxicity of penicillins (as might be more readily equated with chlorinated biphenyls, for example) but rather is a result of the fact that, for some persons with hypersensitivity to penicillins, contact with these residues might pose a life-threatening risk (Hoffman, M. 1998. FSIS, personal communication). Certainly, penicillins are used in human medicine, but the risk to the individual is basically minimized by the patient's knowledge of the intended use and because of physician prescription and oversight. In the case of food residues, the consumer does not usually know what drugs have been used in the food animal from which a product is obtained. Protection is enhanced by assigning a relatively high risk score and allowing a very low level of permitted residue. A new ranking system is being phased in through 1998 that assesses the health risk through a mathematical function that considers the pharmacokinetic distribution and elimination of drugs in animals, as well as the likelihood of residue consumption, and the inherent toxicological properties of compounds and metabolites.

In addition, the evaluation system further refines tolerance levels for different drugs and compounds with regard to slaughter class–compound pairs. The applications and uses of drugs differ and so the chance for residues to occur varies because of differing animal husbandry practices for various species and ages of animals within species. For the purpose of statistical sampling, the numbers of samples and analyses are established to obtain a 95 percent probability of detecting at least 1 violation when 1 percent of the animal population could be theoretically in violation. For example, the number of samples requiring analysis (random sampling) to obtain this 95 percent probability is 299. This

TABLE 5-1   FSIS Animal Drug Residue Test Results

Drug Residue Testing	Samples 1994	1997	Violations 1994	1997	Violation Rate % 1994	1997
Antibiotics						
Monitoring program	8,354	7,375	19	9	0.23	0.12
Enforcement testing	211	118	8	10	3.8	8.4
CAST[a]	65,059	21,045	948	169	1.46	0.803
STOP[b]	102,521	41,995	1,046	292	1.02	0.69
FAST[c]	30,343	255	156,078	1,024	0.84	0.65
Sulfonamides						
Monitoring program	8,098	7,284	23	17	0.28	0.23
Enforcement testing	276	38	98	18	35.5	47.4
SOS[d]	166,091	15,600	104	24	0.06	0.15
Arsenic						
Monitoring program	2,223	1,056	5	6	0.22	0.56
Enforcement testing	66	15	1	0	1.52	0.0
Halofuginone						
Monitoring program	629	1,196	0	0	0.0	0.0
Enforcement testing	10	0	0	0	0.0	0.0
Ivermectin						
Monitoring program	3,926	3,327	7	6	0.18	0.18
Enforcement testing	7	31	0	0	0.0	0.0
Levamisole						
Monitoring program	4,077	3,846	6	0	0.15	0.0
Enforcement testing	59	1	3	0	5.08	0.0
Morantel tartrate	2,478	—[e]	1	—	0.04	—
CHC–COPS[f]						
Monitoring program	9,109	7,409	9	7	0.09	0.09
Enforcement testing	90	298	0	19	0.0	0.06

[a]CAST = Calf antibiotic and sulfonamide test.
[b]STOP = Swab test on premises.
[c]FAST = Fast antimicrobial screen test.
[d]SOS = Sulfa-on-site.
[e]Not done.
[f]CHC–COPS = Chlorinated hydrocarbons and organophosphates.
Source: FSIS 1995, 1998.

increases to 688 if the 99.9 percent probability of detection of one positive in a one percent violative rate and to 13,813 if the desired level of assurance is 99.9 percent in a population with a 0.05 percent violation rate (FSIS 1997).

DRUG RESIDUES IN FISH AND SEAFOOD

The amount of fish and seafood consumed in the United States is modest compared with meat and poultry (about 15.5 pounds per person annually). Much of that fish and seafood is caught rather than farmed. Nevertheless, aquaculture is a growing industry. Five drugs are approved by the FDA for use in aquaculture. Another 4 are approved by the U.S. Department of the Interior's Fish and Wildlife Service for use in hatcheries that supply sport fishing (FWS 1994). However, many more drugs are believed to be used in an extra-label fashion in aquaculture.

Monitoring of animal drug residues in farmed fish and seafood is the responsibility of the FDA Office of Seafood, which began its small monitoring program in 1991. In 1993, that office analyzed 105 samples of domestic and imported salmon and shrimp. Catfish, the largest aquaculture species, was not tested for animal drug residues. Through 1994, the office tested for the presence of two drugs: chloramphenicol in shrimp and oxolinic acid in salmonids. Both are illegal for use in cultured fish. Of 50 samples taken for chloramphenicol testing, 1 violation was found. There also was 1 violative residue of oxolinic acid in 26 samples. In 1995, monitoring of chloramphenicol in shrimp and oxolinic acid in salmonids was again conducted. No violative residues were detected in 36 samples tested for chloramphenicol or in 66 samples tested for oxolinic acid.

The process for choosing which drugs to test involves using the same questions of hazard and exposure as used by FSIS but is much less formal. FDA monitoring of aquaculture products also is constrained by a lack of test methods.

DRUG RESIDUES IN MILK

FDA has the primary responsibility for regulating milk. Its milk safety program relies on participation by state regulatory agencies. The National Conference on Interstate Milk Shipments (NCIMS) is a cooperative program of the states and U.S. Public Health Service for certification of interstate milk shippers. Its procedures, administration, and enforcement actions provide the framework for the nation's Grade A milk safety program (FDA 1995b).

Every tanker-truck milk load entering a dairy processing plant is tested for drug residues. The only official test for detecting drug residues under the Pasteurized Milk Ordinance (PMO) is the *Bacillus stearothermophilus* disk assay. That test is effective in detecting 4 drugs in the penicillin family (β-lactams). However, FDA has approved 53 drugs for use by dairies, including 20 antibiotics.

FDA believes that more than 78 drugs might be used in legal and illegal preparations in dairy cows (GAO 1990). Data from the FDA check ratings (inspections of selected dairy farms and validated state inspection programs) in 1990 and 1991 found 62 drugs not approved for use in dairy cows; 42 drugs were not approved for any use in food animals (GAO 1992).

With the support of NCIMS, FDA initiated the National Drug Residue Milk Monitoring Program (NDRMMP) in February 1991 (FDA 1995b). The program has the following objectives:

• Provide an indication of the animal drug residues that might be present in milk.

• Provide an indication, through follow-up investigations, of the extent to which farmers, distributors, and veterinarians comply with FDA regulations for the proper sale, distribution, and use of drugs in dairy cattle.

• Assist federal, state, and local milk officials in designing educational and enforcement programs by providing information on drug residues in milk.

• Facilitate the transfer of analytical methods and technology from FDA to state and industry laboratories.

The number of samples tested within this program is small relative to the milk supply. In 1993, the program analyzed 357 milk samples for 8 sulfa drugs, 3 tetracyclines, 4 β-lactams, and chloramphenicol (CVM 1993a,b,c; 1994). The tests found only 1 violative residue of a β-lactam and 4 nonviolative residues of sulfadimethoxine.

Violation rates for drugs tested in milk are extremely low. One reason might be that penalties for violations found at the dairies are immediate and severe. Usually, a tanker-truck pools milk from several farms. When a violation is found, further testing is done of samples from each farm. The offending farmer is responsible for finding a site to dump the milk and for reimbursing other farmers for the loss of the load at current prices of $5,000 or more (Carlson 1994).

As of October 31, 1994, all 50 states and Puerto Rico participate in the database program. The database includes results of NDRMMP, as reported by the states. Although all 50 states and Puerto Rico participate in the program, it is important to recognize that the samples and tests reported do not necessarily represent 100 percent of the milk supply from every state because the program is voluntary. However, as state participation in the database program has increased, reporting of the number of samples and tests also has increased.

Between October 1, 1995, and September 30, 1996, 4,565,600 samples of milk were analyzed for animal drug residues. Of these, 5,404 tested positive for a residue. The breakdown of these results by sample source is shown in Table 5–2. The data show that the rate of occurrence of any residues in pasteurized fluid milk is extremely low.

TABLE 5–2   Drug Residue Analysis Results for Grade A and Non-Grade-A Milk

Sample Source	Total Samples	Total Positive Samples	Total Percentage Positive
Grade A			
Bulk Milk			
Pick-Up			
Tanker	3,006,634	3,114	0.104
Pasteurized			
Fluid Milk and			
Milk Products	77,778	0	0
Producer	871,882	1,584	0.182
Other	127,916	43	0.034
Non-grade-A			
Bulk Milk			
Pick-Up			
Tanker	378,145	416	0.110
Pasteurized			
Fluid Milk and			
Milk Products	779	2	0.257
Producer	84,132	233	0.277
Other	18,334	12	0.065
Total	**4,565,600**	**5,404**	*

*The asterisk notes that a summary of the percent positive cannot be provided because there is not uniformity in terms of sampling in the four categories. For example, the PMO sets forth specific sampling requirements for beta-lactam testing as follows:

1. Bulk Milk Pickup Tanker Samples—samples are taken daily on every tanker.

2. Pasteurized fluid milk and milk products—a minimum of four samples must be tested for each product at each plant every six months.

3. Producer—each producer must be tested at least four times every six months.

4. Other—samples are conducted on a random basis.

Source: Adapted from National Milk Drug Residue Data Base Fiscal Year 1996 Annual Report; http://vm.cfsan.fda.gov/~ear/milkrp96.html.

The Grade A Pasteurized Milk Ordinance

The Public Health Service has always held a great interest in dairy products because few foods surpass milk as a single source of dietary elements needed for the maintenance of proper health, particularly in infants and the elderly. Milk also can serve as a vehicle for disease-bearing organisms, and it has been associated with major disease outbreaks.

In recent years, milk and milk products have been associated with less than 1 percent of disease outbreaks due to infected foods and contaminated water. Because of Public Health Service efforts in technical assistance, training, research, standards development, evaluation, and certification, the quality of the nation's milk supply has improved tremendously. Despite the progress, however, occasional milk-borne disease outbreaks still occur, emphasizing the need for continued vigilance at every stage of production (processing, pasteurization, and distribution of milk and milk products). Thus, it is imperative that quality-assurance programs exist that are mutually acceptable to producers and regulatory agencies to ensure the ready availability and safety of milk and milk products.

For example, according to the PMO, every dairy farm milk hauler, milk plant, receiving station, and transfer station is monitored routinely for antibiotic residues. Regulatory agencies inspect each milk tanker-truck at least every 12 months. Similarly, the individual hauler's pick-up and sampling procedures are inspected at least once every 24 months. Every dairy farm and transfer station is inspected at least once every 6 months, and every milk plant and receiving station are inspected at least once every 3 months.

Milk and milk products also are examined. It is the responsibility of the milk hauler to collect a representative sample of milk from each farm bulk tank to determine bacterial counts, somatic-cell counts (SCC, white blood cells found in milk that correlate with udder infection and host response), and cooling temperature. In addition, drug tests on milk from each producer are conducted at least 4 times over a 6-month period. Similarly, bacteria counts, drug tests, coliform determinations, phosphatase tests, and cooling-temperature checks are performed on pasteurized milk and milk products. For the purpose of this discussion, drug-residue testing of milk and milk products will be the central issue, as drug use in food animals is the major concern of the committee.

Unfortunately, some commercially available antibiotic-residue assays may have several procedural drawbacks that could affect conclusions based on these assays. For example, these assays may be performed on tanker-truck milk loads but have never been scientifically validated for such use. Similarly, the use of some assays to trace bulk tank milk back to the dairy farm have never been field tested for such a purpose. Finally, most assays can be performed on milk samples from individual animals but have not been subjected to a stringent validation protocol for this use. The significance of these issues and their implications are difficult to ascertain because much of the "data" are anecdotal in nature. Few verifiable data could be found in the committee's review of this area. Cullor (1992) and Cullor et al. (1994) argued against the use of current antibiotic-residue assays in uncontrolled settings and discussed the consequences of current assay performance.

Drug Residue Testing in Milk

Consumers insist on the production of safe and wholesome dairy products. The veterinary profession has a long history of participating in the development and implementation of medical practices designed to ensure that food safety begins on the dairy farm; this premise is a major focus of dairy production. Thus, animal production food safety is a key understanding between the consumer and the producer. Those who are involved in the production of milk or meat must have the tools and information needed to protect the food chain. However, the necessary tools (reliable antibiotic residue tests) are not available in most cases, and the lack of reliable tests points out a serious need to protect the producer and the consumer in future product development.

The PMO is used as the national standard for milk sanitation to regulate milk and milk products provided by interstate carriers and is recognized by public health agencies, the milk industry, and other organizations. Most important, the PMO is referenced in federal specifications for procurement of milk and milk products. This document is recommended by FDA for adoption by states, counties, and municipalities for improved uniformity in milk-sanitation practices in the United States. Through its adoption, the PMO facilitates the shipment and acceptance of milk and milk products. It defines milk and milk products, prohibits the sale of adulterated and misbranded milk and milk products, requires permits for the sale of milk and milk products, regulates the construction and inspection of dairy farms and milk-processing plants, and provides regulations for the examination, labeling, and pasteurization of milk and milk products and their processing and packaging, distribution, and sale.

CVM sets guidelines for protocols used to evaluate residue assays. An interpretive memorandum (M-a-85) issued in 1994 by the FDA summarizes the in vitro evaluation of β-lactam antibiotic-residue-screening tests (FDA 1997). Various portions of the evaluation were carried out by test sponsors, independent laboratories, and CVM. However, the evaluation protocols did not measure the performance of these tests by using pasteurized milk, mammary-gland secretions from individual cows, or field samples of bulk tank milk.

NCIMS is made up almost exclusively of milk processors, and neither producers nor veterinarians have representation on the executive board of this organization. NCIMS has a laboratory committee that is given information from the CVM protocol and recommends to the executive board whether the assays from CVM's accepted list can be used to conform to the provisions of Appendix N, which deals with drug residue monitoring of the PMO. In addition, processors can choose assays only from the CVM-accepted list to test milk, as prescribed by the PMO. Neither NCIMS nor processors have the authority to test the assays themselves, under their own protocols, or to approve a test kit for use.

Appendix N of the PMO deals with drug residue monitoring and farm surveillance. It was "established to reference safe levels and/or establish tolerances and to assure that milk supplies are in compliance with these safe levels or established tolerances for drug residues in milk." The industry screens all milk collection and transport trucks (called milk tankers) for β-lactam drug residues. Other drug residues are screened by using a random-sampling program for milk tankers. During any consecutive 6 months, at least 4 samples are collected in at least 4 separate months. Samples collected under this random-sampling program are analyzed as specified by FDA.

The testing of milk loads transported by tankers is completed before the milk is processed. Tanker milk samples found to be positive for antibiotic drug residues are retained. The industry records all sample results and retains records for 6 months.

When tanker milk is found to be positive for drug residues, FDA is immediately notified of the results and the ultimate disposition of the raw milk. The individual producer's samples from the tanker milk found to be positive for drug residues are tested to determine the farm of origin. Further pick-ups from that farm are immediately discontinued until subsequent tests are no longer positive for drug residues.

State regulatory agencies monitor industry surveillance activities by making unannounced on-site inspections to collect samples from tanker milk and to review industry records of the random-sampling program. If testing reveals milk positive for drug residues, the milk is removed from the human or animal food chain, except when acceptably reconditioned under FDA compliance policy guidelines.

The regulatory agency immediately suspends the Grade A permit of the responsible producer for a minimum of 2 days or issues an equivalent penalty. On the second occurrence of violative drug residues in a 12-month period, the producer's permit is suspended for a minimum of 4 days or the producer is issued an equivalent penalty, as determined by the regulatory agency. For a third occurrence of violative drug residues in a 12-month period, the suspension of permit is the same as it is for the second occurrence and the regulatory agency initiates administrative procedures to revoke the producer's permit.

The Grade A producer permit can be restored, after the penalty, to a temporary permit if a sample taken from the producer's bulk tank milk is no longer positive for drug residues. In no event may the Grade A permit of the violative producer be reinstated by the regulatory agency unless the responsible producer and a licensed veterinarian have signed a quality-assurance certificate, for display in the milkhouse, which states that the Milk and Dairy Beef Residue Prevention Protocol is in place and is being implemented for the dairy herds from which the adulterated milk, containing violative drug residues, was shipped.

Drug Monitoring in Milk

The influence of regulatory decisions on the fate of collected milk has caused controversy in three areas. First, several commercially available antibiotic test kits are marketed for drug residue detection in milk, and they are not equal in terms of lowest detection limit, repeatability, or specificity. Second, the outcomes of many of these tests are false positive or false negative, particularly at lower limits of assay performance. Third, these tests might be applied differently and tanker milk might not be suitable as a sample source for a given test.

Appendix N to the PMO (FDA 1995b) states that drug residue detection methods are to be evaluated at the safe level and at the tolerance level. As contended by Cullor (1992) and Cullor et al. (1994), it was never the intent, either expressed or implied, that residue-testing methods be "accepted" when they are assay positive, only at several times the established safe or tolerance levels. Unless producers or veterinarians are able to submit a problem at the biennial NCIMS conference and have it addressed, they have little or no input on this important regulatory document.

The PMO dictates that drug residue testing should be performed on raw commingled milk at safe and tolerance levels. CVM has been directed to initiate this evaluation and determine assay acceptance. In response, CVM designed a protocol that permits the acceptance of tests that detect antibiotics in spiked milk samples several-fold below safe or tolerance levels. Next, the NCIMS Board of Directors gives its approval on the basis of the recommendations from its laboratory committee, which obtains information from CVM, which in turn obtains most of its information from kit manufacturers, independent laboratories, or AOAC INTERNATIONAL.

The result is that antibiotic residue assays that are accepted by CVM, certified as performance tested by AOAC INTERNATIONAL, and recommended by NCIMS are used (1) for tanker milk without being scientifically field tested on tanker loads of milk, (2) for tracing back to bulk tank milk without being field tested on bulk tank milk, and (3) on individual animal milk samples without being subjected to the National Mastitis Council's recommended validation protocol.

Unresolved Dairy Testing Issues

Concern exists within the dairy industry that tests for antibiotics in milk are sensitive but largely confounded by variable specificity. As such, Cullor (1992) and Cullor et al. (1994) considered the consequences of false-positive test kit results and summarized the following:

• False-positive test kit results might lead to unwarranted waste of milk and enormous economic losses. (Note: The committee was not able to find data on a rate of true false-positive tests or data on how much milk was discarded because of false positive test results.)

• The dairy industry can be harmed if antibiotic tests that do not adequately identify untreated cows are used indiscriminately to test samples from individual cows. False-positive outcomes create mistrust among consumers, producers, veterinarians, and regulatory personnel, because they are interpreted to mean that bulk tank milk is not monitored adequately for safety.

• False-positive residue results can lead to the inaccurate conclusion that substantial proportions of dairy cows deliver residues into the milk supply every day.

• Despite the dairy industry's efforts to produce a safe and wholesome product, the widely publicized reports of residues in milk, which are based on inappropriately validated and applied technologies, will be the reports that are remembered and responded to by the milk-consuming public.

• Excessive positive assay outcomes, after the recommended withdrawal times have been followed, will result in individual dairy cows being culled from the production line. In the worst case, the false-positive assay outcomes might result in the cows being slaughtered for economic reasons.

• Eventually, this problem will harm international trade because of the belief that too many antibiotics are being administered to animals that are not being detected by the bulk-tank-monitoring system on dairy farms or at meat-processing plants.

Cullor (1992) and Cullor et al. (1994) caution that three salient points be remembered. First, the 1993 Grade A PMO guidelines (Section 6, p. 45, FDA 1995b) state, "In addition, methods which have been independently evaluated or evaluated by FDA and have been found acceptable by FDA for detecting drug residues at current safe or tolerance levels shall be used for each drug of concern." Second, the recent CVM test kit acceptance protocol specifically applies to raw commingled milk (tanker milk), not to bulk tank or milk from individual animals. Third, neither CVM, private testing companies, AOAC INTERNATIONAL, nor test kit manufacturers have evaluated assay performance under field conditions for appropriate examination of commonly tested milk samples (tanker milk, pasteurized milk, bulk tank milk, individual-animal milk, or milk from single-mammary-gland quarters). However, CVM has indicated that some antibiotic-residue test kit manufacturers have made label claims for such use.

The intent of the monitoring system, as viewed by CVM, is to have no false-negative assay outcomes. When implementing this system, false-positive assay outcomes will be automatic. That is acceptable as long as provisions are made to identify the false-positive results and to classify the correct positive samples. In the context of milk residue status, test kit evaluation process should account for bulk tank and tanker-truck samples stratified by SCC, herd size, management practices, and time of year. In addition, other factors, including milk composition, lactoferrin and lysozyme in milk from mastitis-infected cows (Carlsson et al. 1989), and colony-forming units and parity can affect the rate of false-positive results for residue-screening tests (Andrew et al. 1997).

FOOD-BORNE PATHOGENS AND CONTAMINATION OF FOOD

The predominant food-borne infectious organisms cited in surveys (FSIS 1994a, c; 1997) as causing human disease can be present in subclinical as well as active carrier states in slaughter animals. Key organisms are *Salmonella* species, *Campylobacter* species, *Yersinia enterolitica, Listeria* species, *Arcobacter* species, *Aeromonas hydrophila, Escherichia coli* O157:H7, and *Trichinella spiralis.* Other infectious organisms not identified in survey studies that might be present in carrier states in food-producing animals are *Leptospira interrogans, Mycobacterium* species, *Brucella* species, *Coxiella burnetti, Toxoplasma gondii, Cryptosporidium parvum,* and *Cysticercus* species. The use of antibiotic drugs as prophylactic or therapeutic treatment and the use of probiotics (feeding live beneficial microorganisms to animals to maintain or reintroduce balance in gut ecology; see Chapter 8) and vaccinations have been suggested as means of preventing food-producing animals from being carriers of these infectious organisms.

Determination of Pathogens

It is not difficult to determine the cause of "gastric upset" for someone who ate potato salad that was sitting on a table during a summer afternoon softball game. The salad dressing was the probable medium that allowed *E. coli* or *Salmonella* to proliferate throughout the day. It is considerably more difficult to establish the origin of pathogenic or toxic bacteria and microorganisms in meat and milk food that has caused in food-borne disease. Seldom is the level of surface contamination sufficient to cause illness if meat, for example, were to be consumed immediately after slaughter. The greater problem arises when other conditions permit multiplication of the initial contamination. Several factors pertinent to emergence of bacterial contamination of food—food infection— should be considered. Certainly, animals harbor bacteria on their hides, hooves, and within their intestines. Bearing septicemic conditions, clinically healthy animals theoretically produce bacteria-free meat; the internal environment (beyond the lumen of the gut, respiratory, and urogenital tracts) is sterile. Bacteria can contaminate meat in the process of slaughter through contact with the gut lumen contents, through inadvertent contamination of the meat by the meat cutter, or through unsanitary conditions in general, including poor hygiene of food handlers (CDC 1997).

Food-borne disease is an etiologically and epidemiologically difficult area of research. The Centers for Disease Control and Prevention (CDC) estimates that food-borne illness in the United States is often caused by proliferation of pathogenic bacteria in contaminated food (Altekruse et al. 1997). CDC and FSIS have established certain pathogens as sentinel organisms to monitor for food infection because of prevalence, rapid multiplication, ease of transmission, and fundamental difficulty in control containment. Among them are *Campylobacter, E. coli* O157:H7, *Listeria, Salmonella, Shigella, Vibrio,* and *Yersinia.* The food-borne illnesses caused by those pathogens are enteric diseases, and diarrhea and dehydration are the major clinical symptoms. Tables 5–3 through 5–6 summarize the studies of pathogen detection in meat and meat products.

TABLE 5–3   Survey Report of Microbiological Hazards in Swine

	Mean Percentage of Samples Yielding Pathogenic Bacteria in Swine		
Human Pathogen	Carcass	Fresh Meat	Organ Meat
Salmonella spp.	16.2	14.7	30.0
Campylobacter jejuni/coli	10.0	13.4	—[a]
Yersinia enterocolitica	3.7	43.7	21.5
Erysipelothrix rhusiopatheae	—	29.5	—
Arcobacter spp.	—	89.0	—
Aeromonas hydrophila	—	—	—
Listeria monocytogenes	—	34.0	—
Clostridium perfringens	0.0	66.0	12.0
Clostridium botulinum	—	—	—
Bacillus cereus	—	38.0	—
Staphylococcus aureus	100.0	55.0	—
Escherichia coli O157:H7	—	1.5	—

[a]Not tested.

S1   Rasrinaul et al. 1988
S2   D'Aoust et al. 1992
S3   Epling et al. 1993
S4   Saide-Albornez et al. 1992
S5   Barrel 1987
S6   Duitschaever and Butean 1979
S7   Farber et al. 1989
S8   Farber et al. 1988
S9   Lammerding et al. 1988
S10   Madden et al. 1986
S11   Mafu et al. 1989
S12   Tay et al. 1989
S13   Tokumaru et al. 1991
S14   Yadava et al. 1988
S15   Kampelmacher et al. 1963
S16   Epling et al. 1993
S17   Stern 1981
S18   Tokumaru et al. 1991
S19   Bracewell et al. 1985
S20   Rasrinaul et al. 1988
S21   Kwaga et al. 1990
S22   Oosterom 1991
S23   Delmas and Vidon 1985

Ground Meat	Processed Product	Critical Source	Mean References	Prevalence
40.3	35.0	Animal	S1–15	24.1
—	—	Animal	S16–20	12.8
11.9	38.5	Animal	S21–28	27.5
—	—	Animal	S29–30	29.5
—	—	Animal	S31	89.0
100.0	33.0	Animal	S32	66.5
12.0	—	Environment	S33–36	29.6
39.0	81.0	Environment	S37–39	39.6
—	1.0	Environment	S40–41	1.0
—	25.5	Environment	S42	29.6
—	5.5	Human	S43–46	46.0
—	—	Human	S47	1.5

S24   Fukushima 1985
S25   Harmon et al. 1984
S26   Kotula and Sharar 1993
S28   Schiemann 1980
S29   Schiono et al. 1990
S30   Molin et al. 1989
S31   Collins et al. 1993
S32   Palumbo et al. 1985
S33   Johnson et al. 1990
S34   Wang et al. 1993
S35   Pinner et al. 1992
S36   Skovgaard and Norrung 1989
S37   Bauer et al. 1981
S38   Smart et al. 1961
S39   de Guzman et al. 1990
S40   Hauschild and Hilsheimer 1983
S41   Hauschild and Hilsheimer 1980
S42   Konuma et al. 1988
S43   Farber et al. 1987
S44   Ternstrom and Molin 1987
S45   Vorster et al. 1991
S46   Turek et al. 1989
S47   Doyle and Schoeni 1987

TABLE 5–4   Survey Report of Microbiological Hazards in Cattle

| | Mean Percentage of Samples Yielding Pathogenic Bacteria in Cattle | | |
Human Pathogen	Carcass	Fresh Meat	Organ Meat
Salmonella spp.	1.0	7.8	0.0
Campylobacter jejuni	27.0	0.8	12.0
Yersinia enterocolitica	—	2.0	—
Aeromonas spp.	—	—	100.0
Escherichia coli O157:H7	0.2	3.7	0.3
Listeria monocytogenes	4.1	18.2	—
Clostridium perfringens	2.6	25.5	—
Bacillus cereus	—	12.0	—
Staphylococcus aureus	4.2	41.6	72.0

[a]Not tested.

C1	Rasrinaul et al. 1988
C2	D'Aoust et al. 1992
C3	Farber et al. 1988
C4	Tokumaru et al. 1991
C5	Farber et al. 1987
C6	FSIS, 1994C
C7	Garcia et al. 1985
C8	Gill and Harris 1984
C9	Stern 1981
C10	Tokumaru et al. 1991
C11	Rasrinaul et al. 1988
C12	Christopher et al. 1982
C13	FSIS 1994C
C14	Ternstrom and Molin 1987
C15	Palumbo et al. 1985
C16	Hudson and DeLacy 1991
C17	Doyle and Schoeni 1987

In 1996, there were 7,259 laboratory-confirmed, reported cases of diarrheal disease associated with 7 pathogens (FSIS 1997). *Campylobacter, Salmonella,* and *Shigella*, in that order, were isolated as the most commonly encountered bacteria. The joint Sentinel Site Study report (arising from the USDA Pathogen Reduction Task Force 1994) of FSIS, CDC, and FDA showed two patterns of disease emergence: low-level, random occurrences and major outbreaks. Large outbreaks often were traced to nonmeat and nonmilk sources, such as alfalfa sprouts (*Salmonella*), lettuce, and apple cider (*E. coli).*

Simple contamination of the meat, poultry, or seafood and fish might not be

Ground Meat	Processed Product	Critical Source	Mean References	Prevalence
46.0	44.3	Animal	C1–6	27.8
0.0	—[a]	Animal	C7–13	8.6
—	—	Animal	C14	2.0
100.0	12.0	Animal	C15–16	78.0
—	—	Animal	C17–19	1.1
65.6	30.0	Environment	C20-26	29.0
—	—	Environment	C27–29	18.0
20.0	—	Environment	C30	17.3
23.0	73.5	Human	C31–36	48.7

C18   Griffin and Tauxe 1991
C19   FSIS 1994C
C20   Johnson et al. 1990
C21   Grau and Vanderlinde 1992
C22   Wang and Muriana 1994
C23   Vorster et al. 1991
C24   Wang et al. 1993
C25   Pinner et al. 1992
C26   FSIS 1994C
C27   Smart et al. 1961
C28   Ternstrom and Molin 1987
C29   FSIS 1994C
C30   Konuma et al. 1988
C31   Sokari and Anozie 1990
C32   Farber et al. 1987
C33   Ternstrom and Molin 1987
C34   Nwosu 1985
C35   Vorster et al. 1991
C36   FSIS 1994C

significant by itself in contributing to the development of a disease associated with the product. More to the point, the microbial load (the amount of bacteria per gram of product) is critical and is certainly affected by postslaughter practices in storage and handling. Any point in the process of food handling at which the meat or milk can warm to bacteria-proliferating temperatures complicates and escalates the potential for food-borne disease to occur. Similarly, the nature of the finished retail product is a considerable factor in the emergence of food-borne disease. The potential for food infection is greater in ground meat and poultry than it is in an intact muscle product like a steak or chop because of the mixing

TABLE 5–5   Survey Report of Microbiological Hazards in Lamb

	Mean Percentage of Samples Yielding Pathogenic Bacteria in Lamb		
Human Pathogen	Carcass	Fresh Meat	Organ Meat
Salmonella spp.	40.0	0.0	—[a]
Campylobacter jejuni	—	15.0	—
Aeromonas hydrophila	—	53.0	—
Escherichia coli O157:H7	—	2.0	—
Listeria monocytogenes	—	37.0	—
Clostridium perfringens	—	85.0	—

[a] Not tested.

L1   D'Aoust et al. 1992
L2   Farber et al. 1988
L3   Lammerding et al. 1988
L4   Stern 1981
L5   Stern et al. 1984

and spreading of contaminating organisms within and across a greater surface area. Similarly, retail repackaging, transportation to the place of consumption, and cooking habits and preferences all affect the character of disease emergence. Thus, important difficulties arise in tracking down and locating the source of contamination and initiating events that allow the development of food-related disease. Again, the use of antibiotics is thought to be important in reducing the potential bacterial load that might be transferred to meat up to the point of slaughter. Beyond that point, the prior use of antibiotics will not affect proliferation of bacteria in food.

A final word should be said about host susceptibility to disease from microorganisms of animal origin. Disease becomes a relative term if one considers or equates the presence of a bacterium or microorganism with the development of disease. Humans and animals can develop the capacity to resist disease from various organisms as well as different microbial loads. For example, children living in India might not be severely affected by some water-borne microorganisms that would be intolerable to visitors from the West. In the animal world, scavengers eat carcasses of dead, diseased animals and appear to suffer no apparent ill effects. This again reflects the complex interplay between biology, ecology, and culture as it affects clinically significant cases of disease.

Ground Meat	Processed Product	Critical Source	Mean References	Prevalence
75.0	—	Animal	L1–3	47.5
—	—	Animal	L4–5	12.5
82.5	52.3	Animal	L6–8	62.5
—	—	Animal	L9	2.0
—	—	Environment	L10	37.0
—	—	Environment	L11	85.0

L6	Marjeed et al. 1989
L7	Palumbo et al. 1985
L8	Hudson and DeLacy 1991
L9	Doyle and Schoeni 1987
L10	Johnson et al. 1990
L11	Smart et al. 1961

A Nine-Year Survey of Reported Food-Borne Illness

Although the individual incidences of food-related illness is in the millions of cases per year, outbreaks are fewer in number but affect a common population of significant size. Of 4,821 outbreaks of food-borne illness reported from 1983 to 1992 to the CDC (Bryan 1980; Bean and Griffin 1990; CDC 1994), 2,114 were traced to the actual food sources. Pathogens present in meat- or poultry-related products were responsible for 334 (15.8 percent) of the outbreaks traced to the source. Of the 310 outbreaks confirmed to be of animal-product origin, 152 (45.5 percent) were of unknown etiology. CDC reports for 1983 to 1992 included 78 outbreaks traced to milk, ice cream, cheese, and other dairy products. There were 1,061 cases of milk- and dairy-product-borne diseases for the 36 outbreaks from 1988 to 1992. One death was recorded. Large outbreaks of food-borne diseases associated with milk and dairy products are reported in the literature; small outbreaks, unless of unusual etiology, are not reported.

The committee reviewed published reports of international events for 1980 to 1996. An outbreak of gastrointestinal disease affecting at least 110 people in England caused by *Campylobacter jejuni* was associated with drinking inadequately pasteurized milk (Fahye et al. 1996). Seventy-two laboratory-confirmed cases of *Campylobacter jejuni* infection were identified in people who drank unpasteurized milk at a festival in England (Morgan et al. 1994). From Septem-

TABLE 5–6   Survey Report of Microbiological Hazards in Poultry

Human Pathogen	Mean Percentage of Samples Yielding Pathogenic Bacteria in Poultry		
	Carcass	Fresh Meat	Organ Meat
Salmonella spp.	47.4	41.9	52.7
Campylobacter jejuni	66.2	52.7	63.3
Aeromonas hydrophila	98.0	50.0	100.0
Listeria monocytogenes	22.0	23.8	7.0
Clostridium perfringens	79.0	—	—
Bacillus cereus	—	21.5	—
Staphylococcus aureus	—	40.0	—
Escherichia coli O157:H7	—	1.5	—

*a*Not tested.

P1   Kanarat et al. 1991
P2   James et al. 1992
P3   Giese 1992
P4   D'Aoust et al. 1992
P5   Vorster et al. 1991
P6   Berndtson et al. 1992
P7   Lillard et al. 1984
P8   Barrel 1987
P9   Duitschaever and Buteau 1979
P10   Farber et al. 1988
P11   Izat et al. 1989
P12   Lammerding et al. 1988
P13   Tokumaru et al. 1991
P14   Jergklinchan et al. 1994
P15   Lillard 1990
P16   Norberg 1981
P17   Castillo-Ayala 1992
P18   Stern and Line 1992
P19   Slavik et al. 1994
P201   Norberg 1981
P21   DeBoer and Hahne 1990
P22   Harris et al. 1986
P23   Hood et al. 1988
P24   Jones et al. 1991
P25   Marinesca et al. 1987
P26   Flynn et al. 1994

Ground Meat	Processed Product	Critical Source	Mean References	Prevalence
—[a]	56.3	Poultry	P1–16	46.9
—	—	Poultry	P17–32	61.9
—	6.0	Poultry	P33–35	63.5
—	32.5	Environment	P36-48	25.4
—	—	Environment	P47	79.0
—	—	Environment	P48–49	21.5
—	—	Human	P50	40.0
—	—	Human	P51	1.5

P27   Gill and Harris 1984
P28   Kinde et al. 1983
P39   Roberts and Murrell 1993
P30   Shanker et al. 1982
P31   Tokumaru et al. 1991
P32   Christopher et al. 1982
P33   Barnhart et al. 1989
P34   Palumbo et al. 1985
P35   Hudson and DeLacy 1991
P36   Johnson et al. 1990
P37   Wang and Muriana 1994
P38   Vorster et al. 1991
P39   Wang et al. 1993
P40   Kerr et al. 1990
P41   Yarabioff 1990
P42   Wenger et al. 1990
P43   Bailey et al. 1989
P44   Genigeorgis et al. 1990
P45   Genigeorgis 1989
P46   Pinner et al. 1992
P47   Lillard et al. 1984
P48   Konuma et al. 1988
P49   Sooltan et al. 1987
P50   Vorster et al. 1991
P51   Doyle and Schoeni 1987

ber 6 through October 10, 1994, 142 cases of *Salmonella enteritidis* infections in a 3-state area were associated with raw egg contamination of ice-cream mix supplied to a large manufacturer (CDC 1994). In 1989, 164 cases of *Salmonella javiana* and *Salmonella oranienburg* infections in 4 states were associated with mozzarella from a single cheese plant. Those cases were identified in retrospective epidemiological studies (Hedberg et al. 1992). In 1985, a multiple-antibiotic-resistant strain of *Salmonella typhimurium* bypassed faulty pasteurization in a large dairy-processing plant, resulting in an outbreak of more than 1,600 cases traced by the unusual plasmid profile of the organisms (Schuman et al. 1989). From 1980 to 1983 in California, more than one-third of reported cases of *Salmonella dublin* infections were attributed to consumption of raw milk. Among consumers of raw milk, more than 95 percent of reported *S. dublin* infections were associated with drinking contaminated raw milk. A single, major certified dairy in California was associated epidemiologically with that incidence (Richwald et al. 1988).

The shifting patterns of disease outbreak over time as a function of demographics and cultural practices are exemplified by the epidemiology of infections of people with *Brucella melitensis*. Thirty-one cases of infection in residents of a community in Houston, Texas, were traced to unpasteurized goat milk cheese imported from Mexico (Thapar and Young 1986). In a larger study, of the 332 laboratory-confirmed cases of human brucellosis in Texas between 1977 and 1986 (Taylor and Perdue 1989), the patterns of emergence were different between 1977 and 1981 than they were between 1982 and 1986. In the earlier period, 82 percent of the cases were in males and 52 percent of infections were in white people. For the next five years, only 55 percent of the cases were in males and 72 percent of the cases were in people of Hispanic origin. Ingestion of unpasteurized goat milk was reported in 67 percent of the cases between 1982 and 1986.

From the early 1980s to the present, the trend shows that the incidence of microbially related food-borne illness has increased. Generalizations regarding apparent trends need to be made cautiously, because many factors other than the actual number of cases are relevant. For example, reporting of food illnesses has not always been as uniform or widespread as it is now. CDC estimates that only 10 percent of cases are actually reported. Education, awareness, and observation and diagnosis have certainly assisted in increasing the number of food-borne illnesses reported. Similarly, conclusions on a cause-and-effect relationship between antibiotic use in food animals, on-farm food-animal production practices, and the incidence of disease should not be made quickly or in the absence of definitive, trackable proof and data. As seen in Figure 5–1, the incidence of reported cases of food-related illness in all major sentinel organisms has a seasonal component, and the largest number of reported cases of illness occur in July and August. In the United States, ambient environmental conditions are more amenable to increased bacterial proliferation in a shorter time. Those data can be

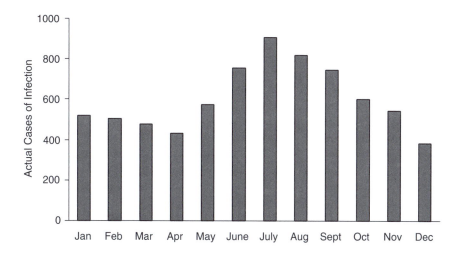

FIGURE 5–1 Seasonality of Reported Cases of Food-Borne Disease as Monitored Across the Seven Sentinel Organisms at All Locations. Source: FSIS 1997.

used as indirect evidence that postproduction practices have an important effect on the number of bacteria entering the food supply. In Minnesota, a state with a relatively high incidence of *Campylobacter* infections, the seasonality of re-ported cases shows a secondary increased incidence of *Campylobacter* reported during winter months, when the outbreak trends would be expected to be low. These cases of *Campylobacter* infections were traced to Minnesotans' vacations in Latin America during the cold Minnesota winter (Smith et al. 1997).

INTEGRATING ISSUES OF RESIDUES AND MICROBIAL CONTAMINATION

Microbial contamination of food is a principal area of food safety for which hazard analysis and critical control points (HACCP) will have a major potential to curb the transfer of microorganisms to humans via food. Issues related to drug residue contamination of animal-derived food products are largely related to the introduction of drugs and compounds into the live animal prior to slaughter or milking. In contrast, microbial contamination of foods, especially where the contamination is animal-feces-related, is an issue at the time of product harvest, and it has tremendous potential for risk to increase with improper food handling prior to consumption. Practical considerations affect the further propensity for organisms to cause disease, including poorly defined interactions of contaminat-ing bacteria with the environment found in the food product (acidity, salinity, cold-storage effects). The magnitude and severity of transference of human pathogens are not inconsequential, and still they are relatively difficult to assess because of a paucity of validated evidence and difficulty in tracking. The extent of the threat might increase or decrease with the identification of solid data to evaluate and draw conclusions. These data will take some time to amass, and recommendations based on the new data might be substantially different from those made today.

A major concern that arises when food-borne bacteria cause illness relates to the potential for a bacterium to become invasive and, therefore, to require medical intervention through the use of antibiotics. Within the context of microbial contamination of food, antibiotic-resistant bacteria constitute a subpopulation of organisms that, when present, can be carried within the food product to pose a formidable challenge to treatment and remediation of disease in humans. Based on the number of reported cases, the threat of disease and illness occurring through food contaminated with microorganisms is much greater than the threat of resistance transfer from animals to humans. To put the comparison of risks into perspective, there are few published reports of resistance transfer from animals to humans, and there are thousands of reported cases and outbreaks of food-related microbial-derived illness in the United States. A significant gap exists in data that could be used to track the occurrence of food-borne bacterial disease and correlate incidents with the presence of antibiotic resistant bacteria. More precisely, the relationship between the actual disease caused by a specific antibiotic-resistant organism needs to be tracked as well as the occurrence where a genetic element of resistance was transferred to bacteria resulting in disease. This is a formidable task, requiring significant financial input and scientific effort. However, if an accurate assessment of the relationship between antibiotic use in food animals, the occurrence of resistance and disease in humans, and the risk to human health are to be established, such data must be collected and analyzed.

According to FDA (CFSAN 1997) and USDA (FSIS 1997), as many as 33 million illnesses and 9,000 deaths occur each year in the United States as a result of food contamination by only 7 pathogens. The yearly medical and productivity costs for those illnesses are estimated to be almost $35 billion. Most of the illnesses arising from contaminated food result in diseases of "inconvenience": Vomiting, diarrhea, and muscle cramping are the symptoms most often observed. Recently, concern about the many microorganisms that infect food is increasing, because new strains of bacteria are being discovered that confound and complicate treatment. Those include the multidrug-resistant forms of *Salmonella* (definitive type DT-104) and forms of *E. coli* not only that have increased intestinal tissue adherence properties but also have the ability to secrete *Shiga*-like toxins (*E. coli* O157:H7).

Achieving the goal of safe food requires a multifocal planning and entails cooperation between individuals and agencies, extending from the farm to the consumer. Achieving the goal was addressed as a national priority by President

Clinton in a report entitled "Food Safety from Farm to Table: A National Food-Safety Initiative," (CFSAN 1997).

As summarized by this report, many levels of responsibility must be functioning simultaneously to keep the food supply safe:

On the Farm	State agencies and EPA oversee the use of pesticides. FDA oversees the use of animal drugs. Animal Plant Health Inspection Service oversees animal and plant disease. The Clean Water Act lessens the environmental burden of animal waste.
At Processing	FDA and USDA monitor the processing of foods to detect residue contamination and microbial pathogens.
Transport and Import	FDA and USDA regulate pertaining to interstate and international food transportation and importation.
Food Services	State and local agencies, FDA, and USDA develop laws for the safe handling and preparation of foods by schools, governing hospitals, restaurants, and so forth.
Water Standards	EPA establishes and maintains water standards, and state and local agencies oversee local standards.
Education	USDA Cooperative State Research, Education and Extension Service (CSREES).
Illness Surveillance	CDC and state health departments.
Food Research	CDC, FDA, ARS, CSREES, and EPA research ways to improve quality control and pathogen and residue detection; HACCP strategies for by-product rendering, slaughter practices, and preparation; and disease prevention strategies.
Consumer	Largely responsible for the safety of the final food as served. Education and awareness can help preserve the integrity of foods. The consumer has the last chance to identify potentially tainted food before it is eaten.

Decreasing the extent and severity of food-related illness is predicated on the establishment of an early-warning system to identify and track the sources of illness. That is a formidable goal and difficult enough to oversee within the U.S. production–consumer system, but it is further complicated by increasing global trade and, perhaps, by inadvertent entry into the United States of contaminated produce from other countries. To accomplish the task, an aggressive plan has been proposed in the National Food Safety Initiative to increase resources for the following:

• Increase food-borne disease surveillance with increased site participation in the National Antimicrobial Susceptibility Monitoring Program–Veterinary Isolates and the Foodborne Diseases Active Surveillance Network (FoodNet, a cooperative project of federal, state, and local agencies with oversight by USDA, FDA, and CDC, that monitors incidences of food-borne illness and the effectiveness of food safety programs to diminish the incidence of food-borne illness).

• Enhance outbreak detection by supporting the development of electronic instrumentation and increased communication between agencies.

• Modernize public health laboratories to increase diagnostic capacity.

• Create a "pathogen fingerprint" database.

• Increase national surveillance of antibiotic resistance, initially concentrating on *Salmonella* and *E. coli* contamination.

• Increase surveillance of human pathogens in food-animal populations, feed, and manure, with special emphasis on identifying the mechanisms of antibiotic resistance.

• Enhance local and state infrastructures to improve detection, evaluation, and response to disease outbreaks.

• Establish a risk assessment consortium to set priorities for research and data collection, serve as a clearinghouse for data, assess effectiveness of current measures, and recommend modifications and amendments to plans.

• Fund the research necessary to establish directives in pathogen avoidance and reduction in food animals, food handling, and storage and cooking, and charge the Office of Science and Technology Policy with coordinating the implementation of these directives in federal programs.

SUMMARY OF FINDINGS AND RECOMMENDATIONS

The committee finds that the general public health is adequately protected by the current system of drug residue surveillance. However, the drug-residue-monitoring system could be improved. There are gaps in testing programs. The number of samples tested is large for meat, poultry, and milk but small for fish. Current incidence of opportunistic pathogen blooms and the consequences for aquatic and human health suggest that putting additional effort into monitoring programs for fish and shellfish would be beneficial.

A serious limiting factor for test programs is the lack of rapid and specific test methods. In general, FDA lacks the analytical methods to test for many extra-label uses of drugs (including human drugs) in food animals. In addition, imported foods might need to be monitored more carefully because of the potential introduction of drug residues and microbial pathogens from countries with farm production practices and quality-control measures that are less stringent than those in the United States. This is a concern because the pharmacokinetics of drug elimination could be different in diseased or recovering animals. Few data are collected that allow comparison of drug metabolism in healthy and diseased animals.

FSIS is planning to devote more resources to the detection and prevention of microbial contamination of meat and poultry products.

Recommendations

• *The committee recommends that more resources be made available for developing appropriate analytical methods for a wider range of drugs. In addition, the committee recommends increasing the specificity of certain tests to reduce the inordinate number of false-positive results, particularly in the inspection of milk.* The high false-positive rate can cause unnecessary dumping of large quantities of milk and it causes unnecessary concern among consumers about the safety of the milk supply.

• *The committee recommends that resources be identified to support the initiatives of programs that monitor residues and microbial contamination.* The private sector should be a partner in this initiative and share in the management and funding of the programs.

• *The committee recommends that further research be pursued to develop more rapid analytical procedures and increased specificity for residue analysis as well as microbial contamination.* Additional research should focus on residue depletion and the pharmacokinetics of drugs in diseased animals.

6

Issues Specific to Antibiotics

The mechanism of action of an antibiotic is the same whether it is administered to a child or a calf. However, access to and choices of antibiotics are far greater if the infection develops in a child than if the calf develops a similar infection. With human health as the standard for all health-related decisions, the cost of developing new medications for human use is of limited consideration, and the development and use of new antibiotics are largely reserved for clinically diagnosable human infections. In the past, a veterinarian might have treated a calf with a preparation specified for human use. Depending on the circumstances, this practice could be considered illegal under the provisions of the Food and Drug Administration (FDA) law governing extra-label use of nonveterinary drugs. Recently, however, modifications in the drug law authorized by Congress legalized and expanded extra-label use of many human drugs for therapeutic purposes in livestock under the supervision of a responsible veterinarian (see Chapter 4). But what are the criteria for deciding whether newly developed antibiotics can or should be used for therapeutic or subtherapeutic treatment in livestock? Given the lack of information and consensus on the appropriate data needed to accurately assess the magnitude of risk to human health in agricultural use of antibiotics, what are the assurances that safeguard humans, animals, and the environment upon whom all medical, veterinary, and animal production drug practices have an effect?

The issues can be summarized as follows:

• The potential for emergence of antibiotic-resistant organisms in animal and human populations from the widespread use of antibiotics in food animals has been documented and has been a reason for concern. The magnitude of the actual animal-to-human transfer problem and associated development of disease is poorly characterized and varies greatly because of food-processing and consumer handling practices that are separate from animal production or antibiotic use in food production.

• Drug discovery and development are fueled by the need to compete with immensely adaptable adversaries, the microorganisms themselves, but the process is lengthy and expensive for manufacturing sponsors. Obtaining regulatory approval also is a time consuming process that can lengthen the time in getting new drugs to market and is expensive.

• Efforts to streamline the government approval process are evolving, and expanding the use of nonveterinary drugs in food animals should increase the number of uses and the availability of these products.

• The world is becoming a global economy, but quality standards vary greatly from one place to another. There is little uniformity in the approach to regulating drug use, and often the lack of approval centers on a socioeconomic concern rather than on concern for human health. As a result, U.S. federal regulatory agencies are reluctant to accept other nations' data to support the approval of a drug. Harmonization efforts could be made to gain acceptance of standardized regulatory approaches and data.

• Are there measures that might be used to better track the potential for a pathogen to emerge as a significant disease threat, particularly as it relates to the development of resistance in humans or animals? How will new infections be controlled in food animals if not with the increased availability of antibiotics?

DEVELOPMENT AND FUNCTIONALITY OF ANTIBIOTIC DRUGS

In general terms, antibiotic drugs are classified into the categories of broad and narrow spectrum (reviewed in Merck Veterinary Manual 1986; Kucers et al. 1997). The nature of the activity spectrum reflects how specific a drug or class of drugs is in terms of its microbial-killing capacity. Broad-spectrum antibiotics are generally effective in killing bacteria or organisms across a range of species. Narrow-spectrum drugs are usually highly selective for a particular species of bacteria, very effective when the identity of the invading organism is suspected or known, and particularly useful when specifically identified as effective against bacteria with known and defined resistance to other antibiotic drugs.

Another feature that affects the broad- or narrow-spectrum attributes is the drug's mode of action (O'Grady et al. 1997). Some antibiotics, such as the penicillins and cephalosporins (called β-lactam antibiotics because of the lactam ring structure), are particularly useful against a variety of organisms. Compounds in this class prevent the proper formation of bacterial cell walls during cell division and function to make the bacteria "leaky" and susceptible to osmotic forces. Because the biochemical paths involved in cell wall synthesis are common to a variety of organisms, these compounds have broad functional applicability. Narrow-spectrum compounds can target biochemical pathways specific to a single type or a few types of microorganisms. The scope of effectiveness of these compounds is limited. Additional layers of classification are related to chemical structure and other aspects of mode of action. In some circumstances, clever chemical modification of parent antibiotic molecules, such as penicillin, can change the spectrum of activity and more narrowly direct targeting for specific types of microorganisms.

Another relevant classification for antibiotic drugs related to mode or mechanism of action is based on the killing capacity of the drug. Bacteri*cidal* drugs have killing capacity and, when administered in therapeutic concentrations, treat infection by actively killing invading organisms (Merck Veterinary Manual 1986; Kucers et al. 1997). In contrast, bacterio*static* drugs prevent the growth of organisms, but do not kill them directly. A key feature of bacteriostatic drugs is that, with the proliferative potential of the organism impaired, the body's natural defense mechanisms can eliminate the disease threat. Sometimes, bactericidal drugs can appear bacteriostatic if effective killing concentrations in blood and tissues are not achieved.

From the standpoint of usefulness, therefore, serious consideration is given to the concentrations necessary for effective action without harming the host. The "therapeutic index" is a measure of the relative toxicity of a drug to a pathogen compared with the toxicity of a drug to an infected host (Grahame-Smith and Aronson 1992). Drugs with high toxicity to pathogens and low toxicity to animals are the most desirable. Therefore, drug developers would capitalize on fundamental biochemical differences between prokaryotes (simple cellular organisms without a membrane-bonded genetic material—bacteria) and eukaryotes (organisms whose cells contain a true nucleus—animal cells) to kill or affect pathogens and minimize danger to the host. Two readily recognizable examples of biochemical differences that might be exploited are the basic differences in cell wall and plasma membrane synthesis that allow β-lactam antibiotics to kill bacteria and be relatively harmless to animal cells and the basic differences in the biochemical composition of protein-synthesizing ribosomes that allow aminoglycoside drugs, such as the streptomycins, to kill organisms by inhibiting prokaryotic protein synthesis, leaving eukaryotic protein synthesis intact (Kucers et al. 1997).

Cell toxicity is just one measure of a drug's potential to harm the host. On a systemic basis, whole-animal responses (for example, allergic reactions) to antibiotics and drugs must be considered. Penicillins are well noted for this problem (Dayan 1993; Grahame-Smith and Aronson 1992). Even though the penicillin molecule is too small to be an effective allergen, its ability to hydrolyze spontaneously in an aqueous environment and covalently cross-link to proteins allows it to function as an immunologically recognizable hapten determinant and thus promote sensitivity to the penicilloyl residue as coupled to a larger protein. When linked to proteins in this fashion, these penicilloyl residues alter the self-recognition of the protein, establishing a "foreign protein" status and eliciting hypersensitivity reactions in the immune system. Finally, compounds with low therapeutic index for internal use might be highly effective as topical preparations and when entry into the body is limited (Grahame-Smith and Aronson 1992; Hardman et al. 1996).

IDENTIFYING AND SCREENING ANTIBIOTICS

Antibiotics are generally sought through initial screening of compounds that occur naturally in nature, particularly in soils. Although these compounds are called antibiotics or antibiotic drugs, they are fundamentally natural products of bacteria, fungi, and molds that are secreted and released into the environment by a species of organism to give it a competitive advantage over other bacteria or molds in its particular ecology. Practically all first-generation antibiotics were developed after isolation of a mold or bacteria that produced a predominant class of antimicrobial product. Around the world, as many as 30,000 species of microorganisms have been isolated from soils and screened for general antimicrobial activity.

Techniques for identifying new antibiotics have changed over the years as information on the mechanisms of actions of different classes of antibiotics has been amassed (Brumfitt and Hamilton-Miller 1988). Older procedures called for enormous batteries of active-culture screenings using live organisms and inoculated flasks of broth or plates of agar. Modern procedures are considerably more automated and mechanistic. Current tests are based on measuring the generalized ability of culture supernatants into which test organisms secrete their antibiotic to inhibit growth of organisms and more specific capacities to affect (inhibit or compete against) a particular biochemical event in a microbial metabolic pathway. Screening often is aimed at a single enzyme target in specific prokaryotic bacteria and fungi.

Discovery of the ability of a compound to affect the proliferation and viability of pathogens allows chemists, with an arsenal of chemical and biochemical modifications, to develop the spectrum of action and a therapeutic index. Chemical properties of naturally occurring antibiotics are often intentionally altered to enhance specific attributes of antibiotics (Drews 1983; Hardman et al. 1996). Starting with the basic chemical structure of a class of drugs, chemists can modify ring structures or add and substitute side-chain molecules to alter relative solubility in aqueous or lipid environments, slow or increase the metabolism and excretion of a drug, and define the site in the body for drug delivery. For example, certain antibiotics have fundamental toxicities if taken internally, but have excellent antibacterial properties. Chemical modification of those compounds can enhance their application as topical or ophthalmic ointments and suspensions. Similarly, chemical modification of sulfa drugs can make them ideal for treating urinary-tract infections, because absorption and excretion patterns after oral administration target antibacterial action at the infection site in the process of drug excretion through the kidneys and bladder. Finally, totally synthetic classes of antibiotic drugs are being developed that are based on the chemical structure and spatial conformation of the antimicrobially active portions of the molecules. An important point regarding the development of synthetic second- and third-generation antibiotics is that the properties of the native parent molecule that confer toxicity to the host can be eliminated even as the desired effects on pathogens are retained.

An interesting development in strategies to increase the efficacy of antibiotic drugs is the concomitant administration of drug metabolism modifiers. In this process, the administration of an additional drug can increase the efficacy of the antibiotic by decreasing inactivation of the antibiotic or by facilitating synergistic drug interactions. For example, some forms of antibiotic resistance develop in bacteria as they acquire properties to degrade a drug enzymatically. In the evolution of bacteria, some have developed the ability to secrete β-lactamase, an enzyme that ruptures the active lactam ring structure of penicillins and inactivates them. Addition of a compound called sublactam, along with ampicillin, provides a competitive inhibitor of the lactamase and arrests the activity of the resistance factor. Another example is the incorporation of trimethaprim with sulfa drugs to increase the bactericidal action of the sulfa.

The animal health pharmaceutical industry also pursues genetic and biochemical strategies to identify compounds with novel mechanisms of action. Several of these compounds are listed below (for reviews see Kucers et al. 1997; Jungkind et al. 1997; St. Georgiev 1998).

• The 8-carbon-sugar keto-deoxy-octulonate (KDO) is unique to Gram-negative bacteria (Garrett et al. 1997). Gram-negative bacteria produce endotoxins, also called lipopolysaccharides, as part of their cell membrane envelopes. An important part of the toxicity of these organisms is conferred through the release of endotoxins, as occurs in septicemia, toxic shock syndrome, and sometimes in food poisoning. Bacteria that make endotoxins synthesize it in a biochemical pathway that uses the enzyme cytidine monophosphate–KDO synthetase. The development of inhibitors of this enzyme could have specificity and selected toxicity against Gram-negative bacteria. The added benefit of this approach to microbial control is that the antibiotic also would limit the toxic endotoxin production and lessen the virulence of the organism and the severity of the host response to infection. That is important because killed bacteria can release endotoxins as they decay. Other compounds that are found to interfere with endotoxin production should have similar merit as antibiotic drugs.

• Novel inhibitors of protein synthesis: Eukaryotic organisms (like humans) and prokaryotic organisms (like bacteria) have fundamental differences in how protein is synthesized in the cells. Proteins are synthesized from the genetic code in the messenger RNA (mRNA) on granules called ribosomes. The ribosomes and mRNA processing differ in people and bacteria, for example. Compounds have been developed that interfere with the association of the bacterial mRNA with the ribosomes, making it impossible for the bacteria to synthesize proteins and thus survive. Antibiotic drugs belonging to this class of compounds, called oxazolidinones, are effective against Gram-positive and Gram-negative organisms.

• DNA gyrase inhibitors: The genetic code of organisms is normally a highly coiled matrix with which enzymes have difficulty interacting. Relaxation of specific regions of the supercoiled DNA in bacteria is accomplished by a class of enzymes called topoisomerases or gyrases. Quinolones inhibit bacterial gyrases, and further chemical modification with bridging to the isothiazole ring increases the gyrase-inhibiting properties. When gyrase is inhibited, the bacteria can no longer perform molecular functions dependent on the unfolding of DNA.

• Bacterial cell division targets: A novel target might exist within the morphogenic system that determines septum formation in bacteria, and a large number of gene products might participate in septum initiation and formation. Septum formation is believed to be easily perturbed. Multiple targets are believed to exist in Gram-negative and Gram-positive bacteria.

• Inhibitors of protein secretion: All bacteria translocate essential proteins outside their cytosol. Selective inhibitors of an enzyme, such as signal peptidase I, which cleaves the signal peptide during translocation of the peptide, would theoretically exhibit broad-spectrum antimicrobial activity.

• Defensins: These are a family of naturally occurring microbicidal peptides found in several major tissues and in circulating immune cells in the body of most animal species. High concentrations of defensins are located in the oral cavity associated with the tongue and other structures. The first antimicrobial peptide, bovine lingual antimicrobial peptide, was isolated from bovine tongue. The antimicrobial mechanism of action of many of these peptides is associated with their basic hydrophobic character, which enables them to penetrate microbial membranes (to the exclusion of eukaryotic membrane penetration), and with the open porous channels that disrupt ion gradients within the bacteria. Many of these peptides are being cloned as the genetic sequences for their structures are discovered. Cloning could facilitate the production of clinically effective defensins as recombinant products.

The use of multiple antibiotics simultaneously has some advantages in specific situations, but knowledge of the mechanism of action of antibiotics is essential for the correct choice to be made. Bactericidal drugs are usually synergistic when coadministered, having efficacy greater than that conferred by single drugs alone, because one drug increases the susceptibility of the organism to the effects of the other. Bacteriostatic drugs are additive in effect. Generally, in multiple-antibiotic therapy, a bacteriostatic drug is never administered simultaneously with a bactericidal drug. Bactericidal drugs often function to kill bacteria during some aspect of replication (from DNA processing to membrane synthesis). For example, penicillins kill replicating bacteria by preventing proper formation of cell walls. Sulfa, a bacteriostatic drug, diminishes the effectiveness of penicillin because sulfa blocks replication. From the standpoint of professional knowledge of modes of action and tissue-specific sites of action, the proper choice of bactericidal or bacteriostatic drugs and routes of body clearance of drugs is critical in special circumstances. Bacteriostatic drugs would be poor choices in animals or humans whose reduced immune capacity makes them unable to effectively destroy the invading pathogens. Similarly, it is imprudent to administer drugs with renal or hepatic toxicity when kidney or liver function is impaired.

BACTERIAL RESISTANCE

Antibiotic drugs are administered to animals and humans to eliminate the threat to internal homeostasis that invading microorganisms present to a host, the result of which is sickness. Since the initial widespread use of antibiotics in the 1940s, situations have been recognized in which an antibiotic has lost its effectiveness in controlling infection, even when the dose is increased. Microorganisms that managed to evolve to escape the action of the drug were called "resistant." The one certainty in the battle against microbial infection is that with time, antibiotic resistance will develop in some population of microorganisms. The question of how this resistance will affect human and animal health is important.

The problem of emergence of bacterial resistance to a drug is a driving force behind the move to increase antibiotic drug discovery and development. Because of increasing development of antibiotic resistance, new antibiotics are considered necessary for animal and human health care personnel to choose from when more traditional therapy would be ineffective. With more choices, a plan of drug administration can be implemented to increase the chances of eliminating an infection caused by an organism resistant to other drugs.

The committee noted in commissioned papers and report presentations that the animal pharmaceutical, production, and health professional organizations are concerned that government restrictions on the use and limited availability of antibiotics is a problem that approaches crisis proportions (AHI 1982; 1992). The immediate consequences of use restrictions are perceived as the loss of strategies and treatments to ensure the health and well-being of animals. Animal health professionals voice concern that the changes in antibiotic sensitivity of animal pathogens has created the potential for disease outbreaks to emerge for which therapeutic treatment is severely challenged. Professionals in human health care share similar concerns and cite the use of antibiotics in animal agriculture as the source of potential drug resistance emergence that would make human treatment more difficult if the patterns of resistance in animal pathogens were to be transferred to humans.

The suggested shortage in antibiotics is not a shortage in the amount available but in the number of classes of newer antibiotics for use in food animals. Three main factors were summarized in the commissioned reports and seen by the committee as reasons for the perceived shortage: (1) the emergence of resistance that compromises the utility of many established and traditional antibiotics for specific applications and pharmacological indications, (2) the federal laws that regulate the legal administration of available drugs to food animals, and (3) the cost per dose to administer many of the new antibiotics and other classes of drugs. The last point is important. For the animal producer, the profit margin is slim after all costs of production are weighed against the sale value of the reared animals. The "traditional" antibiotics continue to be important in livestock production because they are still effective in most applications, and they are profitable even though resistant microorganisms emerge. Manufacturers of those drugs market them relatively inexpensively; new drugs are prohibitively expensive for widespread use in agriculture.

Drug research, development, and approval time and costs, combined with the current problems of antibiotic choice and availability for animals, are believed by some to have far-reaching consequences for the American public. Diseases are appearing in animals and humans for which there are no approved or available treatments. Diseases once thought eradicated are reappearing with the emergence of microbial strains of increased virulence and multiple-drug resistance (for example, *Salmonella* DT-104; see Murray 1991; CDC 1994). Industries that produce sheep, goats, and minor species, such as deer, quail, catfish, exotic and zoo animals, and companion animals, have probably been affected most significantly by the lack of available drug choices. In some instances, the market is so small that no pharmaceutical operation will invest time and money to develop a needed remedy—certainly not within the period in which producers would like the product to be marketed. Several companies are developing and marketing new antibiotics, but industry representatives state that the intended application for these compounds is treatment of human diseases.

It is estimated that it takes 11 years and tens of millions of dollars to bring a new food-animal drug to market. Only 1 compound in 7,500 tested for initial activity reaches the market (AHI 1993). In the process of researching and developing new antibiotic drugs, decisions must be made that affect further development of the product. Drug manufacturers must consider the lifetime of the product (how long it will be on the market and in use before microbial resistance emerges and limits its usefulness), the potency of the compound, the overall cost of production, the size of the antimicrobial spectrum of activity, withdrawal times, marketing advantages, and the potential for bacteria to develop cross-resistance to other compounds in the same class.

ANTIBIOTIC-RESISTANT BACTERIA AND
ANIMAL MANAGEMENT

Continued use of antibiotic drugs in animal feeds or as therapeutic agents in standard agricultural–veterinary practices provides conditions favorable to the selection of antibiotic-resistant bacterial strains in food animals. This selection pressure is enhanced by (1) the large concentration of animals with similar disease susceptibilities and exposure and, thus, similar therapies; (2) the social behavior of livestock, which promotes transmission; (3) poor environmental hygiene, which promotes the survival, reproduction, and transmission of bacteria in water, feed, and bedding; (4) inadequate control over individual dose and treatment duration; (5) the rapid turnover of animal populations, ensuring new groups of susceptible animals if facilities are not disinfected between groups; and (6) the wide movement of carrier animals as breeding and feeding stock.

Antibiotic resistance does not in itself create the ability of bacteria and other organisms to cause disease; it does make treatment of the disease more difficult by increasing morbidity, mortality, and cost. Holmberg et al. (1984a) reported mortality that was 20 times higher for antibiotic-resistant *Salmonella* species than for antibiotic-sensitive species. They also showed that food animals were the source of the bacteria in more than 65 percent of resistant *Salmonella* strains and 45 percent of sensitive strains. The difficulty and the expense of treating resistant infections were discussed in an Institute of Medicine (IOM 1992) summary, "Emerging Infections: Microbial Threats to Health in the United States." As early as 1984, more prudent selection and use of antibiotic drugs as therapeutic agents and production enhancers in animals was recommended (Levy 1984). A detailed review by IOM (1989) of the issue of subtherapeutic use of antibiotic drugs suggested that, even though increased antibiotic resistance was found after use of subtherapeutic antibiotics, no direct evidence showed a definite human hazard.

A microorganism might mutate to develop or otherwise acquire resistance to antibiotic drugs, but there are several factors that determine or influence whether this will result in an increased hazard for humans. First, is the microorganism zoonotic, that is, can a human acquire a disease from the animal? Second, is there a misstep in the normal safety procedures in processing and handling of animal-derived foods that could enhance the risk of transmission of zoonotic microorganisms to humans, whether or not they are resistant to antibiotics? Third, if transmitted to humans from an animal source, is the microorganism more virulent than in its less-antibiotic-resistant form? Fourth, is a zoonotic disease treatable with other antibiotics? Last, are there enough new antibiotics in development to combat resistance built up from past patterns of antibiotic use and abuse? The answers will show whether there is an increased hazard for humans.

Therapeutic applications of antibiotics in fowl and livestock require doses high enough to achieve blood, organ, or tissue concentrations guaranteed to exceed (usually by 4 to 5 times) the minimal inhibitory concentration (MIC, the concentration of an antibiotic that arrests the growth of a particular organism) needed to treat an existing disease. The amount of antibiotic administered to attain MIC will vary according to the clearance rate in the body and the physiological status of the animal. Subtherapeutic concentrations of antibiotics are often administered in the diet or parenterally for more than 2 weeks and can be used at concentrations ranging from 1 to 200 g per ton of feed (Gustafson 1986). When a systemic infection occurs, the usual method is to use large therapeutic doses of antibiotic intramuscularly, intravenously, or by oral bolus to eliminate the invading organism quickly. The published MICs of a given antibiotic vary from organism to organism and within species by strain. According to summarized information on MICs in the Merck Veterinary Manual (1986),

> the reported MIC for a particular bacterial species is not consistent. Methodology, different strains (regional), media used, growth (regrowth) time, bacteriostatic vs. bactericidal concentrations, rate of drug diffusion in the media, and degree of bacterial inhibition required for effective therapy are all significant considerations. It may not even be necessary to maintain inhibitory concentrations of antimicrobial drugs at all times during treatment periods. Persistent antibacterial effects at subinhibitory concentrations, which facilitate removal of affected bacteria by host defense mechanisms, have been demonstrated . . . [for many antibiotics] . . . Organisms damaged by antibiotics are more susceptible to leukocidal activity. (P. 1510)

The last phrase offers some explanation of how subtherapeutic concentrations of antibiotics administered to animals with competent immune systems help the animals fend off disease under current intense production systems (as referenced in Chapter 3).

A detailed discussion of the molecular events and mechanisms of antibiotic resistance is beyond the scope of this report but can be found elsewhere (Hayes and Wolf 1990; Kucers et al. 1997; St. Georgiev 1998). To summarize, resistance of microorganisms to antibiotics develops through several mechanisms (reviewed in Davies and Webb 1998; Hickey and Nelson 1997; O'Grady et al. 1997): (1) when the targeted gene product for the antibiotic's action in the microbe is altered, making the drug incapable of affecting biochemical pathways that otherwise would result in the death or dormancy of a susceptible microbe, (2) when microbes develop enzymatic capability to degrade a drug and lessen its potency, (3) when an altered uptake system prevents entry of the drug into the cell, (4) when a cell develops a mechanism to excrete the drug minimizing its effect, and (5) when the organism can no longer metabolize the drug into the actual inhibitory compound.

Once resistance to an antibiotic is established through the probability of a random mutational event, many genetic aspects of resistance inheritance are chromosomally integrated and as such are passed to subsequent bacterial generations in the process of replication. An additional mechanism of resistance acquisition is the incorporation and expression of resistance genes from one bacterium to another by means of plasmid transfer (Hickey and Nelson 1997). Plasmid transfer between bacteria can be further subdivided into several possible mechanisms. DNA transfer between bacteria can be accomplished by transfer of "free DNA" fragments (a process called transformation), by a form of sexual transfer of genetic material between organisms (conjugation), by phage (bacterial or viral) mediated transfer of genetic material, and by a newly defined class of DNA genes (transposons) easily shuttled between plasmids and chromosomal DNA. Within the nature of bacterial genetics, some organisms can transfer genetic material at higher than normal efficiencies. They are called high-frequency recombinants.

Some aspects of the transmission and development of resistance do warrant comment. A recent review by Levy (1998) summarized the issues he considered relevant to explaining the emergence and escalation of drug resistance emergence and the potential to control it: (1) Given sufficient time and use, resistance at some level will emerge in sensitive organisms. (2) Evidence suggests that resistance may be progressive and can evolve through levels of susceptibility to the drug. (3) There is a propensity for bacteria resistant to one drug to become resistant to others. (4) Once resistance appears, the decline in its frequency is slow. (5) The use of antibiotics by one person affects others in the immediate environment. Levy contends that an effective recourse to the development of resistance is to replace resistant strains with susceptible ones. Although curbing misuse of these drugs in humans and animals will be instrumental in limiting new resistance, education of the public, health professionals (animal and human), and the food animal industry in what constitutes proper use is considered essential.

Multiple-antibiotic resistance can be acquired by bacteria from extra-chromosomal DNA in the form of plasmids. These self-contained pieces of DNA might well represent natural evolution in the sense that many early antibiotics are either derived or modified from natural compounds (Gabay 1994). Resistance to compounds toxic to the biochemical processes of bacteria is a mechanism of survival. Most bacteria do not contain resistant genes, but a small portion of bacteria within a given colony is theorized to have, develop, or acquire resistance. In fact, to date, the true reservoir of bacterial resistance remains unidentified. Until it is defined, the reservoir should be considered ubiquitous.

New data contradict early microbiology dogma that exchange of genetic information occurs only between bacteria of the same species. With greater prevalence of antibiotic-resistant organisms, resistance seems to be transferred not only within species but also between genera. Frieden et al. (1993) described a vancomycin-resistant gene found among *Enterococcus* species and additional reports characterized cross-genera transfer of the resistance to vancomycin both in vitro and in vivo (Leclercq et al. 1989; Patterson and Zervos 1990; Noble et al. 1992). Even more alarming is that certain antibiotics, including the extensively studied tetracycline, can increase the gene-transfer rate of resistant transposons

100-fold (Torres et al. 1991; Davies 1994). Some authors believe that concentrations of antibiotics below the threshold for bacterial growth inhibition stimulate cell-to-cell contact, thereby facilitating direct DNA plasmid transfer of information (Davies 1994). Clinically, multidrug-resistant phenotypes rapidly acquire resistance to newer antibiotics, and that pattern could be profoundly important (Tomasz 1994). Over time, repeated exposure to various antibiotics results in multidrug resistance patterns and the same bacteria acquire resistance to new agents, as has occurred with several *Staphylococcus* species (Koshland 1994).

Further bacterial transfer might occur between animal species—on different farms, far apart—to humans working with animals, and to humans consuming processed food animals (Tauxe et al. 1989). Levy et al. (1986) reported an increased number of tetracycline-resistant *E. coli* in the feces of chickens after only 1 week of feeding with tetracycline-supplemented feeds. Subsequently, in more than one-third of farm family members, 80 percent of the bacterial populations had tetracycline-resistant colonies, compared with 7 percent of the bacterial population in neighbors. No active human infections with tetracycline-resistant organisms were reported. Hummel et al. (1986) found that plasmid-borne resistance to streptothricin was present in *E. coli* from pigs fed nourseothricin, from the employees working with the pigs, and from their family members. They also found the plasmids in fecal samples from asymptomatic humans and from people with active urinary-tract infections, all of whom had no contact with the pig farms but who lived in the region where the drug was used in agriculture. These investigators found no indication of coselection for resistance to other drugs "indispensable for therapeutic use in man," and the authors concluded that the use of this antibiotic in animal husbandry had no clinical implications for human health.

With the occurrence of plasmid transfer across genera, concern must be raised if the patterns of resistance, which occur among the coliforms, are detected as being transferred to other species of bacteria—pathogens in particular. In that case, a serious potential for widespread infection could occur. News stories have reported widespread infections by water- and food-borne organisms that involve a virulent organism that also is resistant to multiple antibiotic drugs (Cohen 1993; Toner 1994; Tillett et al. 1998). Evidence can be cited that resistance and virulence factors can be passed on the same genetic elements (plasmids, etc.) and that the occurrence of this passage is greater than random chance would predict (Kristinsson et al. 1992; Munoz et al. 1992; Tomasz 1994). In this setting, it is plausible that morbidity and mortality would rise sharply and traditional antibiotic therapy would be made more difficult.

SUBTHERAPEUTIC VERSUS THERAPEUTIC USE OF DRUGS

The potential for increasing the growth rate of farm animals with antibiotic agents was first suggested by Moore et al. (1946). Stokstad et al. (1949) demonstrated the growth-promoting properties of supplemental feeding with chlortetra-cycline. Subsequent studies illustrated the beneficial effects of antibiotics in promoting growth in pigs (Cunha et al. 1950), poultry (McGinnis et al. 1950), and calves (Loosli and Wallace 1950). FDA approved the use of penicillin and chlortetracycline as feed additives in 1951 and oxytetracycline in 1953.

The extent and reality of a drug selection pressure depends in part on the concentrations of antibiotics to which bacteria are exposed and whether a concen-tration is achieved that actually can assist in selecting for the proliferation of resistant organisms. For example, for penicillins to work as antibacterials, the bacteria must be in a state of active proliferation and cell wall synthesis, and the concentrations of penicillin must be high enough that they enter the bacteria, bind to the penicillin-binding proteins, and inhibit cell wall synthesis. When penicillin concentrations are below the concentration needed, some degree of partial and residual effect on the bacterial structure facilitates increased phagocytosis of the infecting bacteria by natural host immune cells (Merck Veterinary Manual 1986). Thus, in the mechanism of action of subtherapeutic antibiotics, the interconnec-tivity of drug pharmacology and inherent host immune defenses must be consid-ered.

Eighty-eight percent of antibiotic drugs used in livestock and poultry are used at concentrations below 200 g/ton of feed—that is, at subtherapeutic con-centrations—and typically, the drugs are used for disease prevention or growth promotion (IOM 1989). When considered purely in terms of the amount of drugs used in food animals, the subtherapeutic use of penicillin, tetracycline, and other feed-additive antibiotics (40 percent of antibiotic products in the United States) is viewed as considerable pressure for selection of microorganisms resistant to the mode of action of these drugs.

Antibiotics are used at subtherapeutic concentrations to prevent diseases caused by pathogenic microorganisms and to improve animal performance (en-hance profit, increase rate of weight gain, or improve efficiency of feed use) (Hays 1986). Such concentrations are often used for extended periods and are usually supplied in the diet. There are cases in which the subtherapeutic use of an antibiotic was coincident with the development of resistant populations of bacte-ria, and occasionally these resistant bacteria are transferred to humans, but there is no clear indication that all subtherapeutic antibiotic use causes resistance uni-formly or increases the potential for zoonotic disease. Not all antibiotics are used at the same concentrations as feed additives when used for prophylaxis or growth promotion and certainly not at the same concentrations in all species for which the drug is approved. Data are lacking to specifically address antibiotic use concentrations and the emergence of clinically recognized resistance in patho-gens.

Resistance to antibiotics can sometimes modify some properties of disease-causing bacteria, possibly increasing their virulence or altering their potential to develop resistance to other antibiotics (Fagerberg and Quarles 1979; Hays 1986;

Levy 1998). The more real and more frequently encountered hazard to human health comes from any pathogenic bacteria that can contaminate animal-derived foods, regardless of drug resistance, that proliferates to clinically significant burdens to cause disease either from toxin accumulation in the food or from direct invasive infection. Elimination of resistance would not necessarily reduce the ability of microorganisms to cause disease. Rather, elimination of resistance facilitates the treatment of the disease by making more antibiotics available. However, infection by a proliferating antibiotic-resistant organism does increase the difficulty in using conventional therapy to treat the disease in humans.

Recent examples of human disease associated with animal-derived bacterial infection are illustrated by the outbreaks of severe illness associated with the virulent *E. coli* strain O157:H7 and *Salmonella typhimurium* DT-104. *E. coli* O157:H7 is extremely virulent but not (to date) associated with antibiotic resistance. Whereas the origin of these bacteria is always ultimately animal, some of the most frequent outbreaks have been associated with consumption of nonanimal foods (vegetable and fruit juice). *Salmonella* DT-104, a pathogen of major concern in the United Kingdom, is emerging with increasing frequency in the United States and is associated with multiple-antibiotic resistance (Glynn et al 1998). A summary report by Tauxe (1986) suggests that increased risk in human and animal populations (Hird et al. 1984) to susceptibility to infection with *Salmonella* is associated with recent use of antibiotics within 1 to 4 weeks of exposure.

Epidemiological patterns of occurrence also suggest that household pets are significant reservoirs of these bacteria. This underscores that human behavior is a dynamic factor that must be included in the discussion on risk assessment for disease emergence. When an animal is treated with specific antibiotics, antibiotic resistance does not develop automatically in all species of bacteria that might initially be sensitive. Both the type of antibiotic and the duration of use are important in the patterns of resistance that could develop (Davies and Webb 1998). Some species of bacteria are intrinsically resistant or more susceptible to some antibiotic drugs simply by the mechanism of action of the drug and the physical limitations that the structure of the bacterial cell wall and membrane impose on entry of the drug into the microorganism (Brumfitt and Hamilton-Miller 1988). Penicillins need to enter bacteria to bind to specific penicillin-binding proteins, inhibit proper cell wall synthesis during bacterial proliferation, weaken the cell wall structure, and facilitate lysis of bacteria by osmotic water movement (Merck Veterinary Manual 1986). Thus, the relative susceptibility of *Histomonas influenza, E. coli,* and *Pseudomonas aeruginosa* differ because the bacterial cell wall permeability decreases, respectively. Thus, the concentration gradients (which drive the drug into the bacteria) differ, and the bacterial sensitivity as a function of drug concentration can be affected.

For those populations in which some susceptibility to a given antibiotic exists, relatively low antibiotic concentrations inhibit the antibiotic-susceptible members of the bacterial population. In response to the decreased competition, the resistant bacteria then multiply and increase as a proportion of the total population (Gordon et al. 1959; Kobland et al. 1987).

In some instances, development of resistance is rapid, and high levels of resistance can be attained within a few days. Levy (1992) suggested that, for such a rapid change in emergence of resistance to occur, resistant organisms are probably already present in the original bacterial population. In this situation, only inhibition of the susceptible competitors needs to occur to permit the resistant organisms the opportunity to multiply and become clinically significant (Levy 1992). In other instances, resistance develops after a period in which no effect is apparent (Guinee 1971). That phenomenon might take place when resistant organisms are absent initially but develop within the treated population or are introduced from outside after antibiotic therapy is under way.

Subtherapeutic use of antibiotics as administered in animal feed has been heavily criticized (Levy 1998; Witte 1998): (1) Subtherapeutic use of antibiotics in animal feeds has been blamed as the principal cause of antibiotic-resistant bacteria. (2) If subtherapeutic use were eliminated, the level of resistance of bacteria harbored by animals would be reduced. (3) Reduced resistance to antibiotics in animals would result in an improvement in human health because the potential for transmitting antibiotic-resistant bacteria from animals to humans would be reduced. Such arguments have been advanced for many years, as reviewed by Hays and Black (1989), and were considered more speculation than data-driven fact. In addition, Walton (1986) suggested that their fundamental flaws underscore how inappropriate the recommendations of the Swann committee report (Swann 1969) actually were. Even the requirement for prescription use of antibiotics in the United Kingdom failed to limit the extent of coliform and *Salmonella* resistance (Dupont and Steele 1987). The IOM (1989) report on penicillin and tetracycline use in animals further summarized these lines of evidence, which suggest that the health risk posed to humans in the United Kingdom through the emergence of animal-antibiotic-associated resistance has not been changed substantively by implementation of recommendations in the Swann report. Therapeutic use of drugs continues to contribute to the emergence of antibiotic resistance. In addition, the dynamics of resistance declines are much slower than are the dynamics through which resistance to the use of an antibiotic increases (Langlois et al. 1986; Levy 1998). In the face of stopping antibiotics, resistance levels are slow to decline, and the reasons for this slowness are not well understood and are inadequately addressed in available research reports.

Ahmed et al. (1984) petitioned to ban the subtherapeutic use of penicillin and tetracyclines in animal feeds, citing an imminent hazard to public health. In the petition, they argued that, because therapeutic treatment of animals with antibiotics was episodic and of relatively short duration, it did not contribute significantly, if at all, to the long-term sustained development of antibiotic-resistant bacterial strains in food animals. On that basis, the petition suggested the intermittent use of antibiotics at therapeutic concentrations as an alternative to sub-therapeutic concentrations in animal feeds.

Because of its suggested benefit in limiting the duration and extent of disease-causing bacteria and pathogen shedding (summarized and reviewed in IOM 1980, pp.130–147; 205–220), the use of subtherapeutic drug concentrations has been substantial and has been embraced by, as well as influenced by, the livestock industry (Steele and Beran 1992). The most important benefit has been protection against disease, although the effect has been less pronounced in clean, healthful, and stress-free environments (Hays 1986). Such preventive measures as subtherapeutic drug use reduce shedding of bacteria and subsequent contamination of the environment by pathogens; thus, the occurrence of sporadic or epidemic disease also is reduced in animals that do not receive subtherapeutic doses of drugs. The beneficial effects of subtherapeutic drug use are found to be greatest in poor sanitary conditions (Speer 1982; Zimmerman 1986).

The development of de novo resistance in populations of bacteria in antibiotic-treated animals is influenced by complex interactions between the length of time and the concentrations of the drug to which bacteria are exposed (Baquero and Negri 1997a,b; Baquero et al. 1997). In contrast to the supposed propensity of long-term subtherapeutic doses to promote development of antibiotic-resistant strains of bacteria, short-term therapeutic doses are believed to act rapidly and decisively before being eliminated from the body. Therapeutic doses result in higher plasma and tissue concentrations of antibiotics than are attained with the use of the same antibiotic for growth promotion or disease prophylaxis. Characteristically, therapeutic concentrations are used for shorter times and are administered in the diet or parenterally (Ziv 1986). For example, when a systemic infection occurs, it is normal to use large doses of antibiotic to eliminate the invading organism quickly. Low doses administered over a longer time could favor emergence of resistant organisms (Jukes 1986). However, there remains the nebulous concepts of what constitutes a "low dose" and how long a dose must be present for resistant bacteria to emerge. Tracking resistance emergence is complicated because not all bacterial species or strains have the same limits at which concentration-dependent selections can occur. In addition, because the probability that resistance will emerge is based on the change in development of a favorable mutation, it can rarely be determined how long a drug must be present for the selection to occur.

An interesting relationship in the dynamics between intentional low-level antibiotic use and directed therapeutic use exists in the concentration gradients of antibiotic that form from the site of administration through diffusion and distribution. For in vivo drug distribution within tissues and body compartments, naturally occurring concentration gradients form in the pharmacokinetic processes of delivery, distribution, and elimination (Grahame-Smith and Aronson 1992). Where the elements of drug dose and exposure duration increase the likelihood for resistance to emerge in bacterial populations, these natural gradients might contribute to the localized emergence of resistance (Baquero and Negri 1997a, b; Baquero et al. 1997). The so-called high-level-directed therapeutic drug concentrations can accumulate in tissues locally at relatively low concentrations, and low-level antibiotic uses might be present in pharmacokinetic compartments at concentrations that are too low to select for resistance. This is a complicated interaction, but it serves to demonstrate how reducing the terminology to "therapeutic" and "subtherapeutic" becomes confusing and inappropriate.

Thus, major distinctions between the effects of subtherapeutic and therapeutic antibiotic doses on resistance present themselves in several dimensions, including the temporal aspects of the onset of resistance as well as the propagation and persistence of resistance and the number of resistant organisms maintained in the animal population (IOM 1980). There appears to be no definitive answer regarding whether subtherapeutic or therapeutic antibiotic use in farm animals causes more or less drug resistance. The absolute *number* of antibiotic-resistant isolate bacteria appears to be greater when subtherapeutic doses are used in animal feed than when therapeutic doses are given (IOM 1989). However, Walton (1986) contends that antibiotic concentrations achieved in animals fed antibiotics at many of the subtherapeutic concentrations used in the field do not reach concentrations necessary for the selection of resistant strains.

Therapeutic doses have a greater inhibitory and killing capability than subtherapeutic doses, but Gordon et al. (1959) and Kobland et al. (1987) found that the *proportion* of resistant intestinal bacteria was higher with therapeutic doses than with subtherapeutic doses of antibiotics. In one experiment by Kobland et al. (1987), chickens were fed different amounts of chlortetracycline in the diet and, after 3 days of treatment, were infected artificially with a mixture of sensitive and chlortetracycline-resistant *Salmonella*. In chickens with no chlortetracycline in the diet, elimination of the resistant *Salmonella* was complete 20 days after infection. When chlortetracycline was in the diet, the chickens had not eliminated the chlortetracycline-resistant bacteria by the end of the experiment. Bacteria were eliminated more slowly with therapeutic doses than with subtherapeutic doses. However, by the end of the experiment, the proportion of the chickens still infected with resistant *Salmonella* was lower with therapeutic doses (which were discontinued at the end of day 22) than with subtherapeutic doses (which were supplied continuously throughout the experiment). In the presence of chlortetracycline, the resistant *Salmonella* persisted throughout a substantial portion of the 35- to 56-day life span of broiler chickens.

Another study was made of an isolated herd of swine that had been established by Cesarean section of the sows to avoid contamination of the piglets with antibiotic-resistant and other bacteria at birth (Langlois et al. 1986). After 9 years of intermittent therapeutic use of streptomycin, but no subtherapeutic use of any antibiotic, 73 percent of the fecal coliform bacteria tested were resistant to streptomycin. For pigs, the time from birth to marketing is about 3.5 to 5 months.

Thus, under some circumstances, bacterial resistance from therapeutic use of antibiotics in market pigs might not disappear before slaughter.

One reason for the long residence time of antibiotic-resistant intestinal bacteria is probably continual reinfection and cross-infection of animals from fecal material (Harry 1962) and animal feeds (Durand et al. 1987). Reinfection also might contribute to the development of well-adapted strains that compete with the preexisting nonresistant strains and persist indefinitely. For example, in the herd from the Cesarean-section-derived piglets, 70 percent of the fecal coliform bacteria were found to be resistant to tetracyclines, even though the herd had been kept isolated and no tetracyclines had ever been used (Langlois et al. 1986). The resistance to tetracycline must have been derived from incidental introduction of tetracycline-resistant bacteria, because resistance to streptomycin, which had been used intermittently in therapeutic concentrations, has not been found to confer resistance to tetracycline. In regard to the potential for reinfection, even the most stringent biosecurity measures might be insufficient to guard against incidental introduction of resistant bacteria. For example, manure is a likely reservoir for microorganisms. Passage of microorganisms from farms to people by bird and rodent vectors that scavenge grain from the fecal material as well as agricultural waste runoff and refeeding of animal litter will naturally occur (Haapapuro et al. 1997).

Once an antibiotic has been introduced into animal management practice, either as a subtherapeutic feed application or as a specific therapeutic drug, the emergence of some microbial resistance is highly probable, and cessation of antibiotic use does not significantly alter the pattern of resistance. In swine, the diminution of drug resistance in the gut flora after withdrawal of subtherapeutic concentrations from the feed is not uniform. Antibiotic-resistant flora tend to survive longer in the upper intestinal tract. When such swine are stressed, increased bacterial shedding in the feces includes bacteria from the upper tract (Moro and Beran 1993). Contamination by multiple-drug-resistant *E. coli* was substantially greater in carcasses of swine subjected to preslaughter stress than it was in carcasses with minimized preslaughter stress.

Antibiotic treatment of certain disease entities has led to drug-resistant animal infections, as experienced with a case of *Salmonella typhimurium* (phage type 29) infections in calves (Anderson 1968; Anderson et al. 1975), in which drug-resistant disease transmission was enhanced. In this case, susceptible calves at a facility were exposed under stressful conditions to a multiresistant strain of *Salmonella typhimurium.* Animals were treated ineffectively for salmonellosis and transported to several farms, where they served as sources of infection for other calves, adult cattle, and humans. When the facility where the diseased calves originated ceased operation and the consolidation, exposure, and dispersal of calves ended, the farm outbreaks of salmonellosis decreased.

Results of studies by Endtz et al. (1991) suggest that the emergence of quinolone-resistant strains of *Campylobacter* isolated from humans result from the therapeutic use of these drugs in veterinary medicine. The increased resistance of *Campylobacter* in the animal reservoir could result in treatment failures of enteric diseases if quinolones were to be used in therapy. Based on the time of fluoroquinolones entering the market and on serotyping patterns of emerging resistant bacteria, Endtz et al. (1991) concluded that the animals were more likely the source of resistant strains for humans.

Several reports (CAST 1981; Levy et al. 1986; IOM 1989) have shown that farm workers who have close contact with livestock can acquire, although transiently, antibiotic-resistant intestinal microflora. In addition, evidence indicates that some human diseases from resistant bacteria do occur because of the subtherapeutic use of drugs in animals. The occurrence is rare, and the finding is perhaps confounded by the difficulties associated with identifying and tracking the occurrences. The 1981 CAST report, *Antibiotics in Animal Feeds*, stated that, up to that point, there were only 4 instances (2 in Britain, 1 in Canada, and 1 in the United States) for which there was "evidence linking use of antibiotics in animal agriculture with diseases due to antibiotic-resistant bacteria in humans" (p. 2), and it attributed the incidents to therapeutic rather than subtherapeutic use of antibiotics. Since 1981, many more cases of zoonotic-resistance transfer have been reported. These are summarized in Chapter 3. However, even today we are faced with the challenge of documenting actual cases of resistance transfer from animals to humans in terms of pathogen and nonpathogen transfers. In large part, we do not know the sources or reservoirs for antibiotic-resistant bacteria or their potential to affect the incidence of human disease from antibiotic-resistant bacteria.

Information in the commissioned reviews supplementing the committee's evaluation indicates that some interest is developing in the practice of rotating choices of antibiotics periodically or of using combinations of therapy (such as sulfa antibiotics and trimethoprim) to suppress the rate of the development of drug resistance. This practice might be better implemented if more rapid and extensive surveillance data were generated and used in control strategies.

Cross-resistance among classes of drugs with the same mechanism can have an effect on animal production practices. If one of the macrolide drugs, such as erythromycin, is used to treat a disease over a period, cross-resistance to others (such as tilmicosin or one of the lincosaminides) used in veterinary medicine might be expected to develop (Hickey and Nelson 1997; Levy 1998). Thus, in further treatment of diseases, antibiotics with common resistance patterns would not be the drugs of choice (Jungkind et al. 1997; Kucers et al. 1997).

For therapeutic use, antibiotic drugs should be avoided in instances in which no etiological agent has been isolated from a sick animal, because drug use might select for resistant strains among the resident gut flora. Within 1 week of feeding animals diets supplemented with subtherapeutic concentrations of antibiotic drugs, such as tetracyclines, most gut coliforms become resistant to the drug (Linton et al. 1975). Furthermore, Linton (1977) suggested that the continuous use of antibiotics in pigs leads to the eventual stabilization of resistant organisms in the intestinal tract, and they could become the dominant form of microorganisms. Resistant bacteria can be found in gut flora of farm workers who have close and regular contact with food animals or with antibiotic-enriched feeds and through exposure to the fecally contaminated environment (Levy et al. 1986; Levy 1992). In addition, a given drug should be avoided when the causative organism is known (or is likely) to possess an inducible enzyme or other factor that inactivates the drug. For example, the cephalosporins should not be used to treat an infection caused by an organism that produces an inducible ß-lactamase. Cephalosporins also should be avoided in instances in which a first-generation cephalosporin or a penicillin would be effective. This practice would reduce the use of newer products and subsequently decrease the rate of development of antibiotic resistance to them.

In considering the appropriateness of precautions to lower health risks associated with drug use in animals, the effects of chemical residues must be separated from the biology of microorganisms. Setting appropriate drug withdrawal times is effective in decreasing drug residues and increasing the safety of drug use in food animals. However, withdrawal times are not intended to regulate any effect on residual bacterial populations that might have been affected by the use of the antibiotic. Hays and Black (1989) concluded that resistance of some animal intestinal bacterial flora to certain antibiotic drugs might not disappear from the animal before it is marketed, even though the drugs had not been used during most of the animal's life span.

One recourse and alternative to deal with the problem of resistance is to develop more antibiotic drugs for food animals. The question is whether that strategy resolves the problem or perpetuates it, forcing continued perseverance in the search for new drug alternatives. Regardless of the incidence of drug resistance that arises from the use of antibiotics in food animals, the efficacy of the drugs has remained for disease eradication and growth promotion.

HUMAN AND VETERINARY CLINICAL IMPLICATIONS OF ANTIBIOTIC RESISTANCE

As discussed in Chapter 3, drug resistance can be transferred between animal and human pathogens, or animal and human pathogens could obtain drug resistance from a common pool of resistant organisms in the environment. Pathogenic animal microorganisms might acquire resistance to a variety of antibiotic drugs; the resistant organisms can be transferred to other animals or to humans. Humans can then transfer these drug-resistant pathogens to other humans or back to animals. Additionally, organisms that are neither pathogenic to animals nor to humans might acquire resistance. Human or animal exposure to these nonpathogenic organisms can result in transference of their resistance plasmids to pathogenic organisms. Because of the interrelationship between drug-resistant organisms that infect animals, humans, and the environment, any substantial interference in that cycle might contribute significantly to the overall problem of resistance.

Several reports have described antibiotic drug resistance in food-animal pathogens. Berghash et al. (1983) reported on a study of antibiotic resistance in nonlactating dairy cows that were treated for bovine mastitis. In that study, investigators evaluated the use of dry-cow treatment in 22 dairy herds in New York State. These herds were divided into two groups: one group (12 herds, 365 cows) had antibiotic infusions into the udder at the cessation of each lactation cycle (high-use rate); the other (9 herds, 324 cows) had no use of antibiotics during the nonlactating period (low-use rate). The investigators observed increased resistance to 13 antibiotics in *Streptococcus agalactiae* isolates from the high-use group. These 13 antibiotics were penicillin G, ampicillin, methicillin, cephalosporin C, cephalothin, tetracycline, streptomycin, kanamycin, gentamicin, erythromycin, lincomycin, novobiocin, and chloramphenicol. There was little difference between the two groups in the resistance patterns of the other bacterial species examined.

In another study, Blackburn et al. (1984) described the antibiotic resistance of *Salmonella* isolated from chickens (425 animals sampled), turkeys (749 sampled), cattle (1,307 sampled), and swine (974 sampled) in the United States from October 1981 through September 1982. The study was based on *Salmonella* isolate samples submitted to the National Veterinary Services Laboratory of the USDA Animal and Plant Health Inspection Service (APHIS) for serotyping. In all 3,500 isolates were tested for drug resistance and susceptibility. The drugs tested were ampicillin, chloramphenicol, carbenicillin, cephalothin, erythromycin, gentamicin, kanamycin, neomycin, penicillin G, streptomycin, triple sulfonamides, and tetracycline. High rates of drug resistance were observed. Three cultures were resistant to all the drugs, and 30 percent were resistant to each drug except chloramphenicol, cephalothin, and gentamicin. Multiple resistance was observed in 80 percent of the cultures. Higher percentages were observed in cultures from swine, and more isolates from chickens were resistant to more drugs than were isolates from other domestic animal species sources.

Cases have been documented in which plasmid-resistance patterns were used to epidemiologically trace the animal-to-human transfer of *Salmonella* via tainted hamburger. In a study by Spika et al. (1987), chloramphenicol-resistant *Salmonella newport* was traced through hamburger to dairy herds. This particular study was important because the specific strains of chloramphenicol-resistant *Salmonella newport* found in humans were the same strains that were traced back to the dairy farms. The drug resistance to chloramphenicol from those animal pathogens might have been transferred to humans in the zoonotic transfer of the bacteria from the animals to humans. Furthermore, they showed that the resistance resulted directly from illegal use of chloramphenicol on the farm at which the disease emerged. Chloramphenicol resistance was observed in *Salmonella newport* in a study of California dairies by Pacer et al. (1989). Other animal-to-human transmissions are clearly documented and reproducible (Holmberg et al. 1984a). The interconnectivity of the animal and human ecosystems is clearly demonstrated by Lyons et al. (1980). A drug-resistant *Salmonella heidelberg* was identified and traced from ill veal calves to a farmer, his daughter, her infant, and companion infants in a hospital nursery.

Trimethoprim (TMP) is a synthetic antimicrobial adjunct that is used in human and veterinary medicine against a wide range of bacteria, including *E. coli* and other members of the family *Enterobacteriaceae*. The addition of this compound to a sulfonamide preparation such as sulfamethoxazole (SMX), increases the efficacy of the sulfa by imparting a sequential blockade of bacterial tetrahydrofolate synthesis. The combination is often referred to as a "potentiated sulfonamide." This combination is thought to be a reliable bactericide and less likely to produce resistant organisms. However, studies by Hariharan et al. (1989) showed that *E. coli* in calves and pigs with diarrhea were resistant to this combination of drugs (Table 6–1). What is even more worrisome is the fact that the TMP–SMX resistance found in *E. coli* isolates was accompanied by resistance to 4 other commonly used drugs (Table 6–2). Again, those findings indicate the complexity involved in drug resistance transfer in animal populations and the clinical complications that might result in reduced choices of drugs to use.

In an experimental study, Wray et al. (1990) showed the effects on physical performance and antibiotic sensitivity of gut flora caused by feeding to calves waste milk that contained differing concentrations of antibiotic (as a consequence of cows being treated for mastitis) or an antibiotic-free milk substitute. In the first trial of that study, one-third of the calves were fed waste milk that contained antibiotics, one-third were fed the same milk previously heated and fermented (penicillin concentrations ranged from 0 to 0.24 µg/ml; streptomycin concentra-

TABLE 6–1   *E. coli*[a] Resistance to TMP–SMX

Distribution	Isolates Tested	Resistant Isolates (%)
Porcine	134	52 (39)
Bovine	86	40 (46)
Total	220	92 (42)
Porcine ETEC[b]	88	32 (36)
Bovine ETEC	38	19 (50)

[a]Isolated from calves and pigs with diarrhea.
[b]ETEC = Enterotoxigenic *E. coli*.
Source: Hariharan et al. 1989.

TABLE 6–2　Resistance of TMP–SMX-Resistant
E. coli Isolates to Other Antimicrobial Agents

| Drug | Resistant Isolates (%) | | |
	Total (n^a = 92)	Porcine (n = 52)	Bovine (n = 40)
Tetracycline	98	96	100
Neomycin	80	71	92
Ampicillin	74	67	82
Nitrofurans	30	40	18

[a]n = Number of tested isolates.
Source: Hariharan et al. 1989.

tions were from 0 to 3.8 μg/ml for unfermented and from 0 to 1.8 μg/ml for fermented milk), and one-third were fed a milk substitute that did not contain antibiotics. Fecal *E. coli* were monitored for antibiotic resistance. In the second trial 60 calves were divided into 2 groups, 1 group was fed antibiotic-free milk substitute and the other milk from antibiotic-treated cows (penicillin concentrations ranged from 0.01 to 700 μg/ml). The investigators found streptomycin resistance in calves that were fed antibiotic-contaminated milk, but no resistance developed in the control group. However, a complication in the interpretation of these data was the observation that the milk from treated cows already harbored populations of contaminating bacteria, such as *E. coli*, various *Enterococci*, and some *Staphylococci*, and the patterns of antibiotic resistance and susceptibility of these organisms as they existed in the waste milk were not characterized. Additional antibiotic resistance of *E. coli* strains isolated from calves with enteritis has been reported in many countries, including the United States, Canada, and France (Fairbrother et al. 1978; Coates and Hoopes 1980; Martel et al. 1981; Prescott and Baggot 1993; Prescott et al. 1984) and is summarized in Table 6–3.

Studies of the European experience with the use of antibiotics in veterinary medicine and animal production and surveillance efforts provide an opportunity to observe patterns of bacterial antibiotic resistance. Wray et al. (1993), summarized the emerging trends in England and Wales. Clear increases in bacterial resistance between 1981 and 1989 were evident for some bacteria and some antibiotics, especially ampicillin, chloramphenicol, apramycin and trimethoprim resistance in *Salmonella typhimurium*. (Table 6–4). The authors stated that more than 40 percent of *Salmonella typhimurium* cultures remained sensitive to all antibiotics tested, yet resistance was a rare event in *Salmonella dublin* and *Salmonella enteriditis*. In the *S. typhimurium* isolated from cattle, pigs, poultry and sheep, where increases in resistance were evident, the increases were appar-

TABLE 6–3 Antimicrobial Resistance of *E. coli* Strains Isolated from Enteritis in Calves in the United States, Canada, and France

Antimicrobial Drug	Percentage of Resistant Isolates			
	United States[a]	Canada[b]	United States[c]	France[d]
Cephalothin	20	27	—[e]	—
Ampicillin	59	83	75	89
Chloramphenicol	13	79	22	88
Neomycin	71	79	87	—
Kanamycin	75	77	87	81
Gentamicin	0	1	3	0
Tetracycline	90	100	95	83
Nitrofurazone	6	4	15	40
Triple sulfa	94	95	87	86
TMP–SMX	—	40	3	—

[a]Coates and Hoopes 1980.
[b]Prescott et al. 1984.
[c]Fairbrother et al. 1978.
[d]Martel et al. 1981.
[e]Not tested.

TABLE 6–4 Antibiotic Resistance in *Salmonella* from Animals, Percentage of Cultures Showing Resistance

Antibiotic	Disk Content (μg)	*Salmonella typhimurium*			*Salmonella enteritidis*[a]		
		1981	1989	1990	1988	1989	1990
Ampicillin	10	12	32	30	1	5	4
Chloramphenicol	10	12	23	23	0	0	0
Apramycin	15	0	5	4	0	0	0
Neomycin	10	12	3	2	0	<1	0
Streptomycin	25	ND[b]	22	26	26	1	4
Sulphonamides	500	ND	46	49	2	3	5
Tetracyclines	10	48	50	51	1	6	6
Trimethoprim	25	14	28	28	0	2	4
Furazolidone	15	<1	<1	1	0	<1	<1
Nalidixic acid	30	0	0	<1	0	0	0
Sensitive to all		ND	47	44	97	89	87
Total		1,146	2,151	2,522	585	1,815	3,758

[a]1981: only 28 incidents.
[b]ND = not done.
Source: Wray et al. 1993.

ent in all species (Table 6–5). Resistance to neomycin was the only instance in which decreases were evident. Data from the French experience in resistance surveillance monitoring (Martel and Coudert 1993) demonstrated that the age of the animal population was an important determinant in assessing the emergence of resistance characteristics in animal populations. Resistance emergence in young calves exceeded that of adult animals principally because calf populations are greater recipients of antibiotics because they are more susceptible to bacterial disease than are adult animals. Further summarized by Espinasse (1993), trends in antibiotic resistance before and after 1982 suggest similar increases in antibiotic resistance in food-animal bacteria that were statistically significant for ampicillin and sulfa-trimethoprim and significant decreases in resistance patterns for streptomycin, neomycin, chloramphenicol, and furans.

Reviewing the data from other countries provides the opportunity for some informative comparisons of data and events that affect the resistance–disease issue. However, there are pitfalls that must be avoided or at least accounted for: "The interpretation of data on resistance of bacteria towards antimicrobial drugs is difficult, since both methods applied and interpretation, influence the result." (Wiedmann 1993). For example, care must be exercised in comparing epidemiological data between different countries because the "definition" of resistance varies from country to country as determined by MIC or microbiological breakpoint analysis. The definition of ampicillin resistance in *E. coli* is <2, <4, <8, and <16 mg/ml for Sweden, Germany, the Netherlands, and the United States, respectively (Wiedemann 1993). Functionally, that translates into the observation that only 2 percent of isolated *E. coli* strains are sensitive in Sweden whereas 78 percent of the same strains are called sensitive in the United States. Endtz et al. (1991) reported drug resistance in *Campylobacter* caused by fluoroquinolone use in food animals. Again, the reporting of this emergence of resistance is a function of how the definition of resistance is interpreted and, thus, factors into the human health risk associated with the use of antibiotics in food animals.

CASES TO TEST THE SYSTEM

The future of antibiotic development and use is less than clear. Regulatory issues regarding approval of antibiotics for humans and animals have become more complicated than in the past, largely because of the tremendous capacity for bacteria to adapt to antibiotics and to become more difficult to control. Insight into the complexity of this issue is readily obtained by reviewing the concerns associated with the use of members of the fluoroquinolone class of antibiotics.

Approximately 30 years after the issues that brought attention to the applications and uses of penicillins and tetracyclines in food animals, the controversy has expanded to newer antibiotics. Additional concern for the role of antibiotic use in food animals evolved from the detection of avoparcin (glycopeptide, vancomycin-like) resistant bacteria in manure and in some food products derived from

TABLE 6–5 Antibiotic Resistance in *Salmonella typhimurium* from Animals, Percentage of Cultures Showing Resistance

Antibiotic disk content (μg)	1981				1990			
	Cattle	Poultry	Swine	Sheep	Cattle	Poultry	Swine	Sheep
Tetracylines (10)	55	24	52	43	75	34	75	58
Chloramphenicol (10)	14	<1	24	3	54	2	4	16
Ampicillin (10)	13	2	26	—[a]	67	5	24	42
Neomycin (10)	14	1	26	—	2	<1	4	—
Trimethoprim (25)	16	1	37	29	58	8	34	27
Furazolidone (15)	2	<1	2	—	<1	2	8	—
Apramycin (15)	—	—	—	—	9	<1	3	2
Number of cultures	1146	236	46	35	809	905	115	45

[a]Not tested.
Source: Wray et al. 1993.

chickens and swine in England and Denmark. In addition, a substantive link between the agricultural use of avoparcin in animals and the emergence and transmission of avoparcin–vancomycin-resistant organisms to humans is asserted (Bates et al. 1994; Aarestrup 1995; Witte and Klare 1995; Aaerstrup et al. 1996). The avoparcin concern does not appear to apply in the United States, because such drugs are not approved for use in food animals here. Several European countries also prohibit its use in food animals.

The avoparcin–vancomycin issue is specifically relevant because of several factors. A relatively new class of antibiotics, the naladixic acid derivatives called fluoroquinolones, is coming under scrutiny both here and in Europe for use in food animals. Because of the history of antibiotic issues in the United Kingdom and throughout continental Europe, most of the data cited in the arguments for and against the expanded use of fluoroquinolones in the United States come from public health laboratories in Europe. Resistance to these drugs as well as to others, such as avoparcin, has been monitored for a longer time in Europe than it has in the United States. A logical question is, "If the agricultural use of avoparcin contributed to the emergence of vancomycin resistance in human bacterial isolates, could this occur with the fluoroquinolones?" Analogies between the avoparcin issue and fluoroquinolone use could be drawn, and the importance of public health concerns regarding the emergence of fluoroquinolone resistance in pathogenic bacteria and the zoonotic transmission of these microbes from animals to humans cannot be ignored. It is not known whether this heightened concern is premature, but it substantively shapes and molds the complex arguments that influence the fate of antibiotic development and use in food animals in the United States.

The Fluoroquinolones Issue[1]

Fluoroquinolones are synthetic antimicrobial agents (bacterial gyrase inhibitors) that are structurally associated with naladixic acid (reviewed by Hooper and Wolfson 1993). Effective against a broad range of bacteria, fluoroquinolone antibiotics are useful in the treatment of enteric diseases, and in other countries, they have been used in the prophylaxis and treatment of bacterial diarrhea. Particularly effective in combating infections that are difficult to eradicate, these antibiotics are considered a last line of defense in human medicine in the fight against antibiotic-resistant and difficult-to-manage life-threatening infections.

---

[1]During the course of this study, committee member R. Gregory Stewart changed employment to become affiliated with a pharmaceutical firm that has a drug approval application pending before FDA for a fluoroquinolone antibiotic. As a result, Dr. Stewart excused himself from the committee discussion and deliberations pertaining to this class of antibiotics.

They have added practical considerations of reducing the need, duration, and expense for hospitalization. The β-lactam (penicillin class) or aminoglycoside (gentamicin, tobromycin) antibiotics have resistance factors transmittable by nucleic acid plasmids. In contrast, resistance to fluoroquinolones (naladixic acid derivatives) is mostly associated with random chromosomal mutation in specific bacterial genes, with the resistant phenotype transferred to daughter bacteria in the process of simple multiplication and proliferation under the selection pressure of the drug. While quinolone resistance via plasmid vectors can be demonstrated in the laboratory, this mode of acquisition has not been demonstrated in clinical settings (Hooper and Wolfson 1993).

Two main modes of resistance have been identified for fluoroquinolone drugs in bacteria: reduced binding to and inhibition of DNA gyrases and reduced access to the gyrase inside the bacteria. Eleven specific amino acid substitution mutations in the DNA gyrase GYR-A protein have been documented (Hooper and Wolfson 1993), and the substitution at a specific amino acid site has resulted in different degrees of resistance as estimated by the relative increase in the MICs for naladixic acid (NA) and ciprofloxacin (CIP). Depending on the site of the mutation, MICs are reported to increase from 2.5 to 128 μg/ml and from 4 to 32 μg/ml for NA and CIP, respectively. Additional mutations with correspondingly lesser effects on MIC are reported for mutations in the DNA gyrase B protein and mutations that result in changes in the accessibility of the drug for the target enzyme. Two fluoroquinolone resistance mechanisms in *E. coli* have been identified to account for reduced access to the gyrase enzymes inside bacteria: physical blocking of the entry of the drug into the bacteria at the surface membrane and energy-dependent active excretion of the drug by the bacteria (Piddock 1995).

The position of the mutation and the concurrence of multiple-site amino acid substitutions will affect the clinical significance of the resistance event. Whereas a single mutation event has been suggested to result in relatively low-level fluoroquinolone resistance (MIC <2–4 μg/ml), the development of 2-site mutations, especially in different mechanisms of action, results in high-level resistance (MIC >32 μg/ml) and complicates treatment of incurred disease (Piddock 1995). Similar double mutations resulting in high-level fluoroquinolone resistance have been detected in human and veterinary (cattle) *Salmonella* isolates in Germany (Heisig et al. 1995). In that study the authors suggested that the cattle and human *Salmonella* isolates were identical. They also suggested that human and veterinary reservoirs for this multiple-site-resistant organism exist, although no epidemiological link between them could be established. Dual-mutation high-level quinolone-resistant organism populations also have become established.

In the United States, the FDA Center for Veterinary Medicine (CVM) approved fluoroquinolone antibiotics for use in therapeutic treatment of coliform disease and pasteurellosis in poultry, as directed by prescription by a veterinarian. There is considerable controversy and disagreement among animal and human health care professionals regarding the widespread use of these drugs in food animals. The major argument put forth by the medical community against the use of these drugs in food animals is that the drugs would be needed for humans if resistance to other antibiotics were to become a problem (Levy 1998; IOM 1998). The critics contend that widespread use of fluoroquinolones in food animals, in conjunction with negligent and irresponsible use, would cause fluoroquinolone resistance in organisms to emerge that would pose a significantly increased risk to human health. The concern about greater risk is because of the resistance to fluoroquinolone drugs emerging in organisms such as *Salmonella* DT-104, where resistance to other classes of antibiotics already exists. If realized at the level that some health workers suggest (Threlfall et al. 1996; Glynn et al. 1998), the emergence of fluoroquinolone resistance would make invasive disease by multidrug-resistant microorganisms significantly more difficult to treat. However, Kuschner et al. (1995) described effective therapy against ciprofloxacin-resistant *Campylobacter* with the use of azithromycin, a broad-spectrum, new-generation macrolide (erythromycin-like) antibiotic given to U.S. military personnel stationed in Thailand, where the occurrence of ciprofloxacin resistance in *Campylobacter* is high.

Based on the observed effect of generalized therapeutic use for farm animals in the United Kingdom, Germany, and the Netherlands, many health experts in the United States suggest that further approvals for this drug are not prudent. Therapeutic uses need to be justified, carefully documented, and controlled. Contributing to the disparate views is the definition of resistance. The National Committee for Clinical Laboratory Standards (NCCLS) has established 4 µg/ml concentrations of ciprofloxacin (MIC) as the cutoff to define clinically significant resistance that influences the effectiveness of treatment. The complication in interpretation arises when resistance is assessed in vitro and demonstrated at MICs lower than the NCCLS clinical definition, and when this lower MIC is used to support the emergence of resistance. Thus, defining resistance is critical to documenting changes in the patterns and the magnitude of resistance emergence associated with the use of antibiotics in animal production. It is important to point out that the mere presence of drug resistance does not constitute a clinical threat to human health or drug efficacy for therapeutic remediation of disease. This is true as long as the recommended dose of the drug is well above its MIC.

In the United States, there is currently no significant threat of disease outbreak in humans that can be tracked and associated with the passage of quinolone-resistant organisms from animals to humans. However, because of the relative newness of this drug's use in food animals, FDA and the Centers for Disease Control and Prevention (CDC) (PHS 1995) recommend and support a cautious approach to quinolone use in agriculture, and they are sensitive to the possibility that resistance could become a significant problem in the future.

It was largely outside the charge of this committee to assess the accuracy of the many reports in the literature used to support or refute claims for altered health risk associated with the use of quinolone antibiotics in food animals. To maintain a balance in presenting the views on the issue it is useful to refer to and summarize some of the information available. The work cited in many arguments is published in the peer-reviewed literature and in non-reviewed or critiqued formats and abstracts in scientific society proceedings. Each source of information and opinion serves to shape the character of the issues and controversies surrounding it. The authors' and stakeholders' interpretations of data contribute to the controversy and fuel the arguments that are frequently put forward by opponents to challenge the rigor of the science used in the studies, the statistical robustness of the analysis, or the sizes of the populations studied.

Authors of some scientific publications in the United Kingdom, Spain, and the Netherlands have suggested that the licensing and use of fluoroquinolone drugs for use in animals in those countries was a significant factor in the development of fluoroquinolone resistance in *Campylobacter* and *Salmonella* from food animals (Endtz et al. 1991; Perez-Trallero et al. 1997; Threlfall et al 1996; van den Bogaard et al. 1997). For example, many health officials in federal regulatory agencies look to the data from Europe as evidence that the greater introduction of fluoroquinolone antibiotics into agricultural food-animal applications increases the risk of transfer of fluoroquinolone-resistant pathogens from animals to humans. The magnitude of the reported resistance can be striking as in the case of the *Campylobacter* isolates from humans who suffered from food-borne illness in Spain in 1996. It was reported that more than 80 percent of these isolates were resistant to nalidixic acid (Perez-Trallero et al. 1997), using the NCCLS standard. There is confusion about the definition of resistance used in many of the studies cited and about the current standard for clinically significant resistance levels to fluoroquinolones set by NCCLS at 4 µg/ml. The NCCLS resistance level is 8 to 16 times greater than that assigned by Threlfall et al. (1996), 0.25 to 0.5 µg/ml.

The Animal Health Institute has summarized its position on the relevance of the resistance data in stating that

> Manufacturers believe that these antibiotics are ideally suited for therapeutic use and would serve a critical need in enhancing animal health and contributing to a healthy food supply. . . The issue of antibiotic resistance has been debated for more than 30 years. Studies show that if animal-to-human transfer actually happens, it is a rare occurrence. There is no evidence to show that transferred organisms actually thrive or cause disease in humans. . . . (AHI 1997)

There are in fact several reports of transfer of drug-resistant pathogens from animals to humans (summarized in Chapter 3), and there is evidence that the passage of fluoroquinolone-resistant bacteria from animals to humans is possible, just as is the case for avoparcin-resistant bacteria (Witte and Klare 1995). Two lines of evidence are cited in the scientific literature to substantiate the development of fluoroquinolone resistance in animals and transferred to humans: First, patterns of emergence of fluoroquinolone-resistant *Campylobacter* in the Netherlands in humans and poultry were strongly linked with the introduction of fluoroquinolones in veterinary medicine (Endtz et al. 1991). Second, animals are considered the principal reservoir of the chromosomally encoded, multidrug-resistant *Salmonella* DT-104 and *Campylobacter* (Wall et al. 1995; ERS 1996b; Glynn et al. 1998), and there appear to be cases of fluoroquinolone resistance emerging in these organisms with resistant isolates found in humans. A recent outbreak of 13 cases of food poisoning in the United Kingdom was documented when people contracted a fluoroquinolone-resistant *Salmonella* DT-104 infection from turkeys that had been previously treated with fluoroquinolones. Epidemiological tracking suggested the outbreak was traced directly to the poultry, confirming the potential for transfer of this resistance pattern to humans from animals (Wall, P. 1997, Public Health Laboratory Service, England, personal communication). The critical factor associated with the outbreak, however, was improper thawing of the turkey prior to cooking and subsequent inadequate cooking to kill the proliferating microorganisms. This is another example of the link between the presence of drug-resistant organisms and augmentation of the disease risk being caused, in part, by irresponsible handling of food.

In the U.K. resistance issue, the *Salmonella* DT-104, while significant as a pathogen, is brought into the scenario not as a pathogen as such, but in terms of what it offers as a microbial sentinel to aid in tracking the passage of fluoroquinolone resistance from animals to humans. The United Kingdom is especially interesting to epidemiologists because the use of these drugs in food animals has been approved for a longer time than in other countries and new data are being analyzed that suggest more than a casual link between the use of these drugs in animals and the development of fluoroquinolone resistance in humans. According to the Public Health Laboratory Services of the United Kingdom, the incidence of disease cases in humans by the 5-drug-resistant (ampicillin, chloramphenicol, streptomycin, sulfonamide, tetracycline) *Salmonella* DT-104 increased from 259 in 1990 to 4,006 in 1996 (CDR 1997).

It concerns health officials that, since 1994, resistance to trimethoprim and ciprofloxacin is increasing in a significant proportion of *Salmonella* DT-104 isolates from humans (Threlfall et al. 1998). The increase in ciprofloxacin resistance in human *Salmonella* isolates is shown in Figure 6–1. Approvals for uses of fluoroquinolone antibiotics in food animals in the United Kingdom have continued. Some stakeholders in the United States cite this fact and question FDA for placing a moratorium on further approvals of fluoroquinolone drugs in food animals. FDA has responded that the approval and monitoring processes in the United Kingdom are substantially different from those in the United States.

Treatment of animals with fluoroquinolones is relatively new in the United States, where its use is restricted to poultry. Data on any patterns of emergence of bacterial resistance to fluoroquinolones in animals, and especially data on the resistance in terms of MIC, are few. A recent summary of the surveillance data reviewed by FDA and CDC experts (Glynn et al. 1998) stated that, at the time of the review, there were no isolates of *Salmonella* DT-104 that were resistant to

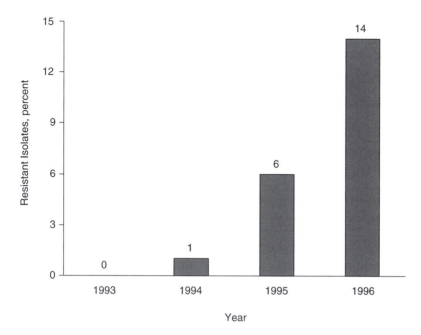

FIGURE 6–1 *Salmonella* DT-104 Ciprofloxacin-Resistant Human Isolates Confirmed in the United Kingdom. Source: CDR Weekly 1997; Wall, PHLS, personal communication.

ciprofloxacin. One isolate was resistant to nalidixic acid, but it did not present the 5-drug resistance pattern typical of *Salmonella* DT-104. The paper concluded that incidences of the 5-drug resistant DT-104 isolates increased from 0.6 percent in 1979 to 34 percent in 1996. Similarly, the paper also stated that the sources for the *Salmonella* DT-104 remained undetermined. The database could not provide evidence that the increase in *Salmonella* DT-104 isolates over the years was related to continued subtherapeutic use of antibiotics in food animals, a combination of subtherapeutic and therapeutic use as factors establishing an environment that could select for these bacteria, or a proliferation and passage of an established population of these organisms persisting perhaps even where antibiotic use is minimal. Furthermore, without data on the relationship between *Salmonella* DT-104 detection in isolates and clinical disease, there is a gap in the information needed to link disease outbreaks to factors that predispose humans to greater risk of infection with this pathogen. However, the absence of detectable fluoroquinolone resistance in *Salmonella* DT-104 in the study isolates serves as a base and timeline from which emergence of fluoroquinolone resistance in bacterial populations can be monitored and referenced.

The final decision for restricted use of fluoroquinolones in food animals in the United States resides with the CVM director, who has restricted further use of these antibiotics in food animals. To assist in the decision-making process, a surveillance board has been established to track and oversee the effect of antibiotics in the development of bacterial resistance. Currently, the oversight of resistance surveillance is in the public sector. Board members are associated with FDA (CVM, Center for Food Safety and Applied Nutrition, Center for Drug Evaluation and Research, and the Office of the Commissioner), USDA (ARS, APHIS, and Food Safety and Inspection Service [FSIS]), CDC, and academic institutions. The project is called "National Surveillance for Antibiotic Resistance in Zoonotic Enteric Pathogens."

In 1996, CDC, FDA, and ARS established the National Antimicrobial Monitoring System to prospectively monitor changes in antimicrobial susceptibilities of zoonotic pathogens from human and animal clinical specimens, from healthy farm animals, and from food-producing animals at slaughter (Tollefson 1996; CDC 1996). The purpose of the program is: (1) to gather data on the extent and trends over time in antimicrobial susceptibility in *Salmonella* and other enteric microorganisms and to monitor several antibiotics for such resistance patterns, (2) to increase the flow of data on resistance emergence in animals and humans, (3) to identify new areas for research, and (4) to prolong the useful life of approved antibiotic drugs. The fluoroquinolones and other standard antibiotics are used as test compounds, with specific bacteria such as *E. coli* and *Salmonella* spp. used as sentinel organisms.

A relevant issue that contributes still further to some aspects of this controversy relates accountability for antibiotic drug use. This probably is more of a problem worldwide than in the United States. It is an understatement to say that this issue is complex. However, the reality is that antibiotics are widely available for use in animals as well as humans through unauthorized routes of distribution. Inappropriate antibiotic use and lack of accountability are insidious and difficult to document. Not only is there a burden of increased risk to human and animal health, but when present and detected as a problem, unorthodox use of antibiotics can skew the interpretation of data and compromise the objectivity of the decision-making process. When a greater-than-expected incidence of resistance to a drug occurs in a population where the regulated use of the drug is weak, how can the source of the problem be accurately assessed? Is it from animal use? Is it from overprescription by licensed practitioners? Is it driven by the illicit-market economics? Unfortunately, assessing the magnitude of the consequences of misuse can be done only retrospectively, usually through epidemiological investigation, when the process has already become an established problem with established health consequences.

In regard to the potential for transfer of resistant organisms from food animals to humans, perhaps increased attention should be given to reducing the incidence of induction and proliferation of resistant organisms on the farm. Strategies should reflect the need to limit the overuse of antibiotics. In addition, the benefit of using antibiotics in managed farm operations should be more widely appreciated. Similarly, consumer education efforts are necessary, so the public will more readily accept modern food safety techniques, such as irradiation and surface sterilization. When properly used, these methods are efficient at stopping the proliferation of microorganisms that can be introduced inadvertently at the time of slaughter (Lagunas-Solar 1995; Osterholm and Potter 1997).

Pharmaceutical developers and manufacturers are watching the fluoro-quinolone resistance and approval issue with great interest because of the ramifi-cations for development of animal antibiotics that will be scrutinized in terms of human or environmental safety. The economic incentive for discovery and intro-duction of new antibiotics could be compromised if human health issues of resistance development and issues of food-animal use and accountability cannot be resolved. This entire issue, driven by elements of disparate views, nonuniform use of definitions and standards, data that are less than clear-cut, and subjective opinion on both sides, is likely to be revisited each time an antibiotic is presented for use in both human medicine and animal agriculture. The importance of resolving these issues rapidly underscores the need for increased communication among stakeholders and for openness in decision making. Much of the burden of weighing the issues and integrating the available surveillance data could be lifted by the development of an oversight board that would collate and integrate infor-mation, without bias, to support science-based regulatory decisions.

The Virginiamycin Issue

The most recent example of agricultural versus human use of antibiotics is just unfolding (Okie 1998). Virginiamycin is an antibiotic that has been used for almost 20 years in the control of infection and growth of swine, cattle, and poultry. Virginiamycin is a member of the streptogramin class of antibiotics. Until recently, streptogramins were not used in human medicine so their use in food animals was of relatively little concern. The recent development of a streptogramin for use in human medicine is hailed as the newest "drug of last resort" to combat life-threatening, drug-resistant infections—vancomycin-resis-tant infections in particular. This is an interesting example of what might be called "reverse concern." Usually, an antibiotic is developed for human use, use for food animals is approved years later, and the debate arises as to the soundness of the decision to approve the drug for animal use, with all of the ramifications of availability, accountability, and resistance emergence. In the case of the strepto-gramins, the approval for use in animals was granted first. Now that a need for use in humans has developed, the question is how much debate will ensue that will challenge the continued use of these drugs in animals.

Approved use of virginiamycin for animal production in the United States, along with an absence of similar or related streptogramin drugs in the human population, offers a unique opportunity to assess some of the controversial issues associated with drug use in food animals.

A human population sampling of bacterial isolates screened for virginiamycin resistance would be a valuable component in a drug resistance database. The general human population should be relatively devoid of streptogramin resistance because it has only recently been approved for human use as a therapeutic drug and its use is not nearly as widespread as is the use of some other drugs, such as the penicillins. The ability to detect specific virginiamycin resistance (as well as MIC) would provide good information on whether prior use of a drug as a feed additive affects human health or threatens the effectiveness of streptogramins for future therapeutic use in humans.

SUMMARY OF FINDINGS AND RECOMMENDATIONS

The presence of antibiotics in the microbial environment constitutes a natural initiating selection pressure that allows bacteria, which have changed phenotypically so that they are less affected by the antibiotic, to survive. The development of antibiotic resistance occurs because populations of microorganisms acquire a beneficial mutation or plasmid transfer and proliferate. The emergence of resistance is highly variable and is affected by intrinsic factors—the antibiotic used, the duration of use, the dose, the bacterial species—as well as extrinsic factors, such as farm hygiene and biosecurity. Antibiotic resistance is an important issue in human and veterinary medicine in part because of the way it is defined. There is conflict in the interpretation of absolute and clinically relevant resistance. How this is defined and exactly what MICs constitute a "resistant" organism are at the heart of the controversy.

Antibiotic drug resistance is increasing in food-animal populations, particularly in bovine, swine, avian, ovine, and catfish species. Similarly, drug resistance is noted in equine, canine, and feline populations. Part of the increase results from greater use of antibiotics in animals, but a large portion of the increase also is the result of significant improvements in surveillance, detection, and screening for antibiotic-resistant organisms. Antibiotic resistance patterns tend to be against more than one drug. Furthermore, resistance has been noted in organisms that are pathogenic in animals only, in zoonotic organisms, and in nonpathogenic organisms. Although little attention had been paid to resistance development in nonpathogenic bacteria (largely because of the difficulty of that task), the occurrence of resistance in these bacteria constitutes a potential area of concern. The exact magnitude and extent of antibiotic drug resistance is difficult to estimate because of a lack of comprehensive surveillance programs in veterinary medicine in the United States and elsewhere and because of the different ways resistance is defined.

A host of clinical complications in veterinary medicine results from the rise of antibiotic drug resistance. Only a small number of antibiotic drugs are approved for use in food-animal species. Therefore, any increase in resistance to these drugs limits practitioners' choices to treat animals or conduct prophylactic programs to improve animal health. The same is true for nonfood animals. Alternative means of controlling or slowing drug resistance must be sought, and research should be encouraged in this area.

Recommendations

• *The committee recommends establishment of an integrated national database to support a rational, visible, science-driven decision-making process and policy development for regulatory approval and antibiotic usage in food-producing animals.*

This will further ensure the safety of these drugs as well as foods of animal origin. The openness and accessibility of this information are critical to the success and validity of decisions that will affect veterinary and human medicine. Information contained in such a database should include the following:

—approved drugs in use and defined MICs that affect the clinical significance of resistance in animals and humans and available resources for treatment;

—volume of usage of approved drugs and incidence of misuse, and resistance patterns in important pathogens and sentinel marker organisms on the farm and at slaughter;

—prevalence of human pathogens in foods of animal origin and the incidence of food-borne infections from food-animal products, with particular reference to resistant organisms.

• *The committee strongly recommends the further development and use of antibiotics in human medicine and food-animal practices have oversight by a panel of experts, interdisciplinary in composition, representing the regulatory agencies and the veterinary–animal health industry, the human medical community, consumer advocates, the animal production industry, researchers, and epidemiologists.*

The mission of this panel would be to undertake scheduled reviews of the data that address the concerns of antibiotic resistance development in animals and humans and to advise regulatory agencies in the development and use of antibiotics in agriculture and human medicine. These tasks require the development of specific databases that encompass surveillance data on antibiotic use and effectiveness patterns, resistance emergence patterns, and trends in sentinel organisms in the United States. Monitoring the data from international sources where a given drug has more history than it has in the United States also would be necessary. The release of data and the ability for others to access them will be important to the oversight process. The private sector and federal regulatory agencies need to share the cost and resources as a part of the resistance-monitoring process. Ultimately, the number of zoonotic-pathogen sentinel organisms will need to be expanded as will the number of antibiotics surveyed. Resistance issues will need to be characterized with regard to the incidence of detectable resistance versus clinically significant, disease-producing resistance, based on minimal inhibitory concentrations. These data should provide a growing base from which to develop models and predict resistance emergence.

• *The committee recommends that basic research, which explores and discovers new or novel antibiotics and mechanisms of action of antibiotics, should receive increased funding.* In particular, funding is needed to develop more rapid and wide-screen diagnostic tests to increase the capability of more accurately tracking emerging trends in antibiotic resistance and zoonotic disease and to transfer this information to the larger database. Funding should come from federal and private sources.

• *The committee recommends that the drug development industry continue to seek new approaches to identify and capitalize on novel microbial–biochemical processes for antibiotic drug development to control the spread of infection.* Because resistance development to one antibiotic poses a significant threat for resistance to emerge against others in the same parent class (cross-resistance), the discovery and development of new classes of antibiotics is essential to ensure infection control in the future.

• *The committee recommends that increased education about issues, practices, and concepts of antibiotics and their uses should be made available in school, industry, home, and professional venues.* The misuse of antibiotics through lack of awareness can no longer be tolerated.

• *The committee recommends the characterization of the relative risk to consumers between chronically ill or carrier food animals and antibiotic resistance in microbes residing in food animals.* Increased educational efforts in this regard and development of strategies for optimizing the balance between the two also are needed.

• *The committee recommends that, to aid in the accountability process, identification of the source of drug resistance would be enhanced substantially by using individual identification systems, such as microchips, in all food animals.*

7

Costs of Eliminating Subtherapeutic Use of Antibiotics

Under current food-animal production practices in the United States, antibiotics are used to treat specific health problems (therapeutic use) and to improve animal performance (subtherapeutic use), as discussed in earlier chapters. Used subtherapeutically, antibiotics result in enhanced growth rates and improved feed efficiency, thereby contributing to lower costs of meat and eggs. However, this practice also is associated with the development of antibiotic-resistant strains of bacteria that contribute to the presence of drug-resistant pathogens in humans, as discussed in Chapters 3 and 6.

It is frequently suggested that, because of the resistance issue, subtherapeutic use of antibiotics should be banned. The main arguments against a ban are that it would cause an economic hardship for livestock and poultry producers and raise costs for consumers. In large part, subtherapeutic feeding of antibiotic drugs is a management tool to prevent infection and to facilitate the use of confinement housing. This practice allows larger numbers of animals to be maintained in a healthy state and at a lower cost per unit to the farmer. If subtherapeutic use of antibiotic agents were eliminated, these production advantages would be reduced or lost and consumers would pay more.

To gauge the cost to consumers of eliminating the subtherapeutic use of antibiotics, the Committee on Drug Use in Food Animals conducted an economic analysis. Under current production practices in the United States, it is difficult to quantify either the probability that subtherapeutic drug use results in human health problems, or the economic value of the current and potential stock of antibiotics. The role of economic analysis is limited to measuring the benefits of subtherapeutic drug use to producers or, alternatively, to identifying the costs incurred if current use of subtherapeutic drugs were prohibited. Ideally, the costs associated with a ban should be compared with the benefits to consumers (valued as the benefits from reduced health problems). Because of the difficulty in measuring economic benefits, only the costs are addressed here. The estimated cost measures can be compared among themselves to elucidate the sensitivity of the results to various assumptions and to provide an understanding of the magnitude of the costs.

CONSIDERATIONS IN DETERMINING THE EFFECT OF A BAN

The best way to determine the economic benefits of subtherapeutic antibiotics is to examine what would occur if the U.S. Food and Drug Administration were to prohibit all forms of subtherapeutic drug use. To make this estimate, several areas must be considered.

Definition of Subtherapeutic Use

If regulators were to decide to limit subtherapeutic drug use, it would become essential to define the difference between therapeutic and subtherapeutic uses more accurately. For a detailed discussion of the different uses, see Chapter 2 and Hays and Black (1989). The current practice of incorporating antibiotics in beef cattle diets in the feedlot is done to prevent liver abscesses and the diseases associated with the stress of moving and commingling animals. Under current regulations, there is little incentive to determine whether such feeding is therapeutic or subtherapeutic, and an argument can be made for either definition. Such feeding is therapeutic in that the incidence of liver abscesses and stress-related diseases would be higher if the drugs were withdrawn. If the symptoms appear after drug withdrawal, the drugs can be used therapeutically. However, a strict interpretation of therapeutic use is to treat a symptom, and if antibiotics are used to prevent a symptom, they are used prophylactically. The argument over definitions is more than one of semantics. The entire beef-feeding industry would be exempt from any ban if the first definition were applied. In the analysis, the strict definition is used, because many of the benefits of subtherapeutic use in poultry and pork industries could also be described as treating symptoms before they develop (that is, before subclinical problems become clinical). This issue is important because it implies that once a subtherapeutic-use ban were in place, there would be strong incentives to restrict therapeutic use.

Measurement Choice

The first effect of any ban on subtherapeutic use of antibiotics would be felt in the animal health industry. In 1995, this industry generated $3.3 billion in sales. In the same year, the human health pharmaceutical industry produced approximately $63 billion in sales. Approximately 62 percent of all animal health products marketed in the United States are used in food-animal production; 38 percent of those products are classified as feed additives and include antibiotics; antibacterial drugs such as sulfonamides, nitrofurans, arsenical compounds, anthelmintics, and coccidiostats; and other pharmaceutical agents such as iono-phores, melengesterol acetate, antioxidants, mold inhibitors, probiotics, and non-antibacterial growth promoters (Richard Carneval, AHI, personal communication 1996). The animal health industry, if asked, could not estimate the reduction in sales it would suffer nor estimate the changes in employment and profits that would occur.

An alternative economic measure would be to enumerate the consequences for farm profits and farm costs. Approximately 100 percent of chickens and turkeys, 90 percent of swine and veal calves, and 60 percent of beef cattle receive diets containing antibiotic drugs during some part of their lives (Manchanda 1994). Thus, it is obvious that most producers find these products useful. One study estimated that subtherapeutic drugs saved the U.S. hog industry approximately $2 billion in annual production costs (Wade and Barkley 1992). However, changes in production costs would not necessarily translate directly into lower profits. First, the cost of the drugs themselves must be considered. For average producers, that amounts to about 3.75 percent of total ration costs, or about 50 percent of the value of the compounds to animal producers (Beran 1987). Second, not all producers rely on these compounds to the same extent. Subtherapeutic antibiotics are most effective in animals under the stress of inadequate nutrition and suboptimal sanitation (Braude et al. 1953). That means the incentive to use these compounds decreases as management practices improve. For example, pork producers who wash hoghouses every time a group of pigs is moved and who move piglets to off-site growing facilities can reduce their reliance on antibiotics (Dial et al. 1992).

Thus, producers who practice good management would not be as greatly affected by a ban as producers who do not. This raises the interesting possibility that a ban on subtherapeutic drug use would actually result in an economic incentive to improve animal care and could result in a more efficient industry in the long term. However, the process required to reach that point would be painful for those producers forced out of business.

Because some producers might actually benefit from a ban on subtherapeutic drug use, the estimate of costs to a typical producer could be misleading. Examples of this can be seen in the successes of specialty producers such as Colemon Natural Beef in Colorado (NRC 1989a). Colemon beef, raised without antibiotic treatments or exogenous growth promoters, costs approximately 25 percent more than conventional beef. Colemon beef is produced for a specific niche market, and farmers pass on the increased production costs to the consumer.

A more viable alternative to cost estimating would be to measure costs to consumers in terms of the higher prices they would pay for meats. This alternative has the advantage of being reasonably representative across all consumer groups. The dollar value expressed on a per capita or per family basis is readily understandable: It is a number anyone can put into perspective. Using a consumer measure also makes sense from an economic perspective, because all changes in production costs must eventually be passed on in output prices in a competitive industry. The effects of a ban on subtherapeutic drug use might need to be offset by technological improvements to obtain equal levels of production. Therefore, costs would increase and meat prices would be higher than they were before the ban.

Viable Antibiotic Substitutes

The studies referenced above assume a worst case, in which the effects of a ban on production are exactly equal to the known production benefits of subtherapeutic use. The rationale for this assumption was suggested in the CAST (1981) report: "Probably most of the economists did not know all the administrative and technical alternatives but expected that the socially optimum restriction would be less than complete elimination. The analyses reviewed did not try to design a socially optimum partial restriction." (P. 39)

A more reasonable assumption would be that the responses of drug companies and the producers cannot be predicted but that some response will occur. As mentioned elsewhere in the CAST report, the response could take the form of different management practices, new products, or even genetic selection. Thus, in a different scenario, only 50 percent of the estimated effect on production is incorporated. (The worst case contains the entire production effect.)

The issue of substitutes for subtherapeutic drug use also gives rise to the question of whether some producers would purchase antibiotics legally but add them illegally to the feed or water. If that occurs on a widespread basis, there would be little effect on output or prices, because illegal use would substitute for legal use. Again, the extent of such activity cannot be predicted, but it should be noted that the incentive to violate the ban would be enormous as long as therapeutic antibiotics were sold without prescription. The issue could become critically important if widespread violations forced a ban on over-the-counter sales of antibiotics. Banning subtherapeutic use of antibiotics without regulating therapeutic use might be impossible. Any attempt to regulate therapeutic use would increase production costs for the U.S. beef and pork industries, because veterinary visits would be required for each diagnosis and prescription. The costs of a ban on over-the-counter sales of antibiotics would possibly be greater than would be the costs of a ban on subtherapeutic drug use.

Total versus Partial Ban

As has become clear in the debate on fluoroquinolone use in animals, any new antibiotics approved for human use will be too expensive for subtherapeutic use in animals. That is an elegant example of the market at work. New antibiotics are pharmacologically valuable because human pathogens have become resistant to the old ones, and by comparison new drugs are quite expensive to manufacture and purchase. The old antibiotics are inexpensive, in part, because they are less useful to humans and also because the manufacturing chemistry is simpler. To some extent, market forces will deter the use of antibiotics in animal feed if human pathogens have not yet developed resistance to these particular drugs. If regulators accept that scenario, then the group of antibiotics in current use will not be banned, and newer, more expensive ones will. In that case, the consequences of any ban would be minimal because they would occur only as animals develop increased resistance to older antibiotics. The rate at which microorganisms in food-animal populations become resistant to antibiotics is slow because of the short lifespans and high turnover of these animal populations (Walton 1986). The food-animal industry could also be expected to take additional steps to avoid multiple-drug resistance as long as the industry knew that replacements would be difficult to obtain. This market-driven solution has much to recommend it. However, the numbers presented in the economic analysis assume that all subtherapeutic use is banned.

Consumer Behavior

It has been argued that the best way to measure the consequences of a subtherapeutic-use ban is at the consumer level. Because information is available at the producer level, some assumptions must be made about how the extra costs would be passed on to consumers. Assumptions also must be made on the responses of consumers to higher prices and to any improvement or reduction in the quality of the meat. Attempts have been made in previous economic analyses to allow consumers to respond to higher prices by reducing consumption and to provide potential responses from retailers and meat processors (Allen and Burbee 1972; Dworkin 1976; Mann and Paulsen 1976; CAST 1981; Wade and Barkley 1992; Gilliam et al. 1993; FSIS 1995a; Office of Technology Assessment, Washington, D.C., unpublished material). To derive the effects of these responses, estimates of consumer–demand elasticity and producer–retail markups must be made. But such estimates are subjective and can vary widely among studies.

A more straightforward approach is to assume that all costs are passed on to consumers and then to measure how much consumers would need to spend to maintain consumption. This measure of consumer costs will slightly overestimate the true cost (by an amount that depends on how meat consumption is affected by prices), but it has the advantage of not depending on elasticity estimates (see Layard and Walters, 1978, p. 147, Figure 5–9). If the effect of a ban were more severe, it might make more sense to build consumer response to higher prices and a production response to lower demand. This would require use of elasticity measures and would make the final results sensitive to these measures. There is no real consensus on the appropriate size of these elasticities, and, given the very small price effect, the committee decided that the elasticity approach would raise more questions than it answered.

A second consideration is whether consumers will pay more for meat that is produced without subtherapeutic antibiotics. In the two most recent studies on this topic (Wade and Barkley 1992; Manchanda 1994), it was assumed that consumption in the United States would increase by 5 percent in response to such a ban. This assumption seems difficult to justify, because no change can be expected in the concentrations of antibiotic residues. The incidence of drug residue violations cited earlier in this report is so low that a ban on subtherapeutic drug use would be unlikely to have any detectable effect (FSIS 1995a). Consequently, the committee concluded that the correct assumption would be that no change in consumption (positive or negative) occurs. That assumption is equivalent to assuming that the positive effect of improved meat quality exactly offsets the negative effect of higher meat prices.

A final part of this question is whether the marketing system itself would pass on the higher costs in terms of cost per pound or in terms of percentage price change. The latter scenario is used in all the previous studies on this topic and implicitly assumes that meat processors and retailers increase their margins on a per-pound basis in response to increases in the prices they pay. This assumption is justified, in part, because the U.S. marketing system works on a percentage-markup basis. This convention is used in the results presented below.

RESULTS OF ECONOMIC ANALYSIS AND CONCLUSIONS

Based on the assumptions discussed above, the committee derived the estimated economic impact of a ban on subtherapeutic use (Table 7–1). Per capita cost is estimated as follows:

$$\text{Per capita Costs} = \%C \times P \times Q$$

Where $\%C$ is %increase in annual production cost, P is retail price, and Q is annual retail quantity sold per capita.

The committee's conclusion is that the average annual per capita cost to consumers of a ban on subtherapeutic drug use is $4.84 to $9.72. The effect of the ban is lowest for poultry prices and highest for beef. That cost seems small; however, assuming a U.S. population of 260 million, the total amounts to about $1.2 billion to $2.5 billion per year. Of course, the higher per capita cost means low-income consumers would spend an even larger proportion of their income on food than would high-income consumers. To determine whether the increase in cost is justified, the amount should be compared with estimated health benefits. Additional costs not included in Table 7–1 are (1) a slight erosion in U.S. export

TABLE 7–1 Approximate Annual Costs of a Ban on Subtherapeutic Antibiotic Use in Four Domestic Retail Markets

Meat	Change in Price ($/lb)		Per Capita Consumption in 1997, Retail Weight (lb)	Extra Cost per Capita per Year ($)		Extra Cost Family of Four per Week ($)		Total National Extra Cost per Year[a] (million $)	
	A[b]	B[c]		A	B	A	B	A	B
Chicken	0.013	0.026	84	1.09	2.20	0.08	0.17	283	572
Turkey	0.015	0.031	18	0.27	0.56	0.002	0.04	70	146
Beef	0.03	0.06	67	2.01	4.02	0.15	0.31	523	1,045
Pork	0.03	0.06	49	1.47	2.94	0.11	0.23	382	764
Total	NA[d]	NA	218	4.84	9.72	0.342	0.75	1,258	2,527

[a]Calculated based on a population of 260 million × column 5 (for scenario A), or 260 million × column 6 (for scenario B).
[b]A = With substitutes. Scenario A assumes that substitutes mitigate the effect by 50 percent.
[c]B = Without substitutes.
[d]Not applicable.
Source: Columns 2 and 3: CAST 1981. Numbers are based on the quantity effects presented in Tables 24 and 25 (that is, a 2.052 percent change in production costs was used) of the CAST report; Column 4: FAPRI 1998; Columns 5–8: Calculated from Columns 2–4.

competitiveness; (2) the personal and financial costs of producers forced out of business; (3) the lower profits and revenues of the companies that manufacture these compounds; and (4) the additional costs that would occur in markets for eggs, dairy, and pet-food, which are not discussed here. The values in Table 7–1 also ignore the possibility that a subtherapeutic-use ban eventually would lead to restrictions on over-the-counter antibiotic sales.

There has not been any previous attempt in the literature to estimate the consequences of an economy-wide ban of subtherapeutic antibiotic use on consumers. Four studies have focused on the economic effects of a ban (Burpee et al. 1978; Wade and Barkley 1992; Gilliam et. al. 1993; Machanda 1994). Those studies present estimates of production cost increases of 4 to 20 percent. Only 2 of the studies (Wade and Barkley 1992; Machanda 1994) attempted to estimate the effect of such a ban on consumers. They were specific to the pork sector and both calculated retail price increases of $0.04 per pound, which is within the range of $0.03 to $0.06 shown in Table 7–1.

A more difficult task would be to estimate the effect of such a ban on the development of new animal drugs by the animal health industry. For example, the animal health industry invested $381 million in research and development: $355 million was spent for internal research and $26 million was invested in external research, primarily at universities. Seventeen percent of the total research and development investment was allocated to feed additives (Richard Carneval, AHI, 1996, personal communication). The reduction in profits and industry confidence that could occur after such a ban would cause a reduction in research and society would lose the research benefits. Although that loss might well be one of the most important consequences of such a ban, it is impossible to put a monetary value on future research, in part because no one knows what drugs would be developed or approved. Because a value cannot be placed on animal drug research, the associated costs are not discussed. That omission means the numbers provided here underestimate the true costs of a ban.

APPENDIX

Technical Notes for Table 7–1

Chicken Data

On the basis of personal communication with Jerry Sell (Iowa State University, 1997), it was assumed that poultry feed conversion efficiency (FCE) changes from 1.85 tons of grain per ton of meat to 1.90 tons of grain per ton of meat, a 2.7 percent increase. This would represent a 1.76 percent increase in total production costs because feed represents 65 percent of producers' total costs. To calculate the expected effect in the scenario without substitutes, this 1.76 percent was multiplied by the 1997 retail price of chicken ($1.46 per pound) to arrive at cost of 2.6 cents per pound. The scenario with substitutes is set equal to one-half of that value. The key point of this substitute scenario is that some substitution will inevitably occur and it will diminish the effect of a ban. Because these substitutions will occur in the future, there is no accurate way to know what they or their likely magnitude will be. The committee used a value of one-half as a crude estimate of the likely effect of substitution.

Turkey Data

For turkeys FCE was assumed to change from 1.68 to 1.75 tons of feed per ton of meat, a 4.2 percent increase. Feed was assumed to represent 70 percent of total production costs. The total cost increase was calculated at 2.94 percent. The 1997 turkey price of $1.05 per pound was then used to calculate a 3.1-cent-per-pound increase in the scenario without substitutes. The value with substitutes was arbitrarily assumed to be one-half of that value.

Beef Data

Personal communications with Richard Cowman (nutrition expert at the National Cattlemen's Beef Association, 1995) indicated that the consequence of a ban would be an increase of $0.06 per pound in the price of beef. However, this expert did not consider that these particular uses stated were subtherapeutic, because the treatments were for preventing liver abscesses and stress-related diseases and, therefore, suggested a zero value. The retail price used was $2.80 per pound to derive a no-substitutes value of 6 cents per pound. The scenario with substitutes was one-half of that value. The analysis assumes that only 60 percent of all beef animals are affected by such a ban.

Pork Data

The pork data are taken from the *Pork Industry Handbook* (1996). The data showed a change in FCE of 6.5 percent for the first 40 pounds of gain and a change of 3.18 percent for the remaining 145 pounds of gain.

The ration costs and FCE for young pigs were $150 per ton and 2.04, respectively. The values for fattening were $120 and 3.0, respectively. These 4 values were used to weigh the changes in feed conversions. The weights were calculated to be 4.3:1. Thus, the 6.5 percent change in FCE in the starter ration came to approximately 19 percent of total ration costs. The 3 percent change was added to the remaining 81 percent. The total change in FCE was, therefore, calculated at 3.6 percent. Assuming that ration costs equal 70 percent of total production costs, the total change in retail prices represent a 2.5 percent increase. The retail price used for 1997 was $2.30 per pound to arrive at a 6-cent-per-pound increase in the scenario without substitutes.

8

Approaches to Minimizing Antibiotic Use in Food-Animal Production

Historical data demonstrate that the intensification of food-animal production in the United States increased with the finding that antibiotics used in one form or another increased productivity by decreasing the incidence and severity of disease (Hays 1986; Cromwell 1991). However, researchers in some European countries suggest that a shift to less intensive rearing and increased attention to hygiene can resolve many of the situations where the disease and stress load on animals might warrant the use of antibiotics and augment the risk to human health (WHO 1997; Witte 1998). There are many differences in the magnitude and scale of animal agriculture between the United States and many European countries. A goal of producing food animals in the United States devoid of antibiotic use might not be realistic now. It would in fact require a total change in the philosophy and the economics of how production animals are raised (Swann 1969; Hays 1986; Walton 1986; ERS 1996c) and a major overhaul of the interactions and interdependencies between animal producers and crop producers (ERS 1996c).

Concerns about the linkage of antibiotic use in food animals to the development of drug resistance in pathogens in animals and, ultimately, in humans have prompted attempts to limit the use of antibiotics in animal production whenever feasible. The use of antibiotics is considered necessary by many proponents to ensure optimal animal health and growth or production efficiency. The therapeutic applications are obvious when faced with the potential losses that can be incurred with the re-emergence of active infection and disease in a herd, flock, or school. If a goal of animal production specialists is to reduce overall use and, certainly, inappropriate use of antibiotics in food animals (NRC 1989a), strategies must be implemented that offset the potential for increased severity and incidence of animal infection. Reducing the use of antibiotics in food animals must benefit human and animal health in reducing the incidence and severity of disease.

Strategies to reduce the extent of therapeutic antibiotic use fall into two categories: prevention of disease and infection and documented diagnosis of the presence of a pathogen and selection of an antibiotic that is effective and thorough in eliminating infection. To end repeated trial-and-error batteries of antibiotics, the bacteria must be sensitive to the antibiotic prescribed. In addition, viral disease should never be confused with bacterial disease.

Curbing the use of antibiotics in subtherapeutic disease prevention and growth promotion might offer the greatest opportunity to reduce the amount of antibiotics used in food animals. Alternative strategies largely will be manifested in the application of appropriate management practices. Appropriate practices will maximize genetic growth or productivity of food-producing animals and provide dietary nutrients in optimal amounts, in proper sequence, and in correct timing to prevent the demands and strains in one physiological system from compromising the functions of others.

The need for antibiotic use in food animals is unlikely to be obviated totally, and strategies involving the prudent and judicious use of antibiotics can have a positive influence on the animal industries. However, what is possible through the integrated use of strategies that are less dependent on antibiotics is an overall reduction in disease incidence. When disease does occur, the duration and severity of illness can be reduced and perhaps more readily managed by selective and appropriate use of antibiotics. The added benefit of maintaining sound immune competence in animals is that the clearance of invading microorganisms can effectively be increased when therapeutic intervention agents are indicated. Ultimately, the hope is that the safety of the food supply will be improved by reducing the adverse consequences of antibiotic overuse, while maintaining high standards of animal welfare, production, and food quality.

Management strategies and preventive-medicine programs that can be used to reduce disease incidence and thus drug use in food-producing animals are as follows: (1) providing stringent controls on hygiene, population dynamics, feed quality, and environmental conditions to prevent or reduce stress; (2) eradicating specific diseases; (3) optimizing nutrition to enhance natural immunity or feeding nutrient regimens as a preventive measure to lessen the consequences of abrupt changes in conditions for animals (for example, transport to feedlots or release onto fresh pasture); (4) breeding for genetically disease-resistant livestock (Axford and Owen 1991); and (5) in some instances, using alternative growth promotants such as cattle anabolics (Rumsey 1988) or somatotropins (NRC 1994), which pose few or no detectable residue problems (Henricks et al. 1983). Some procedures to aid in disease prevention are easily implemented, such as the addition of lime to sawdust bedding to reduce bacterial counts and guard against udder infection in dairy cows (Hogan et al. 1997).

The process of disease eradication is often costly in the short run, but it can be economically justified in specific situations—generally when a public health risk is substantial. The national eradication programs for brucellosis and tuberculosis are examples in which this approach was warranted and successful. However, the eradication of one pathogen might simply lead to its substitution by another (Axford and Owen 1991). In addition, disease that has been eradicated should not be regarded with complacency. Although hog cholera and bovine tuberculosis were successfully controlled in this country, recent data from the U.S. Department of Agriculture's Animal and Plant Health Inspection Service and the Agricultural Research Service suggest that new forms of cholera and tuberculosis might again become a threat to U.S. animal production; they are already a threat abroad. New population dynamics between domestic and wild animals similarly pose a threat to animal production and challenge management strategies.

Extensive research is under way in the agricultural community, which is exploring and refining strategies to maintain or enhance animal productivity and health while decreasing the need for and use of antibiotics. Many of the approaches mentioned below are still being validated with the hope of successful transfer of the technology into animal production.

ANIMAL MANAGEMENT

Management practices encompass a large realm of procedures implemented at various stages in animal production. Although management practices might be considered routine, many have evolved as specific preventive measures to inhibit pathogenic infections and improve animal health and well-being (Swanson 1995). Management practices that have implications for reducing the need for drug use focus on manipulating the animal's environment to reduce stress, introducing hygienic measures to reduce exposure to disease, and developing methods to enhance immunity.

Ambient Temperature and Heat Stress

Animals are more susceptible to disease during periods of environmental stress (Smith and Hogan 1993). Controlling environmental factors can promote host resistance, thereby reducing dependence on antimicrobial agents. Consideration must be given to numerous factors, such as minimizing extremes of temperature and humidity and minimizing social stresses. Fighting with pen-mates, continuous introduction of new animals into a herd or flock, and inadequate space for feeding or sleeping can weaken animals. (Minton et al. 1995; Swanson 1995; Hyun et al. 1998).

Animals subjected to temperature and humidity extremes are less able to resist bacterial challenge. For example, dairy cattle subjected to high temperatures have increased incidences of mastitis. Mastitis is expensive not only because infected cows produce less milk but also because the milk of cows in treatment must be discarded. Dairy animals, which originated in temperate climates, have increased mastitis and somatic-cell counts (SCCs) in tropical environments (Oliver et al. 1956; Roussel et al. 1969; Wegner et al. 1976). Additionally, chronic, perhaps subclinical, infections erupt into obvious disease states more readily in heat-stressed cows than in animals kept in thermoneutral environments (Nelson et al. 1967; Bishop et al. 1980). Therefore, strict mastitis control procedures must be integrated with heat stress management to avoid disease and drug use. The strategies implemented will vary by season and location.

Numerous strategies have evolved to compensate for heat stress, and they are aimed at providing relief to animals to prevent production losses. Evaporative coolers are used to cool poultry, cattle, and swine in areas of low humidity. Design of poultry and swine buildings has evolved to maximize heat loss during high-temperature extremes and to regulate heat loss during cold periods. Moreover, building design can provide uniform distribution of air through all areas of an animal facility. Novel approaches, such as misting the animals with fresh water or providing cooling ponds, relieve animals from heat stress.

Persistent hot weather will cause a drop in milk production, but the decrease will not be as severe if the cows are protected from the sun and provided with high-quality forage. Feed intake varies with ambient temperature, decreasing substantially for animals in hot and humid conditions and resulting in commensurate declines in growth or performance. Animals should be protected from heat as much as possible with natural or artificial shade, especially during persistent hot weather. In field and corral systems, providing shade only over feed mangers and waterers can result in the feeding areas becoming overloaded with manure, because animals remain there for shade. The animals can then become dirty, which for dairy cows can result in mastitis (Smith and Hogan 1993; Roberson et al. 1994). Therefore, additional shaded areas should be provided away from feed.

The use of water mist on heat-stressed cows in corrals was studied for 20 consecutive days at 100°F and above (Shultz et al. 1985; Shultz 1987). In herds with average daily production of 59.4 lb of milk per cow, production losses due to heat were significantly less for misted cows than for cows without access to mist. The use of feed-manger water in California resulted in a marked reduction in deaths of fresh cows that had recent cases of mastitis. It is essential to avoid creating sites that support the growth of mastitis-causing organisms in the environment where cows lie down.

Sprinklers and fanning stations adjacent to milking parlors have been used quite successfully. This method provides evaporative cooling with just enough water to keep the cows' bodies wet, although their udders must be dried before milking to prevent the development of mastitis. The fans help to remove warm, humid air from the body surfaces of cows and help to dry them (Beede et al. 1987). The sprinkler and fan system also was found to reduce body temperature and increase milk yield of cows in Arizona, Florida, and Israel.

Cows can be wet down again in the exit lane of the milking parlor. Spray should cover only the top and sides of the cows so that the germicidal teat dip used after milking is not washed off. Thus, the cows are temporarily relieved from the effects of the sun, and instead of returning immediately to the shade, they follow their normal cool-weather practice of eating and drinking after each milking. That keeps animals on their feet and allows time for teat-duct closure before contact with soil and manure, which can result in intramammary infection. Although the effectiveness of this method of cooling depends on evaporation, it also should work for dairies in more humid areas where evaporative coolers are not practical.

Nutritional measures to alleviate heat stress in ruminants include feeding high-energy rations to reduce excess physiological heat generated by digestion of high-fiber rations. In addition, it is important to avoid handling and milking cows during the hottest part of the day; early-morning and late-evening moving and feeding encourage consumption.

One heat-stress-management strategy for cooling cows and reducing incidence of mastitis involves the use of cooling ponds (Shearer et al. 1987). Florida researchers studied a 1,400-cow dairy that elected to use ponds after comparing costs with other cooling methods and the success of other dairies using them. In the study, 1 group of cows was located in lots with cooling ponds and permanent shade, and the groups with no pond had access to shade structures only. Results showed that cows with access to cooling ponds had significantly less clinical mastitis (9.8 percent vs. 18.6 percent). The authors suggested that the reduction in mastitis was due to enhanced resistance to infection resulting from reduced heat stress as well as to improved udder preparation.

Water quality and availability can offset some of the adverse effects of heat stress. Cows drink about 50 percent more water at 80°F than at 40°F, and they require water to cool themselves in the form of respired moisture and body sweat (Graves 1986). Chilling the drinking water for milking cows during hot weather can help rid cows of the large heat load that they produce and receive from their environment (Lanham et al. 1986). Under conditions of high relative humidity, chilling drinking water to 50°F has helped alleviate heat stress, resulting in increased feed intake, milk yield, and rumen motility, and in decreased respiration and body temperature (Baker et al. 1988). Similarly, evaporative cooling significantly increased reproductive performance and milk production in cows in a hot, dry climate (Ryan et al. 1992; Chen et al. 1993).

A practical application of management strategies and changes to equipment design to combat heat stress in animals is illustrated through management practices being implemented in the broiler industry to facilitate easier drinking for overheated birds. Poultry deaths in the southeastern United States can be devastating during the summer months, and heat stress increases the incidence of disease. The design of poultry waterers can have a significant effect on how heat-stressed birds are able to drink water (May and Lott 1996; May et al. 1997). The consumption of water is not constant during the day and affects the bird's feed consumption patterns and the ability to thermoregulate. In poultry houses, birds need to pant to shed heat. The positioning of waterers, the height of drinking nipples, the drinking process, and panting can become a major problem of coordination for the birds that can result in insufficient intake of water. The problem is associated with reaching for and triggering the nipple waterers, swallowing the water, and panting vigorously.

Overcrowding and Behavioral Stress

Overcrowded animals often must compete for feed, water, and sleeping space and so are more susceptible to disease. Animals that harbor subclinical infections can become chronic shedders of pathogens, which can be transmitted to other animals or to humans through direct contact or through food. Often, constant vigilance by animal caretakers is essential to prevent timid animals from being crowded away from feed and water or from being subjected to fighting. To avoid such problems, animals must be given appropriate space and should be commingled as little as reasonably possible. Sick or weak animals should be housed separately from healthy pen-mates.

In some situations, group feeding results in higher consumption rates than does individual feeding; as a result, overall body-weight gains can be increased. However, competition can result in gorging, particularly by calves fed high-concentrate feeds, which can cause bloating, acidosis, and bacterial imbalances in the rumen and gut. These animals are predisposed to illness and are often treated with additional medicinals and antibiotics.

Vaccination Strategies to Prevent Disease

Traditionally, vaccination has been used to control pathogens that affect agricultural animals. However, the use of vaccines for controlling food-borne pathogens (for example, *Salmonella* in poultry products and *Escherichia coli* O157:H7 in bovine products) is a relatively unexplored method for reducing or eliminating pathogenic bacteria from the food chain.

Vaccination can be a reliable alternative to drug use in the prevention of some diseases in animals. Attenuated live vaccines delivered orally have several distinct advantages over injected vaccines. The vaccine is usually delivered by spray or in drinking water, so needles are not required and animals need not be handled individually. In addition, depending on the life cycle of the parent pathogen, some live vaccines induce humoral, cellular, and mucosal immune responses, because they invade and stimulate the gut-associated lymphoid tissue.

Control of *Salmonella* in poultry with vaccines could be useful for two reasons. First, resistance to antibiotics could be better controlled (Cohen and Tauxe 1986). Second, live attenuated *Salmonella* administered orally elicit cell-mediated mucosal and humoral immune responses, thus making them excellent vaccines (Clements 1987; Curtiss et al. 1993; Griffin and Barrow 1993). Attenuated bacteria also have shown great promise as delivery vehicles for heterologous antigens, such as virulence determinants and epitopes from a variety of mucosal pathogens. Stable expression of heterologous surface-exposed antigens has been achieved in *Salmonella typhimurium* (Curtiss and Kelly 1987; Hassan and Curtiss 1994).

Recent advances in molecular biology and understanding of microbial physiology and pathology have facilitated the development of several well-defined gene deletion mutations in *Salmonella* that result in a virulent immunogenic phenotype. The current approach to attenuation in *Salmonella* species is to introduce mutations that decrease virulence while maintaining the ability to colonize lymphoid tissue, elicit immune response, and maintain genetic stability. This strategy is being used to produce patented live virulent *Salmonella* vaccines to control *Salmonella enteritidis* and *Salmonella typhimurium* in many animal species (Cooper et al. 1994; Hassan and Curtiss 1994, 1996). *Salmonella typhimurium* and other species have been used successfully in model systems to deliver antigens from a variety of mucosal pathogens (Clements 1987; Cardenas and Clements 1993). In addition, several molecular systems have been developed to stabilize the expression of heterologous antigens in vaccine strains (Strugnell et al. 1990a,b, 1992; Morona et al. 1991).

Although most studies have been done in mice with antigens to human pathogens, the results indicate that animal vaccination has significant merit. One important pathogen needing further investigation in this regard is *E. coli*. Various strains of this organism cause economic losses to poultry and swine producers. The O157:H7 strain is a well-known food-borne human health hazard. Morona et al. (1994) showed that *Salmonella typhimurium* vaccine strains expressing relevant *E. coli* fimbrial antigens can elicit antibody responses in pigs comparable to those seen with injected killed vaccines. Other potential pathogen targets for this technology include species of *Campylobacter, Bordetella, Pasteurella, Erysipelothrix, Clostridium, Mycobacterium, Mycoplasma,* and *Eimeria*. A short list of other pathogens from which relevant antigens have been cloned and expressed in *Salmonella* species includes *Salmonella* (Strugnell et al. 1990b) *Echinococcus multilocularis* (Gottstein 1992), and *Bordetella pertussis* (Guzman et al. 1991).

DNA Vaccination

A challenge to animal health experts is the development of proper antigens to use in vaccination programs to prevent the development and spread of disease. Often the use of whole-organism preparations is ineffective because of the similarity in protein antigens among many organisms. In addition, proteins and peptides that are unique to specific pathogen species are often poorly antigenic and ineffective in producing antibodies to protect an animal from a pathogen-specific disease. Recently, experiments were summarized at the International Meeting on Nucleic Acid Vaccines for the Prevention of Infectious Diseases at the National Institutes of Health. In the technique of nucleic acid vaccination, plasmid DNA from a specific pathogen gene is introduced into a host by direct injection, by high-velocity injection using the gene gun, or by oral administration (IMNAVPID 1996). The gene gun is a device in which a 0.22 caliber ammunition blank is used to insert genetic material intracellularly by high-velocity dispersion and cell membrane penetration. Antibodies to the proteins encoded by these DNA fragments that code for the protein are efficiently produced, and the antibody concentration (titer) is roughly proportional to the mass of DNA injected. An important feature of this approach is that the antibody responses are easily manipulated either by coexpression or by the administration of cytokines, such as interleukin-4 (IL-4), IL-6, and interferon-γ (IF-γ). Oral DNA administration is effective in eliciting localized mucosal immune response, where the first site of pathogen interaction might be the mucosal surface itself.

The DNA vaccination, and particularly the use of gene hybrids, presents the opportunity to obtain site-specific immune expression. For example, by fusing a site-specific promoter gene to a desired structural gene, a relatively high expression of the desired antigen can be obtained at a specific site where only the promoter region is activated. Such strategies also could be used in situations where gut-specific antibody production would serve as a first line of defense against a gut pathogen in an animal. An advantage of this approach is that specific base sequences of DNA can be easily and cheaply made to serve as specific antigen stimuli without the need to grow active cultures of organisms and extract proteins (for further detail, see IMNAVPID 1996).

Beneficial Microbial Cultures, Probiotics, and Competitive-Exclusion Alternatives

The disease ramifications associated with microbial contamination of foods are not taken lightly and are the major focus of President Clinton's food safety initiative (CFSAN 1997). As the president stated in a radio address January 25, 1997,

> We have built a solid foundation for the health of America's families. But clearly we must do more. No parent should have to think twice about the juice they pour their children at breakfast, or a hamburger ordered during dinner out.

The chief targets of the initiative are related to bacteria and organisms that enter the food chain from gut and fecal origins from domestic animals. The majority of gut-derived organisms are readily controllable through standard and routine measures established for the food production industries; however, concern heightens when conditions within the animal are right for the emergence of organisms of greater virulence and pathogenicity. Most of the time, proliferation of these undesirable organisms is held in check by the nature of gastrointestinal ecology. This is sometimes called the principle of "competitive exclusion," the ability of a population of beneficial microorganisms to condition the gut and intestinal environment with regard to pH, ionic balance, and selective microbial excretion products and to prevent establishment of pathogenic microorganisms in the gut. An in-depth review of the homeostatis established and maintained in the gut through the proper balance in microbial ecological factors is beyond the scope of this report. However, it is worthwhile to restate that the normal gut microbial population provides a good measure of assurance that inappropriate bacteria find it difficult to establish a clinically significant presence. Under normal circumstances, pathogenic organisms cannot proliferate and are outcompeted by normal flora. Research is demonstrating the effectiveness of feeding live beneficial microorganisms to animals to maintain or reintroduce balance into gut ecology that might have been challenged by the emergence of pathogens (Stark and Wilkenson 1988). The food-animal industry is experiencing an increase in the development of antibiotic-resistant bacteria as well as bacteria that have increased pathogenicity, particularly *Salmonella*, coliforms, and *Campylobacter*. As a result, there is renewed interest in the use of normal gut flora, probiotic, and competitive-exclusion products (CEPs) to reduce gastrointestinal stress and its effects on the animal's performance without resorting to the use of antibiotics. Some proposed benefits of normal gut flora and probiotics are improved survival of newborns, reduction or prevention of diarrhea, increased growth rate, improved feed efficiency, and enhanced immune response (Stark and Wilkenson 1988).

The administration of beneficial microorganisms to animals started in the 1920s, and the name "probiotics" (defined as "for life") was introduced in the 1970s. Feeding beneficial microorganisms to chicks is intended to protect them against colonization by such pathogenic bacteria as *Salmonella* and enterotoxigenic *E. coli* (ETEC) (Nurmi and Rantala 1973). The resident host flora can exclude the newcomer by several mechanisms. Volatile fatty acid production, pH effects, toxic metabolite production, or simple occupation of attachment sites within the gut have been studied and reviewed (Bailey 1987). The most commonly used probiotics are live cultures of 3 to 5 species of lactic-acid-producing bacteria, such as *Lactobacillus acidophilus* or *Streptococcus faecalis*.

In 1989, the U.S. Food and Drug Administration (FDA) required manufacturers of these products to use the term "direct-fed microbial" (DFM) instead of probiotic. DFMs are used to control and promote the proper environmental conditions for establishing an ideal microbial population in an animal's digestive tract. They do not establish or provide the normal gut flora; the animal must obtain flora from its environment. DFM products are regulated by the FDA Center for Veterinary Medicine as food, under the provisions of the Compliance Policy Guide 689.100. Unlike CEPs, the microorganisms administered to animals in DFMs are defined and specified. The organisms used in these products are listed by the Association of American Feed Control Officials. CEPs are unspecified mixtures of live microorganisms isolated from the intestinal tract of animals of different species. Because some of the claims of these products are therapeutic, CEPs are listed as drugs and are regulated as such (CVM 1997a).

Successful antimicrobial plus beneficial microorganism programs have been developed in Europe using quinolone therapy followed by competitive-exclusion microbial cultures to produce *Salmonella*-free broilers. The administration of the proper mix of competitive microorganism cultures also appears beneficial in the control of *Campylobacter fetus* subspecies *jejuni* in young chicks (Soerjadi et al. 1981, 1982).

Scientists researching this interesting form of bioremediation of pathogenic microorganisms suggest that, in animals subjected to stress, the balance between normal and potentially pathogenic bacteria in the intestine is altered (Abe et al. 1995). As a result, the pathogens might proliferate to a population density that permits their emergence within the animal as a disease or be of sufficient numbers to pose a threat to human health if they are contaminants of food. Probiotics, built up by strains of lactic-acid-producing organisms, promote digestive balance by supplementing intestinal microflora with beneficial bacteria, thus creating conditions unfavorable for pathogen growth. Additional mechanisms of action of probiotic microorganisms include production of antimicrobial substances, competition for adhesion receptors in the intestine, competition for nutrients, and immunostimulation, all of which create an environment incompatible for pathogens. Probiotics are used in dairy calf ration supplements as a prophylactic disease control tool against digestive disorders (Stark and Wilkenson 1988). Probiotics also have been shown to improve production performance by increasing average daily gain, feed consumption, and feed efficiency (Abe et al. 1995).

Biosecurity

Biosecurity techniques should be based on an understanding of pathogen transmission. A knowledge of all potential entry routes for pathogens to a herd is an essential prelude to developing a comprehensive biosecurity program. If multiple pathogens with different routes of transmission are listed according to priority for exclusion from a group of animals, a multiple-point biosecurity program is warranted. Dial et al. (1992) summarized several sources in formulating biosecurity policies for swine, but they could be applied to all food animal species:

- Locating herds away from potential sources of infection, including other production facilities, slaughterhouses, sale barns, and roadways.
- Enclosing herds in bird-proof facilities.
- Placing fences around the farm boundaries and placing locks on doors and windows to prevent entry of visitors.
- Prohibiting entry of vehicles used to transport animals, unless they are empty and have been cleaned and disinfected before arrival at the facility.
- Providing secure loading areas that prevent animals from returning to buildings once they have been exposed to trucks.
- Aggressively controlling rodent and fly populations, including the use of weed control and gravel borders to discourage rodents from approaching facilities.
- Excluding cats and dogs from farm complexes.
- Excluding people, including visitors, who are nonessential to farm operations.
- Ensuring that farm personnel do not come in contact with animals outside the herd.
- Establishing a minimum quarantine time for people before they come in contact with livestock.
- Requiring all people to shower before entering farms and providing clothing to wear on farms.
- Ensuring pathogen-free feed sources and instituting methods of delivering feed to farms that closely control the access of potentially contaminated trucks.
- Cleaning outside feed spills to avoid attracting rodents and birds.
- Providing secure manure storage and disposal.
- Promptly disposing of dead animals.
- Moving incoming stock to isolation areas that have separate ventilation and manure removal systems.
- Placing sentinel animals with incoming stock and using diagnostic tests (serological tests or postmortem examination) to detect infection.
- Ensuring that feeds, water, bedding, equipment, and supplies are free of infectious agents.
- Restricting the use of manure-disposal equipment.
- Testing replacement herds for the presence of pathogens.
- Using high-health technologies (for example, artificial insemination, embryo transfer, surgical derivation, and medicated early weaning) to introduce new genetic stock.

Many of these options are based in common sense, but some of the specific elements are difficult to control or implement. The seasonality of biosecurity calls for different measures to be taken at different times of the year. In the fall, wild-animal populations begin to seek additional shelter, warmth, and food, and domestic animal facilities offer much of what those animals seek. In those situations, wild animals can spread disease to domestic populations. Similarly, quarantine, disinfection, and clothing changes are often highly effective measures to counter the spread of potential pathogens. Realistically, few producers have the resources or time to increase their operations to provide for showers and change of clothes every time they enter a different animal facility. If these measures are to be effective, the ease of implementation must be balanced with the return.

Fly Control

Flies are important vectors of bacterial diseases, and biting flies contribute greatly to the stress in cows. Stress can cause a reduction in milk production (Richardson 1987) and a spread in mastitis during warm summer months. Preliminary studies at the Hill Farm Research Station at Louisiana State University, Homer, Louisiana, indicated that flies are instrumental in establishing coagulase-negative staphylococcal teat-canal colonizations in young dairy heifers (Richardson 1987). Such colonizations result in intramammary infections at freshening and persist into lactation. Therefore, fly control is especially important during hot, humid weather when conditions are optimal for multiplication.

The overall presence of ectoparasites can establish conditions in which the stresses on animals are so great that the natural partitioning of nutrients for growth or production is significantly perturbed, and conditions for further disease stress and microbe emergence can be established. Experiments conducted by Cole and Guillot (1987) demonstrated that the excess in energy expenditure of cattle infected with *Psoroptis ovis* was proportional to the area of body surface infected. The data further showed that it was impossible to account for the entire increased energy expenditure by higher feed consumption. Increased energy expenditure from fighting the infection coupled with decreased intake resulted in excessive energy wasting and loss of weight. This is a problem in the modern context of nutrition because it is now realized that the total concept of nutrition is not only what the animal eats, but also how the nutrients are absorbed from the gut and partitioned to different tissues to accomplish specific physiological tasks. This nutrient partitioning is mediated via a complex interaction between the nutrients, the endocrine system, and the immune system, referred to as the endocrine immune gradient (Elsasser et al. 1995, 1997; NRC 1995).

Moisture, Mud, and Manure

If there is a single physical environmental factor that predisposes animals to constant infection and reinfection, it is moisture. Moisture facilitates the development of a proliferative medium to support most microorganisms. Under hot and humid conditions, such factors as rain, mud, manure, and bedding become even more important, because they can increase the number of mastitis and disease-causing organisms present on animals. In this type of environment, disease must be prevented by decreasing exposure to pathogens and increasing animals' resistance to infection. If disease caused by environmental pathogens is a problem, it is imperative that bedding materials be kept as clean and dry as possible. Finely chopped organic bedding materials, such as sawdust, shavings, recycled manure, pelleted corn cobs, peanut hulls, and chopped straw, frequently contain coliforms and streptococci in excess of 1×10^6 colony-forming unit (cfu) per gram and might exceed 1×10^8 cfu/g, a number that often increases mastitis and airborne respiratory disease incidence. Inorganic materials, such as sand or crushed limestone, are preferable to finely chopped organic materials and are recommended to reduce the bacterial load (Hogan et al. 1997).

Enhancing Natural Mediators of Immune Function

Cytokines, the so-called hormones of the immune system, also work in disease prevention and therapy. Cytokines are chemical (peptide) signal molecules that are released from specific or generalized immune cells and nonimmune cells throughout the body to function either at sites remote from the point of origin or locally at the site of origin (Babiuk et al. 1991; Elsasser et al. 1995). Resistance to disease is mediated in part by leukocytes that are directed against microorganisms that enter the body. Cytokines are produced naturally in all animals and function by regulating the activity of leukocytes, monocytes, macrophages, and neutrophils involved in protecting animals from the effects of invading organisms. For example, INF-g modulates phagocytic leukocyte populations. Because INF-γ has been shown to greatly enhance leukocyte ability to destroy bacteria, studies have been conducted to determine whether this cytokine is effective in controlling mastitis in dairy cows. In one investigation (Sordillo and Babiuk 1991), dairy cows given intramammary INF-γ had fewer infected mammary gland quarters, exhibited milder clinical symptoms, and experienced infections of shorter duration (Table 8–1). Success of treatment was attributed to the ability of this cytokine to enhance leukocyte activity and minimize the deleterious effects of bacterial endotoxin. Likewise, Quiroga et al. (1993) found that INF-γ promoted bovine milk neutrophil phagocytic activity in vitro. Prophylactic use of INF-γ shortly before or after calving could reduce the incidence of coliform mastitis, which now occurs frequently in many herds.

Colony-stimulating factors (CSFs) are cytokines required for the proliferation and differentiation of bone marrow stem cells into functional mature leukocytes. Administration of CSFs increases blood leukocyte counts and increases cellular ability to phagocytose and kill disease-causing bacteria.

Granulocyte and macrophage colony-stimulating factor (GMCSF) induces maturation of bone marrow cells into neutrophils and macrophages, and subcutaneous administration to cows before the dry period was found to enhance the

TABLE 8–1 Efficacy of Recombinant Bovine IFN-γ against *E. coli* Mastitis

Treatment Group	Eligible Quarters	Percentage Showing Clinical Signs of Mastitis	Clinical Score[a]	Percentage of Infected Quarters	Percentage Reduction[b]
IFN-γ	24	16.7	1.8	21.4	71.1
Placebo	23	70.0	2.3	74.1	

[a]Clinical scores range from 1 to 5: 1 is normal milk with no quarter swelling; 2 is questionable milk with no quarter swelling; 3 is obvious abnormal milk with no quarter swelling; 4 is abnormal milk with a swollen or tender quarter; and 5 is acute mastitis with systemic involvement (Smith et al. 1985).

[b]Compared with placebo-treated group.

Source: Adapted from Sordillo and Babiuk (1991).

TABLE 8–2 Effect of GCSF on Blood and Milk Leukocyte Profiles and Efficacy against *Staphylococcus aureus* Mastitis

Treatment	Blood Leukocytes (mm^3)	Blood Neutrophils (%)	Milk SCC[a] (1000/ml)	Milk Neutrophils (%)	Reduction[b] (%)
GCSF	30,213	81.3	582	64.4	47
Control	8,675	21.3	261	45.3	

[a]SCC = Somatic cell count.

[b]Compared with control group.

Source: Adapted from Nickerson et al. (1989).

antimicrobial activity of neutrophils (Babiuk et al. 1991). These leukocytes might be more competent in defending the udder during periods when cellular activity is normally compromised; thus, GMCSF might be useful as an alternative to conventional dry-cow antibiotic therapy.

The administration of granulocyte colony-stimulating factor (GCSF) to lactating dairy cows also was found to markedly increase total leukocyte and neutrophil concentrations in blood and milk (Table 8–2). The resulting reduction in new intramammary infections was due to the recruitment of neutrophils that provided a phagocytic line of defense (Nickerson et al. 1989).

In addition to enhancing phagocyte activity, other cytokines regulate the activity of lymphocytes. Local administration of IL-2 to cows at the beginning of the dry period was found to expand lymphocyte populations in mammary tissues and secretions during involution, stimulate the local production of antibodies, and accelerate the involution process, all of which promote resistance to invasive bacteria during the dry period (Nickerson et al. 1993).

Killed Bacterial Adjuvants:
Biomodulation of Cytokine and Immune Function

Further biomodulation of immune system functions might be manipulated by the selective use of specific preparations of bacteria that have inherent adjuvant properties when injected into animals. *Propionibacterium acnes* serves as a general immunostimulant of leukocytes involved in nonspecific resistance to disease. For example, heat-killed cultures and soluble factors of these bacteria stimulate chemotaxis, phagocytosis, and intracellular degradation of bacteria by macrophages and neutrophils (Hogan et al. 1993). The soluble factors produced by *Propionibacterium acnes* can interact directly with cell membranes to alter cellular metabolism or to release cytokines that potentiate defense mechanisms of phagocytes. Cytokines released in response to *Propionibacterium acnes* include INF-γ, GCSF, tumor necrosis factor, IL-1, and IL-2. There are realistic complications and concerns with the implementation of cytokine biomodulation. The endogenous peptides possess considerable cytotoxicity as well as cachectic character when elaborated in states of overproduction (Elsasser et al 1995; 1997). However, modulation effected through localized paracrine (cell-to-cell) cytokine activities could provide the desired immunomodulatory response with minimal toxicity.

NUTRITION

A relationship between nutrition and resistance to infection is becoming increasingly evident (Chandra 1992). Macronutrients and protein and energy relationships are important to proper health status; however, research suggests that the greatest breakthroughs in nutrition and stress management will occur in defining specific micronutrient (trace mineral and antioxidant) requirements (Tengerdy et al. 1981, 1983; Burton and Traber 1990; Burton 1994). The literature contains many reports of altered (improved) immune function associated with changes in dietary components, but much of the work is unrepeatable and, therefore, questionable with regard to the stated conclusions. In addition, the complexity of immune system functions and interactions that appear to be affected by some aspect of nutrition are so extensive that studies performed in vitro on isolated cells or nonspecific blastogenic responses of immune cells do not reflect the nature of the in vivo interactions. In addition, there are few if any substantive in vivo studies that have investigated the relationship between nutrient requirements for optimal animal growth and productivity and those that satisfy the needs of the immune system.

Knowledge of how antioxidants work in nutrition and disease resistance is rapidly increasing. To optimize disease resistance, animal diets should be balanced and formulated for the appropriate stage of growth or production. Although supplementation with antioxidants might reduce adverse cell responses to infection, the therapeutic benefits of nutritional management of clinical disease are not well documented.

The relationship between proper nutrition and resistance to infection is well illustrated in the dairy cow and underscores the need to supplement animal rations with specific micronutrients that promote optimal immune cell function and disease resistance. Finally, management practices must alleviate the detrimental additional effects of the environment to avoid immunosuppression, increased incidence of infection, and, therefore, drug use.

Refined nutrient management could improve growth, feed efficiency, and host response to disease (Elsasser et al. 1995). Diet appears to influence resistance to infection, because specific nutrients are important in endocrine regulation, immune and somatic cell function, antibody production, and tissue integrity. In particular, micronutrient interactions might increase disease resistance through regulating cellular and molecular processes, including membrane flux and integrity, superoxide formation, and leukocyte function (Tengerdy et al. 1981, 1983).

Bovine mastitis is among the most costly diseases to the livestock industry and provides an excellent example of the interaction between nutrition and animal health. Consequently, the potential to modulate mammary resistance to disease by nutritional supplementation has gained widespread interest, aided by the heightened focus on nonantibiotic approaches to infectious-disease control. In dairy cattle, micronutrients increase mammary resistance to infection and therefore decrease the incidence of mastitis (Erskine 1993). Antioxidants, such as selenium and vitamin E are important in immune response to bacterial challenge. Smith et al. (1984) and Hogan et al. (1993) found that dietary supplementation with vitamin E and selenium decreased the incidence and duration of clinical mastitis by producing a more rapid influx of neutrophils into infected mammary glands and increasing intracellular killing of ingested bacteria. Leukocytes are a major defense mechanism of the bovine mammary gland, and nutritional effects on leukocyte function can have a profound effect on mammary immunity. Antioxidants have been shown to be critical to promoting efficient mammary phagocyte killing, and their effects provide evidence of a link between nutrition and mastitis resistance.

Experimental evidence suggests a critical need for antioxidants to support proper bovine phagocytic function. Neutrophils collected from cattle fed diets deficient in copper or selenium have impaired antioxidant enzyme activity and therefore impaired ability to kill ingested bacteria. Vitamin E supplementation of dairy cattle diets enhanced the ability of blood neutrophils to kill ingested *Staphylococcus aureus* and *E. coli*. Likewise, selenium supplementation in dairy cows resulted in mammary neutrophils' increased killing of *Staphylococcus aureus* and *E. coli*, and decreased extracellular hydrogen peroxide production compared

TABLE 8–3   Blood Selenium, GSH-Px, and Serum Vitamin E
of Cows from Low- and High-SCC Herds

Component	Low SCC	High SCC
Blood selenium (mg/ml)	0.133	0.074[a]
Blood GSH-Px (mU/mg of hemoglobin)	35.6	20.2[a]
Serum vitamin E (µg/100 ml)	484.6	421.3

[a] Significantly different (P <0.01)
Source: Adapted from Erskine et al. (1987).

with neutrophils from selenium-deficient cows (Reddy et al. 1986; Hogan et al. 1990; Eicher-Pruiett et al. 1992).

As discussed in Chapter 2, dairy farmers and veterinarians use the presence of immune somatic cells in milk as an indication of the presence of udder infections and mastitis in lactating animals. In 32 Pennsylvania dairy herds, whole-blood concentrations of selenium and activity of the selenium-dependent enzyme glutathione peroxidase (GSH-Px) were higher in herds with low SCCs than in herds with high SCCs (Table 8–3) (Erskine et al. 1987).   Herd prevalence of infection was negatively correlated with blood GSH-Px activity, that is, the higher the GSH-Px activity the lower the prevalence of infection. Weiss et al. (1990) also found that plasma selenium and GSH-Px were negatively correlated with bulk tank milk SCC, and the rate of clinical mastitis was negatively correlated with plasma selenium concentration and vitamin E concentration in the diet. These data suggest that general health of animals can be affected by deficiencies in some aspects of nutrition that compromise an animal's natural ability to fight off invading microorganisms.

Smith et al. (1984) supplemented diets of pregnant heifers with vitamin E (50 to 100 ppm) and selenium (0.3 ppm) 60 days prepartum and throughout lactation. Dietary supplementation reduced staphylococcal and coliform infections at calving by 42.2 percent, and duration of infection by organisms other than *Corynebacterium bovis* was reduced 40 to 50 percent. Clinical mastitis was reduced in early lactation (57.2 percent) and throughout lactation (32.1 percent), and mean SCC was lower. In addition, injection of 50 mg of selenium 3 weeks prepartum decreased new infections at calving. Likewise, Hogan et al. (1993) observed that dietary selenium supplementation resulted in a more rapid influx of neutrophils into infected mammary glands and increased intracellular killing of ingested bacteria. Dietary supplementation with vitamin E resulted in an increased bactericidal activity of neutrophils.

Vitamin A and its precursor, β-carotene, are necessary for the proper function of epithelial cell membranes, and they stimulate cellular and humoral immunity. Chew et al. (1982) showed that cows with lower concentrations of vitamin

A and β-carotene in the blood had more severe mastitis. Vitamin A and β-carotene also reduced the incidence of mammary infection during the early dry period (Dahlquist and Chew 1985) and reduced SCC (Chew and Johnston 1985), although a more recent study (Oldham et al. 1991) found no effect from vitamin A and β-carotene supplementation at concentrations above those recommended by the National Research Council (NRC 1989b).

Leukocytes, particularly activated phagocytes, require antioxidants to achieve efficient performance. The ability of antioxidants to enhance leukocyte function might explain partially their beneficial effect on mammary resistance to disease.

The in vitro killing of *Staphylococcus aureus* by blood neutrophils was enhanced by adding β-carotene to the diet of cows fed rations with low concentrations of β-carotene and no supplemental vitamin A (Erskine 1993).

The use of inorganic trace minerals or organic-complexed minerals to boost health is of considerable interest to producers and feed additive manufacturers. Many reports have been issued on the health benefits of the use of selenium, zinc, copper, and iron. Seldom, however, has research been performed that critically differentiates between the addition of these elements to diets, where the aim is to supplement and remedy a deficiency, and their use in excess of, for example, National Research Council recommendations. However, research examples such as those cited below and previously in this chapter do support the view that mineral supplementation can affect health status of food animals.

Selenium alone or in combination with vitamin E has been effective in reducing the incidence and severity of several reproductive problems in livestock, such as retained placentas, metritis, and other dysfunctions thought to reflect abnormal immune function or a predisposition to infection resulting from the stress of parturition and shift in metabolism to support lactation (Barnouin and Chassagne 1991; Jankowski 1993).

Copper and zinc are essential to immune cell function as the enzyme copper–zinc superoxide dismutase, which is important for production of hydrogen peroxide to destroy engulfed bacteria. Zinc deficiency leads to increased susceptibility to infections in dairy cattle (Miller 1978), and use of organic zinc complexes in the diet has been found to decrease SCC. Kellogg (1990) summarized research with zinc–methionine and showed a significant decrease in SCC with an increase in milk production.

Research indicates that supplemented chromium also might have immuno-stimulating properties and some production-enhancing abilities. Initial effects of supplemental chromium on the immune system were observed in stressed feedlot calves, in which chromium supplementation was associated with lowered morbidity and improved weight gain, feed efficiency, and immune responsiveness. Mallard et al. (1994) showed that cows fed supplemental chromium had a significantly higher number of antibody responses to several antigens and higher lymphocyte proliferation upon mitogen stimulation as compared with nonsupplemented controls. Cows receiving chromium also exhibited higher concentrations of immunoglobin G1 in serum and colostrum. Chromium supplementation was associated with increased milk yield, particularly among primiparous cows. The use of chromium supplementation as a means of increasing animal health must be viewed with some caution. A recent summary of the function of chromium in animal nutrition (NRC 1997) suggests that the data are not strong enough to warrant generalized conclusions regarding chromium and animal health.

Micronutrients also affect optimal disease resistance in pigs (Peplowski et al. 1980), beef cattle (Chew 1987; Erskine et al. 1989), and fish (Durve and Lovell 1982). Pigs fed higher concentrations of vitamin E had increased serum antibody titers against *E. coli* (Ellis and Vorhies 1976). Immunocompetence in beef cattle is enhanced by dietary selenium, iron, copper, and zinc (Chandra and Dayton 1982). Vitamin E has also been found to improve disease resistance in cattle (Erskine 1993). Vitamins have been found to increase immune response in fish (Webster 1991).

Additional research on basic and applied nutritional modulation of animal health should be pursued and research funding should be increased where applicable. Where possible, much of this research should focus on whole-animal approaches to nutritional modulation of health because of the complex interconnectedness of the various components of the immune system. It becomes difficult to assess cause-and-effect relationships where individual components of the immune system are isolates, for example, in in vitro systems, and lose the capability of being modulated by other components of the system.

DISEASE ERADICATION

Some livestock and poultry diseases are so devastating or present such a great public health risk that eradication becomes a viable option. Tuberculosis and brucellosis are approaching complete eradication after many years of testing and slaughter or depopulation programs and long-term national surveillance. More short-term eradication programs, involving complete slaughter of poultry flocks, have made significant progress in eliminating *Salmonella enteriditis* and avian influenza. Other diseases have been virtually eradicated through intensive vaccination programs and the development of breeding stock that is free of specific diseases such as *Salmonella*.

In swine, a program of depopulation and repopulation has been used to improve herd health and productivity and to lower medication use and drug costs (Leman 1988, 1992; McNaughton 1988; Deen 1992). This technique results in an approximate 10 percent improvement in feed efficiency and average daily gain and a 10 to 20 percent increase in pounds of pork marketed annually from each sow (Leman 1992). However, this technique disrupts an enterprise's cash flow and it can be expensive (Kavanaugh 1989; Deen 1992).

GENETICS

Molecular biology approaches can be applied to genetic strategies to enhance selection for advantageous traits, including resistance in livestock to disease. Traditionally, breeding strategies have not been designed to select for host resistance and desirable production traits at the same time. One alternative to the traditional approach is the use of genetic-marker-assisted selection, which offers an opportunity for simultaneous improvement in all the traits.

Selection pressure applied to livestock for economically important traits is often accompanied by increases in stress and disease problems in production environments. Knowledge of the genetic correlation between disease resistance and immune responsiveness traits and production traits will be required to include these traits in livestock selection (Rothschild 1991). Because of the difficulty in measuring disease resistance and immune responsiveness, these traits have been ignored in most selection programs. Breeding for disease resistance also is difficult because resistance is regulated by genes at numerous loci and is greatly influenced by environmental factors.

Heritability estimates (the percentage of variation controlled by genetics) for resistance to most livestock diseases that have been studied are low (Warner et al. 1987; Rothschild 1989). However, genetic variation among animals for disease traits is reasonably large, making breeding for disease resistance possible and justified. New tools of molecular biology make it possible to simultaneously improve production and disease resistance traits. Molecular genotyping techniques allow the detection of DNA polymorphisms. Such polymorphic marker loci can be used in marker-assisted selection. For example, selection for a disease resistance gene, for which there is no direct method of genotyping, can be effected by selection for the appropriate alleles at linked marker loci (Archibald 1991).

A few examples of successful genetic selection strategies already exist for disease resistance in most food-animal species. Broilers are mostly free of Marek's disease and avian leukosis as a result of genetic screening of breeding stock. The use of restriction fragment length polymorphisms to breed for desirable production characteristics and disease resistance is being tested in poultry (Marini 1995). A new DNA test for the porcine stress syndrome (a noninfectious congenital defect) is widely used in the pork industry to eliminate animals with that syndrome from the breeding herd. Dairy breeders can use a DNA-based test to detect and remove carriers of bovine leukocyte adhesion deficiency. The Ndama breed of cattle in West Africa is resistant to trypanosomiasis, and genetic research is under way to transfer this trait to other cattle. Research on the major histocompatibility complex in humans and laboratory animals has been fruitful. In the cow, that complex is known as the bovine lymphocyte antigen (BoLA) complex, and much progress has been made in understanding how it promotes disease resistance. Associations between specific BoLA alleles and mastitis, tick resistance, enzootic leukosis, milk fat, milk protein, and weight gain have been reported (Stear et al. 1985). A Canadian study reported a significant influence of specific BoLA class I alleles on traits with economic importance, such as disease-treatment costs (Batra et al. 1989).

Breeding programs for dairy cows have resulted in great genetic improvement for milk yield but have led to increased susceptibility to mastitis, because thus far, the correlation between milk yield and disease resistance is negative. Simulation studies showed that breeding programs based on milk and butterfat production increased the number of cases of clinical mastitis per cow per year by 0.02, resulting in a loss of 180 kg of milk per lactation and a cost of approximately $50.00 (Standberg and Shook 1989).

Genetic variation in resistance of cows to mastitis can be used in selection programs to improve disease resistance. However, it is long-term process that must be cost effective if it is to be a part of disease control programs. Shook (1989) organized the approaches to disease control according to priority and, within a category of preventive measures, listed genetic improvement last—after eradication, sanitation, and enhancement.

Biochemical markers can be used to predict susceptibility to mastitis. For example, the M-blood-group system might be closely linked to the BoLA system, and the presence of the M-blood-group system was found to be associated with increased incidence of mastitis (Larsen et al. 1985). Jensen et al. (1985) observed that cows carrying the M-factor (M/M and M/–) appeared to exhibit higher frequencies of mastitis than did cows that lack that factor. Likewise, Walawski et al. (1993) found higher SCCs in M-positive cows than in M-negative cows.

Enhancing immunity also could offer alternatives to the use of antibiotics in food animals. Animals vary in their ability to resist, control, or reject infections. The complex interactions between a pathogen, the environment, and the host are controlled by many genes. Only a small number of the genes that control the variations and the specificity or quality of immune responses have been identified and characterized. Strains selected for resistance to one pathogen or for a high immune response potential are not necessarily resistant to all pathogens. Genetics can control the response to infection in 3 ways: by controlling innate immunity, by determining the specificity of acquired responses, and by affecting the magnitude of the acquired immune response (Doenhoff and Davies 1991). Those mechanisms and the genetics controlling them can be exploited with the use of molecular biology approaches to develop more effective biological products and immune-enhancing strategies.

RECOMMENDATIONS

• *The committee recommends increased investment of research funds on the influence of nutrition and other management practices on immune function and disease resistance in all species of food animals.* Such investment, aimed particularly toward whole-animal studies, could significantly increase our understanding of this complex issue. Specifically, there is great need to define the effect of meeting requirements in states of deficiency, to refine the effect of supplementing beyond the state of adequate growth requirement, and to further refine the requirements for growth and productivity in contrast to those needed for optimal immune function.

Of particular importance is the identification of feeding strategies that decrease or prevent the development of stress-related disease opportunities by specific use of diets or diet ingredients in anticipation of stresses—such as shipping, weaning, and group penning—that animals might experience. In addition, increases in private and public funding and conduct of research in the identification of nutrient–gene interactions that modulate immune function will enhance our ability to determine how nutrient components can be helpful in mitigating challenges to animal health.

- *The committee recommends increased research funding for development of new vaccination techniques and a better understanding of the biochemical basis for antibody production and manipulation in vivo.*

New strategies for vaccination regimens offer promise to allow the host animal to develop its own biological response to control pathogens, and research funding should underwrite this approach. Likewise, research on integrating the immune and production responses, including genetic selection, will benefit the quest to reduce dependence on drug use to maintain production capabilities. Genetic selection, molecular genetic engineering of food animals for disease resistance, and immune enhancement could increase the efficiency of milk and meat production. However, use of such strategies will not reduce the reliance on drugs in livestock production in the immediate future. Research efforts also are needed in gene mapping, development of molecular techniques, and genetic evaluation of food-producing animals.

References

Aarestrup, F. M. 1995. Occurrence of glycopeptide resistance among *Enterococcus faecium* from conventional and ecological poultry farms. Microbial Drug Resistance 1: 255–257.

Aarestrup F. M., P. Ahrens, M. Madsen, L. V. Pallesen, R. L. Poulsen, and H. Westh. 1996. Glycopeptide susceptibility among Danish *Enterococcus faecium* and *Enterococcus faecalis* isolates of animal and human origin and PCR identification of genes within the vanA cluster. Antimicrobial Agents and Chemotherapy 40(8):1938–1940.

Abe, F., N. I. Ishibashi, and S. Shimamura. 1995. Effect of administration of bifidobacteria and lactic acid bacteria to newborn calves and piglets. J. Dairy Sci. 78: 2838–2846.

Agrimetrics Associates. 1994. Summary of data compiled for the National Academy of Science/National Research Council Joint Panel on Animal Health and Veterinary Medicine. Chester, Virginia: Agrimetrics Associates, Inc.

AHI (Animal Health Institute). 1982. Animal Drug Lag. Alexandria, Virginia: Animal Health Institute.

AHI (Animal Health Institute). 1992. Animal Drug Availability: Current Impediments and Recommendations. Alexandria, Virginia: Animal Health Institute.

AHI (Animal Health Institute). 1993. New Drug Availability: Policy Recommendations of the Animal Health Institute. Alexandria, Virginia: Animal Health Institute.

AHI (Animal Health Institute). 1994. Understanding The Animal Drug Availability Crisis—Facts to remember. Alexandria, Virginia: Animal Health Institute.

AHI (Animal Health Institute). 1997. General Information: Summary of the antibiotic resistance issue. [Online]. Available: http://www.ahi.org/.

AHI (Animal Health Institute). 1998. General Information: Antibiotics Info Kit. [Online]. Available: http://www.ahi.org/info/general/antibiotics.htm. [3 June].

Ahmed, A. K., S. Chasis, and B. McBarnette. 1984. Petition of the Natural Resources Defense Council, Inc. to the Secretary of Health and Human Services requesting immediate suspension of approval of the subtherapeutic use of penicillin and tetracyclines in animals feeds. New York: Natural Resources Defense Council.

Allen, G., and C. Burbee. 1972. Economic consequences of the restricted use of antibiotics at subtherapeutic levels in broiler and turkey production. Washington, D.C.: U.S. Department of Agriculture, Commodity Economics Division, Econ. Res. Serv., November.

Altekruse, S. F., M. L. Cohen, and D. L. Swerdlow. 1997. Emerging foodborne diseases. Emerg. Infect. Dis. 3(3):285–293.

Amabile-Cuevas, C. 1993. Origin, Evolution, and Spread of Antibiotic Resistance Genes: Molecular Biology Intelligence Unit. Austin: R. G. Landes Company; Boca Raton, Florida: Distributed worldwide by CRC Press.

Anderson, E. S. 1968. The ecology of transferable drug resistance in the enterobacteria. Ann. Rev. Microbiol. 22:131.

Anderson, E. S., G. O. Humphreys, and G. A. Willshaw. 1975. The molecular relatedness of R. factors in enterobacteria of human and animal origin. J. Gen. Microbiol. 91:376.

Andrew, S. M., R. A. Frobish, M. J. Paape, and L. J. Maturin. 1997. Evaluation of selected antibiotic residue screening tests for milk from individual cows and examination of factors that affect the probability of false-positive outcomes. J. Dairy Sci. 80:3050-3057.

Andrus, D. F., and L. D. McGilliard. 1975. Selection of dairy cattle for overall excellence. J. Dairy Sci. 58(12):1876–1879.

APHIS (Animal and Plant Health Inspection Service). 1993. Beef Cow/Calf Health and Productivity Audit, Part I: Beef Cow/Calf Herd Management Practices in the United States. U.S. Department of Agriculture, Washington, D.C.

Archibald, A. L. 1991. Molecular biological approaches and their possible applications. Pp. 100-122 in Breeding for Disease Resistance in Farm Animals, J. B. Owen, ed. United Kingdom: CAB International, Redwood Press.

Axford, R. F. E., and J. B. Owen. 1991. Strategies for disease control. Pp. 3-9 in Breeding for Disease Resistance in Farm Animals, J. B. Owen, ed. United Kingdom: CAB International, Redwood Press.

AVMA (American Veterinary Medical Association). 1998. Caring for Animals: 1998 AVMA Directory and Resource Manual. Schaumburg, Illinois: American Veterinary Medical Association.

Babiuk, L. A., L. M. Sordillo, M. Campos, H. P. Hughes, A. Rossi-Campos, and R. Harland. 1991. Application of interferons in the control of infectious diseases of cattle. J. Dairy Sci. 74(12):4385–4398.

Bailey, J. S. 1987. Factors affecting microbial competitive exclusion in poultry. Food Technology 41:88–92.

Bailey, J. S., D. L. Fletcher, and N. A. Cox. 1989. Recovery and serotype distribution of *Listeria monocytogenes* from broiler chickens in the southeastern United States. J. Food Prot. 52:148–150.

Baker, C. C., C. E. Coppock, J. K. Lanham, and D. H. Nave. 1988. Chilled drinking water effects on lactating Holstein cows in summer. J. Dairy Sci. 71(10):2699–2770.

Baquero, F., and M. C. Negri. 1997a. Strategies to minimize the development of antibiotic resistance. J. Chemother. 9(Suppl. 3):29–37.

Baquero, F., and M. C. Negri. 1997b. Selective compartments for resistant microorganisms in antibiotic gradients. Bioessays. 19(8):731–736.

Baquero, F., M. C. Negri, M. I. Morosini, and J. Blazquez. 1997. The antibiotic selective process: concentration-specific amplification of low-level resistant populations. Ciba. Found. Symp. 201:93–105; discus. 105–111.

Barkema, A., and M. L. Cook. 1993. The changing U.S. pork industry: A dilemma for public policy. Econ. Rev. Kansas City, Missouri 78(2):49–65.

Barnhart, H. M., O. C. Pancorbo, D. W. Dreesen, and E. B. Shotts, Jr. 1989. Recovery of *Aeromonas hydrophila* from carcasses and processing water in a broiler processing operation. J. Food Prot. 52:646–649.

Barnouin, J., and M. Chassagne. 1991. An aetiological hypothesis for the nutrition-induced association between retained placenta and milk fever in the dairy cow. Ann. Rech. Vet. 22:331–334.

Barrel, R. A. E. 1987. Isolations of *Salmonella* from humans and foods in the Manchester area: 1981–1985. Epidem. Infect. 98:277–284.

Bassi, L., and G. Bolzoni. 1982. Immunosuppression by Rifamycins. Pp. 12–20 in The Influence of Antibiotics on the Host-Parasite Relationship. H. U. Eickenberg, H. Hahn, and W. Opferkuch, eds. New York: Springer-Verlag.

Bates, J., J. Z. Jordens, and D. T. Griffiths. 1994. Farm animals as a putative reservoir for vancomycin-resistant enterococcal infection in man. J. Antimicrobial Chemotherapy 34: 507–516.

Batra, T. R., A. J. Lee, J. S. Gavora, and M. J. Stear. 1989. Class I alleles of the bovine major histocompatibility system and their association with economic traits. J. Dairy Sci. 72(8):2115–2124.

Bauer, F. T., J. A. Carpenter, and J. O. Reagan. 1981. Prevalence of *Clostridium perfringens* in pork during processing. J. Food Prot. 44:279–283.

Bauman, D. E., R. G. Vernon. 1993. Effects of exogenous bovine somatrotropin on lactation. Rev. Nutr. 13:437–461.

Bean, N. H., and P. M. Griffin. 1990. Food-borne disease outbreaks in the U.S., 1973–1987: Pathogens, vehicles, and trends. J. Food Prot. 53(9):804–817.

Beede, D., D. Bray, and R. Bucklin. 1987. Plan your strategies for beating summer heat. Hoard's Dairyman 132:495.

Beisel, W. 1988. The effects of infection on growth. Pp. 395-408 in Biomechanisms Regulating Growth and Development, Vol. 12. Boston, Massachusetts: Kluwer Publishing.

Bender, F. E., and E. T. Mallinson. 1991. Healthy birds are lower cost birds. Broiler Industry January: 62–64.

Beran, G. W. 1987. Use of drugs in animals: an epidemiologic perspective. Pp. 3–27 in Proceedings of the Symposium on Animal Drug Use—Dollars and Sense. Rockville, Maryland: Center for Veterinary Medicine.

Berghash, S. R., J. N. Davidson, J. C. Armstrong, and G. M. Dunny. 1983. Effects of antibiotic treatment of nonlactating dairy cows on antibiotic resistance patterns of bovine mastitis pathogens. Antimicrob. Agents Chemother. 24(5):771–776.

Berndtson, E., M. Tivemo, and A. Engvall. 1992. Distribution and numbers of *Campylobacter* in newly slaughter broiler chickens and hens. Int. J. Food Microbiol. 15:45–50.

Bingen, E. H., E. Denamur, N. Lambert-zechovsky and J. Elion. 1991. Evidence for the genetic unrelatedness of nosocomial vancomycin-resistant *Enterococcus faecium* strains in a paediatric hospital. J. Clin. Microbiol. 29: 1888–1892.

Bishop, J. R., A. B. Bodine, and J. J. Janzen. 1980. Sensitivities to antibiotics and seasonal occurrence of mastitis pathogens. J. Dairy Sci. 63(7):1134–1137.

Black, W. D. 1984. The use of antimicrobial drugs in agriculture. Can. J. Physioc. Pharmacol. 62:1044–1048.

Blackburn, B. O., L. K. Schlater, and M. R. Swanson. 1984. Antibiotic resistance of members of the genus *Salmonella* isolated from chickens, turkeys, cattle, and swine in the United States during October 1981 through September 1982. Am. J. Vet. Res. 45(6):1245–1249.

Boeckman, S., and K. R. Carlson. 1995. Milk and dairy beef residue prevention protocol: 1996 producer manual. Schaumburg, Illinois: Agri-Education, Inc.

Borrie, P., and J. Barrett. 1961. Dermatitis caused by penicillin in bulked milk supplies. Bri. Med. J. 2:1267. Page 3–25;

Boykin, C. C., H. C. Gilliam, and R. A. Gustafson. 1980. Structural characteristics of beef cattle raising in the United States. Ag. Econ. Rep. U.S. Dep. Agric. (450). 11 pp.

Bracewell, A. J., J. O. Reagan, J. A. Carpenter, and L. C. Blankenship. 1985. Incidence of *Campylobacter coli/jejuni* on pork carcasses in the northeast Georgia area. J. Food Prot. 48:808–810.

Braude, R., S. K. Kon, and J. W. G. Porter. 1953. Antibiotics in nutrition. Nutr. Abstr. Rev. 23:473–495.

Brumfitt, W., and J. M. T. Hamilton-Miller. 1988. The changing face of chemotherapy. Postgrad. Med. J. 64:552–558.

Bryan, F. L. 1980. Food-borne diseases in the United States associated with meat and poultry. J. Food Prot. 43:140–150.

Brynes, S. D., and M. S. Yong. 1993. Harmonization of Tolerances Under the Free Trade Agreement Between the United States and Canada, Proceedings of the EuroResidue II Conference on Residues of Veterinary Drugs in Food, The Netherlands, May 3–5.

Bugos, G. E. 1992. Intellectual property protection in the American chicken-breeding industry. Business History Review 66: 127–167.

Buntain, B., J. Day, S. Boeckman, D. Breiner, S. Harper, A. Hentschl, D. E. Johnson, C. Kuhlman, C. Langrehr, and D. Morse. 1993. A Subcommittee Review of the Quality Assurance Initiative: Implementation Issues From the Implementation and Communication Subcommittee of the Drug Residue Committee. Pp. 144–146 in Proceedings Annual Meeting of the National Mastitis Council, Inc. Arlington, Virginia: Natl. Mastitis Council.

Burke, J. P., and S. B. Levy. 1985. Summary report of worldwide antibiotic resistance: International task forces on antibiotic use. Rev. Infect. Dis. 7(4):560–564.

Burpee C. et al.. 1978. Economic Effects of a Prohibition on the use of Selected Animal Drugs. No. 414. Washington D.C.: U.S. Department of Agriculture.

Burton, G. W. 1994. Vitamin E: molecular and biological function. Proc. Nutr. Soc. 53(2):251–262.

Burton, G. W., and M. G. Traber. 1990. Vitamin E: antioxidant activity, biokinetics, and bioavailability. Ann. Rev. Nutr. 10:357–382.

Calnek, B., H. J. Barnes, C. W. Beard, W. M. Reid, and H. W. Yoder (Eds.). 1991. Diseases of Poultry. Ames, Iowa: Iowa State Univ. Press.

Cardenas, L., and J. D. Clements. 1993. Development of mucosal protection against the heat stable enterotoxin (ST) of *E. coli* by oral immunization with a genetic fusion delivery by a bacterial vector. Infect. Immun. 61:4629–4636.

Carlson, G. S. 1994. Milk testing for antibiotics overlooked in BST controversy. Feedstuffs 66(14):4.

Carlsson, A., L. Bjorck, and K. Persson. 1989. Lactoferrin and lysozyme in milk during acute mastitis and their inhibitory effect in Delvotest® P. J. Dairy Sci. 72:3166.

CAST (Council for Agricultural Science and Technology). 1981. Antibiotics in Animal Feeds. Report No. 88, Ames, Iowa: Council for Agricultural Science and Technology.

Castillo-Ayala, A. 1992. Comparison of selective enrichment broths for isolation of *Campylobacter jejuni/coli* from freshly deboned market chicken. J. Food Prot. 55:333–336.

CDC (Centers for Disease Control and Prevention). 1994. Addressing Emerging Infections Disease Threats: A Prevention Strategy for the United States. Atlanta, Georgia: U.S. Department of Health and Human Services, Public Health Service. 46 pp.

CDC (Centers for Disease Control and Prevention). 1996. Notice to readers: establishment of a national surveillance program for antimicrobial resistance in *Salmonella*. MMWR 45:110–111.

CDC (Centers for Disease Control and Prevention). 1997. Foodborne bacterial diseases—general information. [Online]. Available: http:www.cdc.gov/ncidod/diseases/bacter/foodborn.html. Dec. 1.

CDR (Communicable Disease Report). 1997. Investigating *Salmonella typhimurium* DT104 infections. CDR Weekly. 7(16):1.

CFSAN (Center for Food Safety and Applied Nutrition). 1997. Food safety from farm to table: national food safety initiative, Report to the President, May. Washington, D.C.: U.S. Food and Drug Administration, U.S. Department of Agriculture, U.S. Environmental Protection Agency, and Centers for Disease Control and Prevention.

Chalker, R. B., and M. J. Blaser. 1988. A review of human salmonellosis: III. Magnitude of *Salmonella* infection in the United States. Rev. Infect. Dis. 10(1):11–124.

Chandra, R. K., and D. H. Dayton. 1982. Trace element regulation of immunity and infection. 2(6):721–733.

Chandra, R. K. 1992. Nutrition and immunoregulation. Significance for host resistance to tumors and infectious diseases in humans and rodents. J. Nutr. 122(Suppl. 3):754–757.

Chaperon, E. A. 1982. Suppression of Lymphocytes by Cephalosporins. Pp. 22–30 in The Influence of Antibiotics on the Host-Parasite Relationship. H. U. Eickenberg, H. Hahn, and W. Opferkuch, eds. New York: Springer-Verlag.

Chen, K. H., J. T. Huber, C. B. Theurer, D. V. Armstrong, R. C. Wanderley, J. M. Simas, S. C. Chan, and J. L. Sullivan. 1993. Effect of protein quality and evaporative cooling on lactational performance of Holstein cows in hot weather. J. Dairy Sci. 76: 819–825.

Chew, B. P. 1987. Immune function: vitamin A and beta carotene on host defense. J. Dairy Sci. 70:2832–2843.

Chew, B. P., and L. A. Johnston. 1985. Effects of supplemental vitamin A and β-carotene on mastitis in dairy cows. J. Dairy Sci. 68(Suppl. 1):191.

Chew, B. P., L. L. Hollen, J. K. Hillers, and M. L. Herlugson. 1982. Relationship between vitamin A and beta-carotene on blood plasma and milk and mastitis in Holsteins. J. Dairy Sci. 65(11):2111–2118.

Christopher, F. M., G. C. Smith, and C. Vanderzant. 1982. Examination of poultry giblets, raw milk and meat for *Campylobacter fetus* subsp. *jejuni*. J. Food Prot. 45:260–262.

Clements, J. D. 1987. Use of attenuated mutants of *Salmonella* as carriers for delivery of heterologous antigens to the secretory immune system. Pathol. Immunopathol. Res. 6:137–146.

Clifton-Hadley, F. A. 1983. *Streptococcus suis* type 2 infections. Br. Vet. J. 139(1):1–5.

Coates, S. R., and K. H. Hoopes. 1980. Sensitivities of *Escherichia coli* isolated from bovine and porcine enteric infections to antimicrobial antibiotics. Am. J. Vet. Res. 41(11):1882–1883.

Cohen, M. L. 1993. Infectious disease: New and forgotten risks. Health and Environment Digest 7(7):1–4.

Cohen, M. L., and R. V. Tauxe. 1986. Drug-resistant *Salmonella* in the United States: An epidemiologic perspective. Science 234:964–969.

Cole, N. A., and F. S. Guillot. 1987. Influence of *Psorptes ovis* on the energy metabolism of heifer calves. Vet. Parasitol. 23:285–295.

Collins, C. I., I. V. Wesley, and E. A. Murano. 1993. Incidence of *Arcobacter* spp. in ground pork. Pp. 22–23 in Proceedings of the Food Safety Consortium Annual Meeting, Kansas City.

Colwell, M., and L. Brooks. 1994. Megatrends in *Salmonella* isolation over a 17 year period. In Proceedings of 131st Annual Meeting of the American Veterinary Medical Association, Annual meeting of the American Association of Avian Pathologists, July 9–13, San Francisco, California: Abstract published on p. 123.

Compendium of Veterinary Products. 1993. K. Bennett, ed. Port Huron, Michigan: North American Compendiums.

Cooper, G. L., L. M. Venables, M. J. Woodward, and C. E. Hormaeche. 1994. Vaccination of chickens with strain CVL30, a genetically defined *Salmonella enteriditis* aroA live oral vaccine candidate. Infect. Immunol. 62:4747–4754.

Cooper, S. 1991. Bacterial Growth and Division: Biochemistry and regulation of prokaryotic and eukaryotic division cycles. New York: Academic Press, Inc.

Corry, J. E. L., M. R. Sharma, and M. L. Bates. 1983. Detection of antibiotic residues in milk and animal tissues: Fermentation failure due to residues. Pp. 349–370 in Antibiotics: Assessment of Antimicrobial Activity and Resistance. A. D. Russell, ed. New York: Academic Press.

Cromwell, G. L. 1991. Antimicrobial agents. Pp. 297–314 in Swine Nutrition. E. R. Miller, D. E. Ullrey, and A. J. Lewis, eds. Stoneham, Massachusetts: Butterworth-Heinemann.

Cullor, J. S. 1992. Cowside testing for antibiotic residues: problems and solutions. P. 153 in Proceedings 31st Annual Meeting of the National Mastitis Council, Arlington, Virginia. Madison, Wisconsin: National Mastitis Council.

Cullor, J. S., A. van Eenennaam, I. Gardner, L. Perani, J. Dellinger, W. L. Smith, T. Thompson, M. A. Payne, L. Jensen, and W. M. Guterbock. 1994. Performance of various tests used to screen antibiotic residues in milk samples from individual animals. JAOAC Int. 77(4):862–870.

Culotta, E. 1994. Funding crunch hobbles antibiotic resistance research. Science 264:362–363.

Cummings, T. S., B. L. McMurray, and Y. M. Saif. 1995. Minimum inhibitory concentrations of Clostridium perfringens isolates from necrotic enteritis outbreaks to virginiamycin, penicillin, bacitracin, and lincomycin. Pp. 92–93 in Proceedings of the 44th Western Poultry Disease Conference, Mar. 5–7, Sacramento, California. Davis, California: University of California.

Cunha, T. J., G. B. Meadows, H. M. Edwards, R. F. Sewell, C. B. Sharvet, A. M. Pearson, and R. S. Glasscock. 1950. Effect of aureomycin and other antibiotics on the pig. J. Anim. Sci. 9:653.

Curtiss, R., and S. M. Kelly. 1987. Salmonella typhimurium deletion mutants lacking adenylate cyclase and cyclic AMP receptor are avirulent and immunogenic. Infect. Immunol. 55:3035–3043.

Curtiss, R., S. M. Kelly, and J. O. Hassan. 1993. Live oral avirulent Salmonella vaccines. Vet. Microbiol. 37(3–4):397–405.

CVM (Center for Veterinary Medicine). 1984. Extra-label Drug Use Guideline. Washington, D.C.: U.S. Food and Drug Administration.

CVM (Center for Veterinary Medicine). 1993a. National Drug Residue Milk Monitoring Program, Quarterly Reports. April 19. Washington, D.C.: Food and Drug Administration.

CVM (Center for Veterinary Medicine). 1993b. National Drug Residue Milk Monitoring Program, Quarterly Reports. July 20. Washington, D.C.: Food and Drug Administration.

CVM (Center for Veterinary Medicine). 1993c. National Drug Residue Milk Monitoring Program, Quarterly Reports. October 12. Washington, D.C.: Food and Drug Administration.

CVM (Center for Veterinary Medicine). 1994. National Drug Residue Milk Monitoring Program, Quarterly Reports. February 3. Washington, D.C.: Food and Drug Administration.

CVM (Center for Veterinary Medicine). 1997a. CVM policy on competitive exclusion products. [Online]. Available: http://www.cvm.fda.gov/fda/infores/updates/compexcl.html.

CVM (Center for Veterinary Medicine). 1997b. Food and Drug Administration Center For Veterinary Medicine Strategic Plan. [Online]. Available: http://www.cvm.fda.gov/fda/director/plannar.html#vision.

D'Aoust, J. Y., A. M. Sewell, and E. Daley. 1992. Inadequacy of small transfer volume and short (6 hr) selective enrichment for the detection of foodborne Salmonella. J. Food Prot. 55:326–328.

Dahlquist, S. P., and B. P. Chew. 1985. Effects of vitamin A and β-carotene on mastitis in dairy cows during early dry period. J. Dairy Sci. 68:(Suppl. 1):91.

Davies, J. 1994. Inactivation of antibiotics and the dissemination of resistance genes. Science 264:375–382.

Davies, J., and V. Webb. 1998. Antibiotic resistance in bacteria. Pp. 239 in Emerging Infections: Biomedical research reports. R. M. Krause, ed. New York: Academic Press.

Dayan, A. D. 1993. Allergy to antimicrobial residues in food: Assessment of the risk to man. Vet. Microbiol. 35: 213–226.

de Guzman, A. M. S., B. Micalizzi, C. E. Torres Pagano, and D. F. Giménez. 1990. Incidence of Clostridium perfringens in fresh sausages in Argentina. J. Food Prot. 53:173–175.

DeBoer, E., and M. Hahne. 1990. Cross contamination with *C. jejuni* and *Salmonella* spp. from raw chicken products during food preparation. J. Food Prot. 53:1067–1068.

Deen, J. 1992. An evaluation of depopulation and repopulation of swine herds using production driven cash-flows. Pp. 49–58 in Proceedings Special Preconvention Seminar of the American Association of Swine Practitioners: A treatise on depopulation/repopulation technologies. American Association of Swine Practitioners. Perry, Iowa.

DeGeeter, M. J., G. L. Stahl, and S. Geng. 1976. Effect of lincomycin on prevalence, duration, and quantity of *Salmonella typhimurium* excreted by swine. Am. J. Vet. Res. 37:525–529.

Delmas, C. L., and D. J. Vidon. 1985. Isolation of *Yersinia enterocolitica* and related species from foods in France. Appl. Environ. Microbiol. 50:767–771.

Dewdney, A. D., and R. G. Edwards. 1984. Penicillin hypersensitivity; is milk a significant hazard? J. R. Soc. Med. 77: 866–877.

Dewdney, J. M., L. R. Maes, F. Blane, F. P. Scheid, T. Jackson, S. Lens, and C. Verschueren. 1991. Risk assessment of antibiotic residues for beta-lactams and macrolides in food products with regard to their immunoallergic potential. Food Chem. Tox. 29: 477–483.

Dial, G. D., B. S. Wiseman, P. R. Davies, W. E. Marsh, T. W. Molitor, R. B. Morrison, and D. G. Thawley. 1992. Strategies employed in the U.S.A. for improving the health of swine. Pig News and Information 13(3):111–123.

Doenhoff, M. J., and A. J. S. Davies. 1991. Genetic improvement of the immune system: possibilities for animals. Pp. 24–53 in Breeding for Disease Resistance in Farm Animals, J. B. Owen, ed. United Kingdom: CAB International, Redwood Press.

Doyle, M. P., and J. L. Schoeni. 1987. Isolation of *Escherichia coli* O157:H7 from retail fresh meats and poultry. Appl. Environ. Microbiol. 53:2394–2396.

Drews, J. 1983. Experimental models relevant for therapy. Pp. 49-55 in Decision Making in Drug Research. F. Gross, ed. New York: Raven Press.

Duitschaever, C. L., and C. Buteau. 1979. Incidence of *Salmonella* in pork and poultry products. J. Food Prot. 42:662–663.

Dupont, H. L., and J. H. Steele. 1987. Use of antimicrobial agents in animal feeds: implications for human health. Rev. Infect. Dis. 9(3):447–460.

Durand, A. M., M. L. Barnard, M. L. Swanepoel, and M. M. Engelbrecht. 1987. Resistance to various antibiotics of *Salmonella* and *Escherichia coli* isolated from registrable farm feeds. The Onderstepoort J. Vet. Res. 54(1):21–26.

Durve, V. S., and R. T. Lovell. 1982. Vitamin C and disease resistance in channel catfish (Ictalurus punctatus) asorbic acid. C. J. Fish. Aquat. Sci. J. Can. Sci. Halieutiques. Aquat. 39(7)948–951.

Dworkin, F. H. 1976. Some Economic Consequences of Restricting the Subtherapeutic Use of Tetracyclines in Feedlot Cattle and Swine. OPE Study 33. Washington, D.C.: Food and Drug Administration.

Easmon, C. S. F., and A. M. Desmond. 1982. The effect of subinhibitory antibiotic concentrations on the opsonization, uptake, and killing of bacteria by human neutrophils. P. 202 in The Influence of Antibiotics on the Host-Parasite Relationship. H. U. Eickenberg, H. Hahn, and W. Opferkuch, eds. New York: Springer-Verlag.

Eicher-Pruiett, S. D., J. L. Morril, F. Blecha, H. H. Higgins, N. V. Anderson, P. G. Reddy. 1992. Neutrophil and lymphocyte response to supplementation with vitamins C and E in young calves. J. Dairy Sci: 75(6):1635–1642.

Ellis, R. P., and M. W. Vorhies. 1976. Effect of supplemental dietary vitamin E on the serologic response of swine to an *Escherichia coli* bacterin. J. Am. Vet. Med. Assoc. 168(3):231–232.

Elsasser, T. H., N. C. Steele, and R. Fayer. 1995. Cytokines, Stress, and Growth Modulation. Pp. 261–290 in Cytokines in Animal Health and Disease, M. J. Myers, and M. P. Murtaugh, eds. New York: Marcel Dekker, Inc.

Elsasser, T. H., S. Kahl, N. C. Steele, and T. S. Rumsey. 1997. Nutritional modulation of somatotropic axis-cytokine relationships in cattle: A brief review. Comp. Biochem. Physiol. A. Physiol. 116(3):209–221.

Endtz, H. P., G. J. Ruijs, B. van Klingeren, W. H. Jansen, T. van der Reyden, and R. P. Mouton. 1991. Quinolone resistance in *Campylobacter* isolated from man and poultry following the introduction of fluoroquinolones in veterinary medicine. J. Antimicrob. Chemother. 27:199–208.

Epling, L. K., J. A. Carpenter, and L. C. Blankenship. 1993. Prevalence of *Campylobacter* spp. and *Salmonella* spp. and the reduction effected by spraying with lactic acid. J. Food Prot. 56:536–537.

ERS (Economic Research Service). 1994. Using Historical Information to Identify Consumer Concerns about Food Safety. Technical Bulletin No. 1835. Washington, D.C.: U.S. Government Printing Office.

ERS (Economic Research Service). 1996a. Agricultural Outlook. June/AO-230. Washington D.C.: Economic Research Service Publications.

ERS (Economic Research Service). 1996b. Bacterial Foodborne Disease: Medical Costs and Productivity. Agricultural Economic Report No. 741. Washington, D.C.: U.S. Government Printing Office.

ERS (Economic Research Service). 1996c. Farm Business Economics Report. Washington D.C.: U.S. Department of Agriculture.

Erskine, R. J. 1993. Nutrition and mastitis. Vet. Clin. North Am. Food Anim. Pract. 9(3):551–560.

Erskine, R. J., R. J. Eberhart, L. G. Hutchinson, and R. W. Scholz. 1987. Blood selenium concentrations and glutathione peroxidase activities in dairy herds with high and low somatic cell counts. J. Am. Vet. Med. Assoc. 190(11):1417–1421.

Erskine, R. J., R. J. Eberhart, P. J. Grasso, and R. W. Scholz. 1989. Induction of *Escherichia coli* mastitis in cows fed selenium-deficient or selenium-supplemented diets. J. Am. Vet. Res. 50(12):2093–2100.

Espinasse, J. 1993. Responsible use of antimicrobials in veterinary medicine: perspectives in France. Vet. Microbiol. 35:289–301.

Fagerberg, D. J., and C. L. Quarles. 1979. Antibiotic feeding, antibiotic resistance and alternatives. Somerville, New Jersey: American Hoechst Corp. Animal Health Division. 91 pp.

Fahye, T., D. Morgan, C. Gunneburg, G. K. Adak, F. Majid, and E. Kaczmarski. 1996. An outbreak of *Camplyobacter jejuni* enteritis associated with failed milk pasteurisation. J. Infect. 31(2):137–143.

Fairbrother, J. M., P. L. McDonough, and S. J. Shin. 1978. A survey of drug resistance in *Escherichia coli* isolated from neonatal calves in New York State from 1976 to 1978. Pp. 515–524 in Proceedings of the Second International Symposium on Neonatal Diarrhea, Oct. 3–5. S. D. Acres, ed. Saskatoon, Canada: VIDO.

FAO/WHO (Food and Agriculture Organization/World Health Organization). 1961. Evaluation of the Carcinogenic Hazards of Food Additives: 5th report of the Joint FAO/WHO Expert Committee on Food Additives. Technical Report Series No. 220. Geneva, Switzerland: World Health Organization. 33 pp.

FAO/WHO (Food and Agriculture Organization/World Health Organization). 1988. Evaluation of Certain Veterinary Drug Residues in Food. Technical Report Series No. 763. Rome, Italy: Food and Agriculture Organization. 40 pp.

FAPRI (Food and Agricultural Policy Research Institute). 1994. FAPRI 1994 U.S. Agricultural Outlook, Staff Report #1-94. Ames, Iowa: Iowa State University.

FAPRI (Food and Agricultural Policy Research Institute). 1998. FAPRI 1998 U.S. Agricultural Outlook, Staff Report #1-98. Ames: Iowa State University.

Farber, J.M., and J.I. Speirs. 1987. Monoclonal antibodies directed against the flagellar antigens of *Listeria* species and their potential in EIA-based methods. J. Food Prot. 50(6):479–484.

Farber, J. M., S. A. Malcolm, K. F. Weiss, and M. A. Johnston. 1988. Microbiological quality of fresh and frozen breakfast-type sausages sold in Canada. J. Food Prot. 51:397–401.

Farber, J. M., G. W. Sanders, and M. A. Johnston. 1989. A survey of various foods for the presence of *Listeria* species. J. Food Prot. 52:456–458.

Farber, T. M. 1995. Current Testing Procedures for Residues and Contaminants, Drug Metabolism Rev. 27(4):543–548.

FDA (Food and Drug Administration). 1992. Approved Drugs for Food Fish Aquaculture. Food and Drug Administration, Center for Veterinary Medicine, Communications and Education Branch, HFV-12. Washington, D.C.: Government Printing Office.

FDA (Food and Drug Administration). 1995a. Drugs Approved for Use in Aquaculture, Center for Veterinary Medicine, U.S. Food and Drug Administration. Revised June, 1995 [Online]. Available: http://www.fda.gov:80/cvm/fda/infores/other/aqua/appendixa.html

FDA (Food and Drug Administration). 1995b. Grade A Pasteurized Milk Ordinance as modified by IMS–a–39. Washington, D.C.: Government Printing Office.

FDA (Food and Drug Administration). 1997. Interpretive memorandium M–a–85 Revision #6. [Online]. Available: http://vm.cfsan.fda.gov/~ear/m-a-85-6.html.

FDA (Food and Drug Administration). 1998a. Approved Animal Drug List (Green Book). Available: http//www.fda.gov/cvm/fda/greenbook/greenbook.html.

FDA (Food and Drug Administration). 1998b. Organizational Structure of CVM within DHHS. Available: http//www.fda.gov/dvm/fda/aboutcvm/dvmorg.html; May.

Federal Register. 1996. Extra-label Drug Use in Animals; Final Rule. 21 CFR Part 530. 61(217):57731–57746.

Feed Additive Compendium. 1995. Minneapolis: Miller Publishing Co.

Feed Additive Compendium. 1997. Minneapolis: Miller Publishing Co.

Feedstuffs. 1996. Passage of animal drug availability bill to be applauded. 68(41):10.

Filali, E., J. G. Bell, M. El Houadfi, M. B. Huggins, and J. K. A. Cook. 1988. Antibiotic resistance of *Escherichia coli* isolates from chickens with colisepticemia in Morocco. Comp. Immunol. Microbiol. Infect. Dis. 11:121–124.

Fitzpatrick, S. C., S. D. Brynes, and G. B. Guest. 1995. Dietary intake estimates as a means to harmonization of maximum residue levels for veterinary drugs. I. Concept. J. Vet. Pharmacol. Therap. 18:325–327.

Fleming, A., ed. 1950. Penicillin: Its practical application. Second ed. St. Louis, Mo.: The C. V. Mosby Company.

Florey, H. W. 1945. The use of microorganisms for therapeutic purposes. Bri. Med. J. Nov. 10:635-642.

Flynn, O. M. J., I. S. Blair, and D. A. McDowell. 1994. Prevalence of *Campylobacter* species on fresh retail chicken wings in Northern Ireland. J. Food Prot. 57:334–336.

Frappaolo, P. J. 1986. Risks to human health from the use of antibiotics in animal feeds. Pp. 100–113 in Agricultural Uses of Anitbiotics. W. A. Moats, ed. Washington, D.C.: American Chemical Society.

Fraunfelder, R. R., G. C. Bagby, Jr., and D. J. Kelly. 1982. Fatal aplastic anemia following topical administration of ophthalmic chloramphenicol. Am. J. Ophthalmol. 93(3):356–360.

Fredeen, H. T., and B. G. Harmon. 1983. The swine industry: changes and challenges. J. Anim. Sci. 57(suppl. 2):100–118.

Frieden T. R., S. S. Munsiff, D. E. Low, B. M. Willey, G. Williams, Y. Faur, W. Eisner, S. Warren, and B. Kreiswirth. 1993. Emergence of vancomycin-resisistant *Enterococci* in New York City. Lancet 342:76–79.

Friedman, M.A. 1997. Statement before Subcommittee on Agriculture, Rural Development, and Related Agencies; Committee on Appropriations, United States Senate. May 1, 1997, Washington, D.C.

FSIS (Food Safety and Inspection Service). 1992. Domestic Residue Databook: National Residue Program. Washington, D.C.: U.S. Department of Agriculture.

FSIS (Food Safety and Inspection Service). 1993a. Report of the Secretary of Agriculture to the U.S. Congress, 1992. U.S. Department of Agriculture, Washington, D.C. 62 pp.

FSIS (Food Safety and Inspection Service). 1993b. Proceedings of the World Congress on Meat and Poultry Inspection. Washington, D.C.: U.S. Department of Agriculture.

FSIS (Food Safety Inspection Service). 1993c. Domestic Residue Databook: National Residue Program. Washington, D.C.: U.S. Department of Agriculture.

FSIS (Food Safety Inspection Service). 1994a. Domestic Residue Databook: National Residue Program. Washington, D.C.: U.S. Department of Agriculture.

FSIS (Food Safety Inspection Service). 1994b. National Residue Program Plan. Washington, D.C.: U.S. Department of Agriculture.

FSIS (Food Safety Inspection Service). 1994c. Nationwide Beef Microbiological Baseline Data Collection Program: Steers and Heifers. Washington, D.C.: U.S. Department of Agriculture.

FSIS (Food Safety Inspection Service). 1995a. Domestic Residue Databook: National Residue Program. Washington, D.C.: U.S. Department of Agriculture.

FSIS (Food Safety Inspection Service). 1995b. FSIS, FDA, CDC, State Health Departments Collaborate on Foodborne Illness Project. [Online]. Available: http://www.usda.gov/agency/fsis/joint/html.

FSIS (Food Safety Inspection Service). 1997. The Establishment and Implementation of an Active Surveillance System for Bacterial Foodborne Diseases in the United States. Washington, D.C.: U.S. Department of Agriculture.

FSIS (Food Safety Inspection Service). 1998. Domestic Residue Databook: National Residue Datebook: National Residue Program. Washington, D.C.: U.S. Department of Agriculture.

Fukata, T., Y. Hadate, E. Baba, and A. Arakawa. 1991. Influence of bacteria on *Clostridium perfringens* infections in young chickens. Avian Dis. 35(1):224–227.

Fukushima, H. 1985. Direct isolation of *Yersinia enterocolitica* and *Yersinia pseudotuberculosis* from meat. Appl. Environ. Microbiol. 50:710-712.

FWS (Fish and Wildlife Service). 1994. Approved Fish and Wildlife Service INADs as of May 13. Washington, D.C: U.S. Department of the Interior.

Gabay, J. E. 1994. Ubiquitous natural antibiotics. Science 264(5157):373–374.

GAO (U.S. General Accounting Office). 1990. FDA surveys not adequate to demonstrate safety of milk supply. GAO/RCED–91–26:3.

GAO (U.S. General Accounting Office). 1992. FDA strategy needed to address animal drug residues in milk. U.S. General Accounting Office GAO/RCED–92–209:46.

Garcia, M. M., H. Lior, R. B. Stewar, G. M. Ruckerbauer, J. R. R. Trudel, and A. Skliarevski. 1985. Isolation, characterization and serotyping of *Campylobacter jejuni* and *Campylobacter coli* from slaughter cattle. Appl. Environ. Microbiol. 49:667–672.

Garrett, T. A., J. L. Kadrmas, and C. R. H. Raetz. 1997. Identification of the gene encoding the *Escherichia coli* lipid A 4'-kinase. Facile phosphorylation of endotoxin analogs with recombinant LpxK. J. Biol. Chem. 272(35):21855–21864.

Genigeorgis, C. A. 1989. Present state of knowledge on staphylococcal intoxication. Intl. J. Food Microbiol. 9:327–360.

Genigeorgis, C. A., P. Oanca, and D. Dutulescu. 1990. Prevalence of *Listeria* spp. in turkey meat at the supermarket and slaughterhouse level. J. Food Prot. 53:282–288.

Giese, J. 1992. Experimental process reduces *Salmonella* in poultry. Food Technol. 46:112.

Gill, C. O., and L. M. Harris. 1984. Hamburgers and broiler chickens as potential sources of human *Campylobacter* enteritis. J. Food Prot. 47:96–99.

Gilliam, H. C., J. R. Martin, W. C. Bursch, and R. B. Smith. 1993. Economic consequences of banning the use of antibiotics at subtherapeutic levels in livestock production. Departmental Technical Report No. 73–2. College Station: Texas A&M University.

Gillissen, G. J. 1982. Influence of Cephalosporins on humoral immune response. Pp. 5–10 in The Influence of Antibiotics on the Host-Parasite Relationship. H. U. Eickenberg, H. Hahn, and W. Opferkuch, eds. New York: Springer-Verlag.

Glynn, M. K., Bopp, C., Dewitt, W., Dabney, P., Mokhtar, and Angulo, F.J. 1998. Emergence of multidrug-resistant *Salmonella enterica* serotype *typhimurium* DT-104 infections in the United States. N. Engl. J. Med. 338:1333–1338.

Gordon, R. F., J. S. Garside, and J. F. Tucker. 1959. Emergence of resistant strains of bacteria following the continuous feeding of antibiotics to poultry. Pp. 347–349 in Proc. XVIth Intl. Vet. Cong.

Gottstein, B. 1992. Molecular and immunological diagnosis of echinococcosis. Clin. Microbiol. Rev. 5(3):248–261.

Grahame-Smith, D. G., and J. K Aronson. 1992. Clinical Pharmacology and Drug Therapy, 2nd ed. New York: Oxford University Press.

Grau, F. H., and P. B. Vanderlinde. 1992. Occurrence, numbers, and growth of *Listeria monocytogenes* on some vacuum-packaged processed meats. J. Food Prot. 55:4–7.

Graves, R. E. 1986. You can help cows keep working in the heat. Hoard's Dairyman 131:560.

Griffin, H. G., and P. A. Barrow. 1993. Construction of an aroA mutant of *Salmonella* serotype *galinarum*: Its effectiveness in immunization against experimental fowl typhoid. Vaccine 4:457–462.

Griffin, P. M., and R. V. Tauxe. 1991. The epidemiology of infectious *Escherichia coli* O157:H7, other enterhemorrhagic *E. coli*, and the associated hemolytic uremia syndrome. Epidemiol. Rev. 13:60–98.

Guinee, P. A. 1971. Prevalence of extrachromosomal drug resistance. Bacterial drug resistance in animals. Ann. N.Y. Acad. Sci. 182:40–51.

Gustafson, R. H. 1986. Antibiotics use in agriculture: An overview. Pp. 1–6 in Agricultural Uses of Antibiotics. W. A. Moats, ed. Washington, D.C.: American Chemical Society.

Gutzmann, F., H. Layton, K. Simkins, and H. Jarolmen. 1976. Influence of antibiotic-supplemented feed on the occurrence and persistence of *Salmonella typhimurium* in experimentally infected swine. Am. J. Vet. Res. 37:649–655.

Guzman, C. A., M. J. Walker, M. Rhode, K. N. Timmis. 1991. Direct expression of *Bordetella pertussis* filamentous hemagglutinin in *Escherichia coli* and *Salmonella typhimurium* aroA. Infect. Immunol. 59(10):3787–3795.

Haapapuro, E. R., N. D. Barnard, and M. Simon. 1997. Review—Animal waste used as livestock feed: Dangers to human health. Preventive Medicine 26:599–602.

Hancock, D. L., J. F. Wagner, and D. B. Anderson. 1991. Effects of estrogens and androgens on animal growth. Pp. 255–297 in Growth Regulation in Farm Animals: Advances in meat research, vol. 7. A. M. Person and T. R. Dutson, eds. Elsevier Applied Science.

Hand, W. L., N. L. King-Thompson, T. H. Steinberg, and D. L. Hand. 1989. Interactions between antibiotics, phagocytes, and bacteria. P. 4 in The Influence of Antibiotic on the Host-Parasite Relationship, Vol. 3. G. Gillissen, W. Opferkuch, G. Peters, and G. Pulverer, eds. Berlin, Germany: Springer-Verlag.

Hansen, L. B., R. W. Touchberry, C. W. Young, and K. P. Miller. 1979. Health care requirements of dairy cattle. II. Nongenetic effects. J. Dairy Sci. 62:1932–1940.

Hardman, J. G., L. E. Limbird, P. B. Molinoff, R. W. Ruddon, A. G. Gilman, eds. 1996. The Pharmacological Basis of Therapeutics, 9th ed. New York: McGraw-Hill.

Hariharan, H., J. W. Bryenton, J. St.Onge, J. R. Long, and M. O. Ojo. 1989. Resistance to trimethoprim-sulfamethoxazole of *Escherichia coli* isolated from pigs and calves with diarrhea. Can. Vet. J. 30(4):348–349.

Harmon, M. C., B. Swaminathan, and J. C. Forrest. 1984. Isolation of *Yersinia enterocolitica* and related species from porcine samples obtained from an abattoir. Appl. Bacteriol. 56:421–427.

Harris, N. V., D. Thompson, D. C. Martin, and C. M. Nolan. 1986. A survey of *Campylobacter* and other bacterial contaminants of pre-market chicken and retail poultry and meats, King County, Washington. Am. J. Public Health 76: 401–406.

Harry, E. G. 1962. The ability of low concentrations of chemotherapeutic substances to induce resistance in *E. coli*. Res. Vet. Sci. 3:85–93.

Hassan, J. O., and R. Curtiss. 1994. Development and evaluation of an experimental vaccination program using a live avirulent *Salmonella typhimurium* strain to protect chickens against challenge with homologous and heterologous *Salmonella* serotypes. Infect. Immunol. 62:5519–5527.

Hassan, J. O., and R. Curtiss. 1996. Effect of vaccination of hens with an avirulent strain of *Salmonella typhimurium* on immunity of progeny challenged with wild-type *Salmonella* strains. Infect. Immunol. 64:938–944.

Hauschild, A. H. W., and R. Hilsheimer. 1980. Incidence of *Clostidium botulinum* in commercial bacon. J. Food Prot. 43:564–565.

Hauschild, A. H. W., and R. Hilsheimer. 1983. Prevalence of *Clostidium botulinum* in commercial liver sausage. J. Food Prot. 46:242–244.

Hayenga, M., V. J. Rhodes, J.A. Brandt, and R. E. Deiter. 1985. The U.S. Pork Sector: Changing Structure and Organization. Ames: Iowa State University Press.

Hayes, J. D., and C. R. Wolf. 1990. Molecular mechanisms of drug resistance. Biochem. J. 272(2):281–295.

Hays, V. W. 1986. Benefits and risks of antibiotics use in agriculture. Pp. 74–87 in Agricultural Uses of Antibiotics. W. A. Moats, ed. Washington, D.C.: American Chemical Society.

Hays, V. W., and C. A. Black. 1989. Pp. 1–10 in Antibiotics for Animals: the Antibiotic-resistance Issue. Council for Agricultural Science and Technology. Ames, Iowa.

Hedberg, C. W., J. A. Korlath, J. Y. D'Aoust, K. E. White, W. L. Schell, M. R. Miller, D. N. Cameron, K. L. MacDonald, and M. T. Osterholm. 1992. A multistate outbreak of *Salmonella javiana* and *Salmonella oranienburg* infections due to consumption of contaminated cheese. J. Am. Med. Assoc. 268(22):3203–3207.

Heisig, P., B. Kratz, E. Halle, Y. Gräser, M. Altwegg, W. Rabsch, and J. P. Faber. 1995. Identification of DNA gyrase A mutations in ciprofloxacin-resistant isolates of *Salmonella typhimurium* from men and cattle in Germany. Microb. Drug Res. 1:211–218.

Henricks, D. M., S. L. Gray, and J. L. B. Hoover. 1983. Residue levels of endogenous estrogens in beef tissues. Pp. 233–248 in Anabolics in Animal Production: Public health aspects, analytical methods and regulation. E. Meissonnier, ed. Paris: Office International des Epizooties.

Hickey, S. M., and J. D. Nelson. Mechanisms of antibacterial resistance. 1997. Chap. 1 in Advances in Pediatrics®, Vol. 44. Barness, L. A., D. C. DeVivo, M. M. Kaback, G. Morrow III, F. A. Oski, and A. M. Rudolph, eds. Chicago, Ill.: Mosby-Year Book, Inc.

Hill, J. R., and J. E. T. Jones. 1984a. An investigation of the causes and of the financial loss of rejection of pig carcasses and viscera unfit for human consumption. I: Studies at one abattoir. Br. Vet. J. 140(6):450–457.

Hill, J. R., and J. E. T. Jones. 1984b. An investigation of the causes and of the financial loss of rejection of pig carcasses and viscera unfit for human consumption. II: Studies at seven abattoirs. Br. Vet. J. 140(6):558–569.

Hird, D. W., M. Pappaioanou, and B. P. Smith. 1984. Case-control study of risk factors associated with isolation of *Salmonella saintpaul* in hospitalized horses. Am. J. Epidemiol. 120:852.

Hogan, J. S., W. P. Weiss, and K. L. Smith. 1993. Role of vitamin E and selenium in host defense against mastitis. J. Dairy Sci. 76(9):2795–2803.

Hogan, J. S., W. P. Weiss, and K. L. Smith. 1997. Bacteria counts in sawdust bedding. J. Dairy Sci. 80 (8):1600–1605.

Hogan, J.S., K. L Smith, W.P. Weiss, D. A. Todhunter, and W. L. Schockey. 1990. Relationships among vitamin E, selenium, and bovine blood neutrophils. J. Dairy Sci. 73;2372–2378.

Holmberg, S. D., M. T. Osterholm, K. A. Senger, and M. L. Cohen. 1984a. Drug-resistant *Salmonella* from animals fed antimicrobials. N. Engl. J. Med. 311:617.

Holmberg, S. D., J. G. Wells, and M. L. Cohen. 1984b. Animal-to-man transmissions of antimicrobial-resistant *Salmonella*: Investigations of U.S. outbreaks, 1971–1983. Science 225:833–835.

Hood, A. M., A. D. Pearson, and M. Shahmat. 1988. The extent of surface contamination of retail chickens with *C. jejuni* serogroups. Epidem. Invest. 100:17–25.

Hooper, D. C., and J. S. Wolfson. 1993. Mechanisms of bacterial resistance to quinolones. Pp. 97–103 in Quinonlone Antimicrobial Agents, 2nd ed. Hopper, D. C., and J. S. Wolfson, eds. Washington, D.C.: American Society for Microbiology.

Houston, D. L. 1985. Science and the necessity of *Salmonella* control. Pp. 1–6 in Proceedings of the International Symposium on *Salmonella*, July 19–20, 1984, New Orleans, La., G. H. Snoeyenbos, ed. Kennett Square, Pa.: American Association of Avian Pathologists.

Hudson, J. A., and K. M. DeLacy. 1991. Incidence of motile *Aeromonas* in New Zealand retail foods. J. Food Prot. 54:696–699.

Hummel, R., H. Tschape, and W. Witte. 1986. Spread of plasmid-mediated nourseothricin resistance due to antibiotic use in animal husbandry. J. Basic Microbiol. 26:461–466.

Hurt, C., K. A. Foster, J. E. Kadlec, and G. F. Patrick. 1992. Hog industry evolution. Feedstuffs 64:18 (August 24).

Hyun, Y., M. Ellis, G. Riskowski, R.W. Johnson. 1998. Growth performance of pigs subjected to multiple concurrent environmental stressors. J. Anim. Sci. 76(3):721–727.

IMNAVPID (International Meeting Nucleic Acid Vaccines For the Prevention of Infectious Diseases). 1996. Abstracts from meeting, February 5–7, Bethesda, Maryland: National Institutes of Health.

IOM (Institute of Medicine). 1980. The Effects on Human Health of Subtherapeutic Use of Antimicrobials in Animal Feeds. Washington, D.C.: National Academy Press.

IOM (Institute of Medicine). 1989. Human Health Risks with the Subtherapeutic Use of Penicillin or Tetracyclines in Animal Feed. Washington, D.C.: National Academy Press.

IOM (Institute of Medicine). 1992. Emerging Infections: Microbial Threats to Health in the United States. Washington, D.C.: National Academy Press. 312 pp.

IOM (Institute of Medicine). 1998. Antimicrobial Resistance: Issues and Options. Washington, D.C.: National Academy Press.

Izat, A. L., C. D. Druggers, M. Colberg, M. A. Reiber, and M. H. Adams. 1989. Comparison of the DNA probe to culture methods for the detection of *Salmonella* on poultry carcasses and processing waters. J. Food Prot. 52:564–570.

Jacks, T. M., C. J. Welter, G. R. Fitzgerald, and B. M. Miller. 1981. Cephamycin C treatment of induced swine *Salmonellosis*. Antimicrob. Agents Chemother. 19:562–566.

Jackson, E. R. 1993. The proper use and benefits of veterinary antimicrobial agents in practice in cattle. Vet. Microbiol. 35:349–356.

James, W. O., R. L. Brewer, J. C. Prucha, W. O. Williams, and D. R. Parham. 1992. Effects of chlorination of chill water on the bacteriologic profile of raw chicken carcasses and giblets. J. Am. Vet. Med. Assoc. 200:60–63.

Jankowski, J. M. 1993. The effect of antepartum doses of selenium-vitamin E combinations on the incidence of puerperal disorders in cattle. Tier. Prax. 21:111–116.

Jensen, N. E., P. Madsen, B. Larsen, O. Klastrup, S. M. Nielsen, and P. S. Madsen. 1985. Heritability of and markers of resistance against mastitis in the Danish RDM breed. Kieler Milchwirtschaftliche Forschungsberichte 37:506–509.

Jergklinchan, J., C. Koowatananukul, K. Daengprom, and K. Saitanu. 1994. Occurrence of *Salmonellae* in raw broilers and their products in Thailand. J. Food Prot. 57:808–810.

Johnson, J. L., M. P. Doyle, and R. G. Cassens. 1990. *Listeria monocytogenes* and other *Listeria* spp. in meat and meat products: a review. J. Food Prot. 53:81–91.

Jones, F. T., R. C. Axtell, D. V. Rives, S.E. Scheidler, J. R. Taver, R. L. Walker, and M. J. Wineland. 1991. A survey of *Campylobacter jejuni* in modern broiler production and processing systems. J. Food Prot. 54:259–262.

Jukes, T. H. 1986. Effects of low levels of antibiotics in livestock feeds. Pp. 110–126 in Agricultural Uses of Anitbiotics. W. A. Moats, ed. Washington, D.C.: American Chemical Society.

Jungkind, D. L., J. E. Mortensen, H. S. Fraimow, and G. B. Calandra, eds. 1997. Antimicrobial Resistance: A crisis in health care. New York: Plenum Press.

Kampelmacher, E. H., P. A. M. Guinee, K. Hofstra, and H. Van Keulen. 1963. Further studies on *Salmonella* in slaughterhouses and in normal slaughter pigs. Zentrabl. Veterinaermed. Reihe B. 10:1–9.

Kanarat, S., P. Harupathanapanich, P. Tongra-Are, and W. Chaisrisongkram. 1991. *Salmonella* serotypes in frozen chicken meat. 29th Kasetsart. Univ. Annual Conference, Feb. 4–9.

Kavanaugh, N. T. 1989. Improving herd health by depopulating and restocking M.D. stock: Planning the programme. Pp. 19–39 in Proceedings Minnesota Swine Herd Health Programming Conference. College of Veterinary Medicine, University of Minnesota, St. Paul, Minnesota. Perry, Iowa: American Association of Swine Practitioners.

Kellogg, D. W. 1990. Zinc methionine affects performance of lactating cows. Feedstuffs 62:1–3.

Kerr, K. G., N. A. Rotowa, P. M. Hawkey, and R. W. Lacey. 1990. Incidence of *Listeria* spp. in precooked, chilled chicken products as determined by culture and enzyme-linked immunoassay (ELISA). J. Food Prot. 53:606–607.

Kidd, A. R. 1994. The potential risk of effects of antimicrobial residues on human gastrointestinal microflora. Vet. Rec. 137(19):496.

Kimberling, C., ed. 1988. Jensen and Swift Diseases of Sheep. 3rd edition, Malvern, Pennsylvania: Lea and Febiger.

Kinde, H., C. A. Genigeorgis, and M. Pappaioanou. 1983. Prevalence of *Campylobacter jejuni* in chicken wings. Appl. Environ. Microbiol. 45:1116–1118.

Kingman, S. 1994. Resistance a European problem, too. Science 264:363–365.

Klasing, K. C., D. E. Laurin, R. C. Peng, and D. M. Fry. 1987. Immunologically mediated growth depression in chicks: Influence of feed intake, corticosterone and interleukin-I. J. Nutr. 117:1629–1637.

Knutson, J. 1993. Meat and Poultry Facts. Washington, D.C.: American Meat Institute.

Kobland, J. D., G. O. Gale, R. H. Gustafson, and K. L. Simkins. 1987. Comparison of therapeutic versus subtherapeutic levels of chlortetracycline in the diet for selection of resistant *Salmonella* in experimentally challenged chickens. Poult. Sci. 66:1129–1137.

Koch, R. M., and J. W. Algeo. 1983. The beef cattle industry: changes and challenges. J. Anim. Sci. 57(suppl. 2):28–43.

Konuma, H., K. Shinagawa, M. Tokumara, Y. Onoue, J. S. Konno, N. Fujino, T. Shigehisa, H. Kurata, Y. Kuwabara, and C.A.M. Lopes. 1988. Occurrence of *Bacillus cereus* in meat products, raw meat and meat product additives. J. Food Prot. 51:324–326.

Koshland, D. E., Jr. 1994. The biological warfare of the future. Science 264:327.

Kotula, A. W., and A. K. Sharar. 1993. Presence of *Yersinia enterocolitica* serotype 0:5,27 in slaughter pigs. J. Food Prot. 56:215–218.

Kotula, A. W., and N. J. Stern. 1984. The importance of *Campylobacter jejuni* to the meat industry: A review. J. Anim. Sci. 58:1561–1566.

Kristinsson, K. G., M. A. Hjalmarsdottir, and O. Steingrimsson. 1992. Increasing penicillin resistance in *Pneumococci* in Iceland. Lancet 339:1606–1607.

Kucers, A, S. M. Crowe, M. L. Grayson, and J. F. Hoy. 1997. The Use of Antibiotics: A clinical review of antibacterial, antifungal, and antiviral drugs, 5th edition. Victoria, Australia: Butterworth Heinemann.

Kunin, C. M. 1983. Antibiotic resistance—a world health problem we cannot ignore. Ann. Intern. Med. 99:859–860.

Kunin, C. M. 1993. Resistance to antimicrobial drugs—A worldwide calamity. Ann. Intern. Med. 118:557–561.

Kuschner, R.A., A. F. Trofa, R. J. Thomas, C. W. Hoge, C. Pitarangsi, S. Amato, R. P. Olafson, P. Echeverria, J. C. Sadoff, and D. N. Taylor. 1995. Use of azithromycin for the treatment of *Campylobacter enteritis* in travelers to Thailand, an area where ciprofloxacin resistance is prevalent. Clin. Infect. Dis. 21(3):536–541.

Kwaga, J., J. O. Iversen, and J. R. Saunders. 1990. Comparison of two enrichment protocols for the detection of *Yersinia* in slaughtered hogs and pork products. J. Food Prot. 53:1047–1049.

Lagunas-Solar, M. C. 1995. Radiation processing of foods: an overview of scientific principles and current status. J. Food. Prot. 58:186–192.

Lammerding, A. M., M. M. Garcia, E. D. Mann, Y. Robinson, W. J. Dorward, R. B. Truscott, and F. Tihiger. 1988. Prevalence of *Salmonella* and thermophilic *Campylobacteria* in fresh pork, beef, veal, and poultry in Canada. J. Food Prot. 51:47–52.

Langlois, B. E., K. A. Dawson, G. L. Cromwell, and T. S. Stahly. 1986. Antibiotic resistance in pigs following a 13-year ban. J. Anim. Sci. 62(Suppl. 3):18–32.

Lanham, J. K., K. Z. Milam, and C. E. Coppock. 1986. Cool water may help solve hot-weather problems. Hoard's Dairyman 131:546.

Larsen, B., N. E. Jensen, P. Madsen, S. M. Nielsen, O. Klastrup, and P. S. Madsen. 1985. Association of the M blood group system with bovine mastitis. An. Blood Groups Biochem. Gene. 16(3):165–173.

Lasley, F. A. 1983. The U.S. Poultry Industry. Agric. Economics Report No. 502. Washington, D.C.: U.S. Department of Agriculture.

Lasley, F. A., W. L. Henson, and H. B. Jones. 1983. The U.S. Turkey Industry. Agric. Economics Report No. 525. Washington, D.C.: U.S. Department of Agriculture.

Layard, P. R. G., and A. A. Walters. 1978. Microeconomic Theory. New York: McGraw-Hill Book Company. 498 pp.

Leclercq, R., E. Derlot, M. Weber, J. Duval, and P. Courvalin. 1989. Transferable vancomycin and teicoplanin resistance in *Enterococcus fascicium*. Antimicrob. Agents Chemother. 33:10–15.

Leman, A. 1988. Repopulation strategies and costs. Pp. 251–254 in Proceedings Minnesota Swine Herd Health Programming Conference. College of Veterinary Medicine, University of Minnesota, St. Paul, Minnesota. Perry, Iowa: American Association of Swine Practitioners.

Leman, A. 1992. The decision to repopulate. Pp. 9–12 in Proceedings Special Preconvention Seminar of the American Association of Swine Practitioners: A treatise on depopulation/ repopulation technologies. Perry, Iowa: American Association of Swine Practitioners.

Levy, S. B. 1984. Playing antibiotic pool: time to tally the score. N. Engl. J. Med. 311:663–665.

Levy, S. B. 1992. Antibiotics, animals, and the resistance gene pool. Pp. 137–156 in The Antibiotic Paradox. New York: Plenum Press.

Levy, S. B. 1998. Multidrug resistance – A sign of the times. N. Engl. J. Med. 338:1376–1378.

Levy, S. B., G. B. Fitzgerald, and A. B. Macone. 1986. Changes in intestinal flora of farm personnel after introduction of a tetracycline-supplemented feed on a farm. N. Engl. J. Med. 295:583–588.

Lillard, H. S. 1990. The impact of commercial processing procedures on the bacterial contamination and cross contamination of broiler carcasses. J. Food Prot. 53:202–204.

Lillard, H. S., D. Hamm, and J. E. Thomson. 1984. Effect of reduced processing on recovery of foodborne pathogens from hot-boned broiler meat and skin. J. Food Prot. 47:209–212.

Linton, A. H. 1977. Antibiotics—animal and man—An appraisal of a contentious subject. In: Antibiotics and Antibiosis in Nature. Woodbine, ed. Pp. 315–343. Butterworth, Inc., Woburn, Massachusetts.

Linton, A. H., K. Howe, and A. D. Osborne. 1975. The effects of feeding tetracycline, nitrovin, and quindoxin on the drug resistance of *E. coli-aerogenes* bacteria from calves and pigs. J. Applied Bacteriol. 38: 255–261.

Loosli, J. K., and H. D. Wallace. 1950. Influence of APF and aureomycin on the growth of dairy calves. Proc. Soc. Exp. Biol. Med. 75:531–533.

Lyons, R. W., C. L. Samples, H. N. DeSilva, K. A. Ross, E. M. Julian, and P. J. Checko. 1980. An epidemic of resistant *Salmonella* in a nursery: Animal-to-human spread. J. Am. Med. Assoc. 243:546–547.

Mackinnon, J. D. 1993. The proper use and benefits of veterinary antimicrobial agents in swine practice. Vet. Microbiol. 35: 357–367.

Madden, R. H., B. Hough, and C. W. Gillespie. 1986. Occurrence of *Salmonella* in porcine liver in Northern Ireland. J. Food Prot. 49:893–894.

Mafu, A. A., R. Higgins, M. Nadeau, and G. Cousineau. 1989. The incidence of *Salmonella, Campylobacter* and *Yersinia enterocolitica* in swine carcasses and the slaughterhouse environment. J. Food Prot. 52:642–645.

Mallard, B. A., D. N. Mowat, K. Leslie, X. Chang, and A. Wright. 1994. Immunomodulatory effects of chelated chromium on dairy health and production. Pp. 69–76 in Proceedings Annual Meeting of the National Mastitis Council, Inc., Arlington, Virginia. Perry, Iowa: American Association of Swine Practitioners.

Manchanda, S. 1994. Economic Comparison of Alternatives to Sulfamethazine Drug Use in Pork Production. M. A. thesis. Iowa State University.

Mann, T., and A. Paulsen. 1976. Economic Impact of restricting feed additives in livestock and poultry production. Am. J. Agric. Econ. 58:47–53.

Marinesca, M., R. Festy Derimay, and F. Megraud. 1987. High frequency of *Campylobacter coli* from poultry meat in France. Eur. J. Food Microbiol. 6:693–695.

Marini, P. J. 1995. Nicholas turkey breeder to use molecular techniques. Feedstuffs March 7, 1995.

Marjeed, K., A. E. Egan, and I. C. MacRae. 1989. Enterotoxigenic aeromonads on retail lamb meat and offal. J. Appl. Bacteriol. 67:165–170.

Martel, J. L. and M. Coudert. 1993. Bacterial resistance monitoring in animals: The French national experiences of surveillance schemes. Vet. Microbiol. 35: 321–338.

Martel, J. L., M. Contrepois, H. C. Dubourguier, J. P. Girardeau, Ph. Gouet, C. Bordas, F. Hayers, A. Quilleriet-Eliez, J. Ramisse, and R. Sendral. 1981. Fréquence de l'antigène K99 et antibiorésistance chez *Escherichia coli* d'origine bovine en France. Ann. Rech. Vet. 12(3):253–257.

May, J. D., and B. D. Lott. 1996. Water management for best performance with broilers. Poultry Digest 8:12–14.

May, J. D., B. D. Lott, and J. D. Simmons. 1997. Water consumption by broilers in high cyclic temperatures: Bell versus nipple waterers. Poultry Sci. 76:944–947.

McGinnis, J., L. R. Berg, J. R. Stern, R. A. Wilcox, and G. E. Bearse. 1950. The effect of aureomycin and streptomycin on growth of chicks and turkey poults. Poult. Sci. 29:771(Abstr.).

McNaughton, C. L. 1988. Guidelines for depopulation and repopulation of swine herds. *Compendium for the Continuing Education of the Practicing Veterinarian* 10(10):1233–1239.

Merck Veterinary Manual. 1986. A Handbook of Diagnosis, Therapy, and Disease Prevention and Control for the Veterinarian. Rahway, N.J.: Merck Publishing Group.

Miles, A. M., and H. J. Barnes. 1995. Use of *Escherichia coli* model to compare immune function in turkeys. Pp. 89–90 in Proceedings of the 44th Western Poultry Disease Conference, Mar. 5–7, Sacramento, California. Davis, California: University of California.

Miller, W. J. 1978. Dairy Cattle Feeding and Nutrition. New York: Academic Press.

Minton, J.E., J.K. Apple, K.M. Parsons, F. Blecha. 1995. Stress-associated concentrations of plasma cortisol cannot account for reduced lymphocyte function and changes in serum enzymes in lambs exposed to restraint and isolation stress. J. Anim. Sci. 73(3):812–817.

Molin, G., O. Soderlind, J. Ursing, A. Norrung, A. Ternstrom, and C. Lowenhielm. 1989. Occurrence of *Erysipelothrix rhusiopathiae* on pork and in pig slurry, and the distribution of specific antibodies in abattoir workers. J. Appl. Bacteriol. 67:347–352.

Moore, P. R., A. Evenson, T. D. Luckey, E. McCoy, C. A. Elvehjem, and E. B. Hart. 1946. Use of sulfasuxidine, streptothricin, and streptomycin in nutritional studies with the chick. J. Biol. Chem. 165:437–441.

Morgan, D., C. Gunneberg, D. Gunnell, T. D. Healing, S. Lamerton, N. Soltanpoor, D. A Lewis, and D. G. White. 1994. An outbreak of *Campylobacter* infection associated with the consumption of unpasteurized milk at a large festival in England. Eur. J. Epidemiol. 10(5): 581–585.

Moro, M. H., and G. W. Beran. 1993. Effects of environmental stress on the antimicrobial drug resistance of *Escherichia coli* of the intestinal flora of swine. Pp. 26–27 in Proceedings of the Annual Symposium of the Food Safety Consortium, Oct. 20–21, Kansas City, Missouri.

Morona, R., J. Yeadon, A. Considine, J. K. Morona, and P. A. Manning. 1991. Construction of plasmid vectors with a non-antibiotic selection system based on *Escherichia coli* thyA+ gene: Application to cholera vaccine development. Gene 107:139–144.

Morona, R., J. K. Morona, A. Considine, J. A. Hackett, L. Van Den Bosch, L. Beyer, and S. R. Attridge. 1994. Construction of K88- and K99-expressing clones of *Salmonella typhimurium* G30: immunogenicity following oral administration to pigs. Vaccine 12(6):513–517.

Muirhead, S. 1998. Future goal is definition of 'prudent use' for antimicrobials. Feedstuffs 70(17):1–5.

Mulligan, L. T. 1995. New toxicological testing approaches based upon exposure/activity/availability assessments. Drug Metabol. Rev. 27(4):573–579.

Munoz, R., J. M. Musser, M. Crain, D. E. Briles, A. Marton, A. J. Parkinson, U. Sorensen, A. Tomasz. 1992. Geographic distribution of penicillin-resistant clones of *Streptococcus pneumoniae*: Characterization by penicillin-binding protein profile, surface protein A typing, and multilocus enzyme analysis. Clin. Infect. Dis. 15:112–118.

Murray, B. 1991. New aspects of antimicrobial resistance and the resulting therapeutic dilemmas. J. Infect. Dis. 163:1185–1194.

Murray, P. R. 1994. Antimicrobial susceptibility in tests: testing methods and interpretive problems. Pp. 15–24 in Antimicrobial Susceptibility Testing: Critical issues for the 90s. J. A. Poupard, L. R. Walsh, and B. Kleger, eds. New York: Plenum Press.

NAS (National Academy of Sciences). 1969. The use of drugs in animal feeds. Proceedings of a symposium. Washington, D.C.: National Academy of Sciences.

National Library of Medicine. 1994. Medline Express 1966–July 1994. Washington, D.C.: National Library of Medicine.

National Milk Residue Data Base Fiscal Year 1996 Annual Report. Available: http://vm.cfsan.fda.gov/~ear/milkrp96.html.

National Performance Review. 1995. President Clinton.

NCBA (National Cattlemen's Beef Association). 1995. Cattle and Beef Handbook—Facts, Figures, and Information.

NCBA (National Cattlemen's Beef Association). 1997. The Beef Handbook—NCBA (National Cattlemen's Beef Association). 1997. The Beef Handbook—Food Safety. [Online]. Available: http://www.beef.org./beef_handbook/nca47410.html.

Nelson, F. E., J. D. Schuh, and G. H. Stott. 1967. Influence of season on leukocytes in milk. J. Dairy Sci. 50:978.

Neu, H. C. 1992. The crisis in antibiotic resistance. Science 257:1064–1073.

Newton, J. E. 1982. Intensive Arable Systems. Pp. 377–399 In: Sheep and Goat Production. I. E. Coop, ed., Amsterdam: Elsevier.

Nickerson, S. C., W. E. Owens, and J. L. Watts. 1989. Effects of recombinant granulocyte colony-stimulating factor on *Staphylococcus aureus* mastitis in lactating dairy cows. J. Dairy Sci. 72:3286–3294.

Nickerson, S. C., W. E. Owens, and R. L. Boddie. 1993. Effect of a *Staphylococcus aureus* bacterin on serum antibody, new infection, and mammary histology in nonlactating dairy cows. J. Dairy Sci. 76:1290–1297.

Noble, W. C., Z. Vitani, and R. G. Cree. 1992. Co-transfer of vancomycin and other resistance genes from *Enterococcus faecalis* NCTC 12201 to *Staphylococcus aureus*. FEMS Microb. Lett. 72:195–198.

Norberg, P. 1981. Enteropathogenic bacteria in frozen chicken. Appl. Environ. Microbiol. 42:32–34.

North, M. O. 1984. Commercial Chicken Production Manual. 3rd edition. Westport, Conn.: AVI Publishing.

NPPC (National Pork Producers Council). 1994. 1993–1994 Pork Facts. Des Moines, Iowa.

NPPC (National Pork Producers Council). 1997. Pork Quality Assurance: A program of America's Pork Producers. Des Moines, Iowa: National Pork Producers Council in cooperation with the National Pork Board.

NRC (National Research Council). 1980. The Effects on Human Health of Subtherapeutic Use of Antimicrobials in Animal Feeds. Washington, D.C.: National Academy of Sciences.

NRC (National Research Council). 1985. Meat and Poultry Inspection: The Scientific Basis of the Nation's Program. Washington, D.C.: National Academy Press.

NRC (National Research Council). 1988. Designing Foods: Animal product options in the marketplace. Washington, D.C.: National Academy Press.

NRC (National Research Council). 1989a. Alternative Agriculture. Washington, D.C.: National Academy Press.

NRC (National Research Council). 1989b. Nutrient Requirements of Dairy Cattle, 6th ed. Washington, D.C.: National Academy Press.

NRC (National Research Council). 1994. Metabolic Modifiers: Effects on the Nutrient Requirements of Food Producing Animals. Washington, D.C.: National Academy Press.

NRC (National Research Council). 1995. Building a North American Feed System. Washington, D.C.: National Academy Press.

NRC (National Research Council). 1997. The Role of Chromium in Animal Nutrition. Washington, D.C.: National Academy Press.

Nurmi, E., and M. Rantala. 1973. New aspects of *Salmonella* infection in broiler production. Nature 214:210.

Nwosu, V. C. 1985. Prevalence of coagulace-positive *Staphylococcus* in market meats. Awka. J. Food Prot. 48:603–605.

O'Grady, F., R. G. Finch, H. P. Lambert, and D. Greenwood, eds. 1997. Antibiotic and chemotherapy: anti-infective agents and their use in therapy, 7th ed.. New York: Churchill Livingstone.

Okie, S. 1998. New antibiotic offers hope against resistance. *The Washington Post, Tuesday*, 10 March, Health section, p 7.

Oldham, E. R., R. J. Eberhart, and L. D. Muller. 1991. Effects of supplemental vitamin A or beta-carotene during the dry period and early lactation on udder health. J. Dairy Sci. 74:3775–3781.

Oliver, J., F. H. Dodd, and F. K. Neave. 1956. Udder infections in the dry period. The effect of teat disinfection at drying off on the incidence of infections in the early dry period. J. Dairy Res. 23:212–216.

Oosterom, J. 1991. Epidemiological studies and proposed preventive measures in the fight against human salmonellosis. Intl. J. Food Microbiol. 12: 41–52.

Opara, O. O., L. E. Carr, E. Russek-Cohen, C. R. Tate, E. T. Mallinson, R. G. Miller, L. E. Stewart, R. W. Johnston, and S. W. Joseph. 1992. Correlation of water activity and other environmental conditions with repeated detection of *Salmonella* contamination on poultry farms. Avian Dis. 36: 664–671. Published erratum appears in Avian. Dis. 1993 37:635.

Osterholm, M. T., and M. E. Potter. 1997. Irradiation pasteurization of solid foods: taking safety to the next level. Emerging Infectious Dis. 3(4):575–577.

OTA (U.S. Congress, Office of Technology Assessment). 1991. U.S. Dairy Industry at a Crossroad: Biotechnology and Policy Choices—Special Report, OTA-F-470. Washington, D.C.: U.S. Government Printing Office.

OTA (Office of Technology Assessment). 1995. Impacts of Antibiotic Resistant Bacteria. OTA-H-629. Washington, D.C.: U.S. Government Printing Office.

Pacer, R. E., J. S. Spika, M. C. Thurmond, N. Hargrett-Bean, and M. E. Potter. 1989. Prevalence of *Salmonella* and multiple antimicrobial-resistant *Salmonella* in California dairies. J. Am. Vet. Med. Assoc. 195(1):59–63.

Palumbo, S. A., F. Maxion, A. C. Williams, R. L. Buchanan, and D. W. Thayer. 1985. Starch-ampicillin agar for the quantitative detection of *Aeromonas hydrophila*. Appl. Environ. Microbiol. 50:1027–1030.

Parker, C. F., and A. L. Pope. 1983. The U.S. Sheep Industry: Changes and Challenges. J. Anim. Sci. 57: Suppl. 2:75–99.

Patterson, J. E., and M. J. Zervos. 1990. High-level gentamicin resistance in *Enterococci*: Microbiology, genetic basis, and epidemiology. Rev. Inf. Dis. 12:644–652.

Peplowski, M. A., D. C. Mahan, F. A. Murry, A. L. Moxon, A. H. Cantor, K. E. Ekstrom. 1980. Effect of dietary and injectable vitamin E and selenium in weanling swine antigenically challenged with sheep red blood cells. J. Anim. Sci. 51:344–351.

Perez-Trallero, E., F. Otero, C. Lopez-lopategui, M. Montes, J. M. Garcia-Arenaana, and M. Gomariz. High prevalence of ciprofloxacin resistant *Campylobacter jejuni/coli* in Spain. 1997. P. 49 in Abstracts of the 37th Interscience Conference on Antimicrobial Agents and Chemotherapy, Sept. 28–Oct. 1, Toronto, Canada. Washington, D.C.: American Society for Microbiology.

Peters, J. H., C. R. Gordon, E. Lin, C. E. Green, and C.A. Tyson. 1990. Anaphylaxis to penicillin in a frozen dinner. Ann. Allergy 52: 342–343.

Philpot, W. N., and S. C. Nickerson. 1992. Mastitis: Counter Attack. Naperville, Ill.: Babson Bros. Co. 150 pp.

PHS (Public Health Service). 1995. Update on fluoroquinolones. FDA Bet. 10(40). [Online]. Available: http://www/cvm/fda/gov/fda/infores/fdavet/1996/1195fdavet.html.

Piddock, L. J. V. 1995. Mechanisms of resistance to fluoroquinolones: State-of-the art, 1992–1994. Drugs 49(Suppl. 2):29–35.

Pinner, R. W., A. Schuchat, B. Swaminathan, P. S. Hayes, K. A. Deaver, R. E. Weaver, B. D. Pikaeves, C. V. Broome, and J. D. Wenger. 1992. Role of foods in sporadic listeriosis. II. Microbiologic and epidemiologic investigation. J. Am. Med. Assoc. 267:2046–2050.

Pork Industry Handbook. 1996. West Lafayette, Indiana: Purdue University Cooperative Extension Service.

Prescott, J. F., and J. D. Baggot, eds. 1993. Antimicrobial Therapy in Veterinary Medicine. Second ed. Ames: Iowa State University Press. 612 pp.

Prescott, J. F., V. P. Gannon, G. Kittler, and G. Hlywka. 1984. Antimicrobial drug susceptibility of bacteria isolated from disease processes in cattle, horses, dogs and cats. Can. Vet. J. 25:289–292.

Quiroga, G. H., W. E. Owens, and S. C. Nickerson. 1993. Response of heifer mammary gland macrophages and neutrophils to interferon-gamma stimulation *in vitro*. Can. J. Vet. Res. 57:212–214.

Raemdonck, D. L., A. C. Tanner, S. T. Tolling, and S. L. Michener. 1992. *In vitro* susceptibility of avian *Escherichia coli* and *Pasteurella multocida* to danofloxacin and five other antimicrobials. Avian Dis. 36(4):964–967.

Rasrinaul, L., O. Suthienkul, P. O. Echeverria, D. N. Taylor, J. Sevantana, A. Banglrakulnonth, and U. Leromboon. 1988. Foods as a source of enteropathogens causing childhood diarrhea in Thailand. Am. J. Trop. Med. Hyg. 39:97–102.

Reddy, P. G., J. L. Morrill, H.C. Minocha, M. B. Morrill, A. D. Dayton, and R A. Frey. 1986. Effect of supplemental vitamin E on the immune system of calves. J. Dairy Sci. 69:164–171.

Richardson, C. W. 1987. Hot weather and the dairy cow. Dairy News in Oklahoma. Cooperative Extension Service 38(4).

Richwald, G. A., S. Greenland; B. J. Johnson, J. M. Friedland, E. J. Goldstein, D. T. Plichta. 1988. Assessment of the excess risk of *Salmonella dublin* infection associated with the use of certified raw milk. Public Health Rep. 103(5):489–493.

Riley, L. W., M. L. Cohen, J. E. Seals, M. J. Blaser, K. A. Birkness, N. T. Hagrett, S. M. Martin, and R. A. Feldman. 1984. Importance of host factors in human salmonellosis caused by multiresistant strains of *Salmonella*. J. Infect. Dis. 149(6):878–883.

Roberson, J. R., L. K. Fox, D. D. Hancock, J. M. Gay, and T. E. Besser. 1994. Ecology of *Staphylococcus aureus* isolated from various sites on dairy farms. J. Dairy Sci. 77(11):3354–3364.

Roberts, T., and K. D. Murrell. 1993. Economic losses caused by food-borne parasitic diseases. Pp. 51–75 in Proceedings of an International Symposium on Cost-Benefit Aspects of Food Irradiation Processing. International Atomic Energy Agency.

Rogers, R. T. 1993. Broilers—Differentiating a commodity. Pp. 3–32 in Industry Studies. L. L. Tuetsch, ed. Englewood Cliffs, New Jersey: Prentice-Hall.

Rothschild, M. F. 1989. Selective breeding for immune responsiveness and disease resistance in livestock. Ag. Biotech News Info. 3:355–360.

Rothschild, M. F. 1991. Selection under challenging environments. Pp. 73–85 in Breeding for Disease Resistance in Farm Animals, J. B. Owen, ed. United Kingdom: CAB International, Redwood Press.

Roura, E., J. Homedes, and K.C. Klasing. 1992. Prevention of immunologic stress contributes to the growth-permitting ability of dietary antibiotics in chicks. J. Nutr. 122(12):2383–2390.

Roussel, J. D., J. A. Lee, J. F. Beatty, and I. H. Ghols. 1969. Effects of thermal stress on somatic cell count, milk constituents, and blood cells [abstract]. J. Dairy Sci. 52:562.

Rumsey, T. S. 1988. Chemicals for regulating animal growth and production. Pp. 91–108 in: Beltsville Symposia in Agricultural Research. VIII. Agricultural Chemicals of the Future. J. L. Hilton, ed. Totowa, NJ: Rowman and Allanheld.

Ryan, D. P., M. P. Boland, E. Kopel, D. Armstrong, L. Munyakazi, R. A. Godke, and R. H. Ingraham. 1992. Evaluating two different evaporative cooling management systems for dairy cows in a hot, dry climate. J. Dairy Sci. 75:1052–1059.

Saide-Albornez, J.J., C. L. Knipe, E. A. Murano, and G. W. Beran. 1992. Identification of five pathogenic bacteria on pork carcasses processed at three Iowa packing plants. Pp. 31–35 in Proceedings of the Food Safety Consortium Annual Meeting, Kansas City.

Savage, D. C. 1977. Immunological interactions between the host and its microbes in bay animals. Microbial ecology of the gastrointestinal tract. Ann. Rev. Microbiol. 31:107–113.

Schiemann, D. A. 1980. Isolation of toxigenic *Yersinia enterocolitica* from retail pork products. J. Food Prot. 43:360–365.

Schiono, H., Hayashidani, H., Haneko, K. I., Ogawa, M., and M. Muramatsu. 1990. Occurrence of *Erysipelothrix rhusiopathiae* in retail raw pork. J. Food Prot. 53:856–858.

Schuman, J. D., E. A. Zottola, and S. K. Harlander. Preliminary characterization of a food-borne multiple-antibiotic-resistant *Salmonella typhimurium* strain. 1989. Appl. Environ. Microbiol. 55(9):2344–2348.

Schwartz, K. J. 1991. Salmonellosis in swine. Compend. Contin. Educ. Pract. Vet. 13:139–147.

Schwartz, H. J., and T. H. Sher. 1984. Anaphylaxis to penicillin in a frozen dinner. Ann. Allergy 52:342–343.

Scott, F.W. 1987. Principles of food animal drug use. In: Animal Drug Use: Dollars and Sense. Symposium proceedings. Pp.121–125. Department of Health and Human Services Publication # (FDA) 88–6045. Center for Veterinary Medicine, Rockville, Maryland.

Scroggins, C. D. 1988. Stepping stone or stumbling blocks: A consumer perspective of animal drug use. In: Animal Drug Use: Dollars and Sense. Department of Health and Human Services Publication # 88.6045. Pp. 53–58. Center for Veterinary Medicine. Rockville, Maryland.

Settepani, J. A. 1984. The hazard of using chloramephenicol in food animals. J. Am. Vet. Med. Assoc. 184(8):930–931.

Shah, P. M., V. Schafer, and H. Knothe. 1993. Medical and veterinary use of antimicrobial agents: Implications for public health. A clinician's view on antimicrobial resistance. Vet. Microbiol. 35:269–274.

Shanker, S., Rosenfield, J.A., Davey, G.R., and T. C. Sorrel. 1982. *Campylobacter jejuni*: Incidence in processed broilers and biotype distribution in human and broiler isolates. Appl. Environ. Microbiol. 43:1219–1220.

Shearer, J. K., D. R. Bray, F. C. Elvinger, and P. A. Reed. 1987. The incidence of clinical mastitis in cows exposed to cooling ponds for heat stress management. Pp. 66–70 in Proceedings Annual Meeting of the National Mastitis Council, Inc. Arlington, Virginia. Perry, Iowa: American Association of Swine Practitioners.

Shepard, M. L., P. W. Carr, and V. M. Loomis, eds. 1992. Handbook of Approved New Animal Drug Applications in the United States. Dallas, TX: Shortwell and Carr, Inc.

Shook, G. E. 1989. Selection for disease resistance. J. Dairy Sci. 72(5):1349–1362.

Shultz, T. A. 1987. Manger misters fight summer heat stress. Hoard's Dairyman 132:407.

Shultz, T. A., L. S. Collar, and S. R. Morrison. 1985. Corral manger misting effects on heat stressed lactating cows. J. Dairy Sci. 68(Suppl. 1):239.

Skovgaard, N., and B. Norrung. 1989. The incidence of *Listeria* spp. in faeces of Danish pigs and in minced pork meat. Intl. J. Food Microbiol. 8:59–63.

Slavik, M.F., J. W. Kim, M. D. Pharr, D. P. Raben, S. Tsai, and C. M. Lobsinger. 1994. Effect of trisodium phosphate on *Campylobacter* attached to post-chill chicken carcasses. J. Food Prot. 57:324–326.

Smart, J. L., T. A. Roberts, M. F. Stringer, and N. Shah. 1961. The incidence and serotypes of *Clostidium perfringens* on beef, pork, and lamb carcasses. J. Appl. Bacteriol. 24:235–242.

Smith, K. E., J. Besser, J. Bender, J. Hogan, C. Hedberg, K. MacDonald, M. Osterholm. 1997. Quinolone-Resistant *Campylobacter jejuni* Infections in Minnesota Residents. In Abstracts of the 37th Interscience Conference on Antimicrobial Agents and Chemotherapy, Sept. 28–Oct. 1, Toronto, Ontario. American Society for Microbiology.

Smith, K. L., J. H. Harrison, D. D. Harrison, D. D. Hancock, D. A. Todhunter, and H. R. Conrad. 1984. Effect of vitamin E and selenium supplementation on incidence of clinical mastitis and duration of clinical symptoms. J. Dairy Sci. 67(6):1293–1300.

Smith, K.L., Todhunter, D.A. and P.S. Schoenberger, 1985. Environmental mastitis: cause, prevalence, prevention. J. Dairy Sci. 68:1531.

Smith, K. L., and J. S. Hogan. 1993. Environmental mastitis. Vet. Clin. North Am. Food Anim. Pract. 9(3):489–498.

Soerjadi, A. S., G. H. Snoeyenbos, and O. M. Weinack. 1982. Intestinal colonization and competitive exclusion of *Campylobacter fetus* subsp. *jejuni* in young chicks. Avian Dis. 26:520–524.

Soerjadi, A. S., S. M. Stehman, G. H. Snoeyenbos, O. M. Weinack, and C. F. Smyser. 1981. Some measurements of protection against paratyphoid *Salmonella* and *Escherichia coli* by competitive exclusion in chickens. Avian Dis. 25(3):706–712.

Sokari, T. G., and S. O. Anozie. 1990. Occurrence of enterotoxin producing strains of *Staphylococcus aureus* in meat and related samples from traditional markets in Nigeria. J. Food Prot. 53:1069–1070.

Somogyi, A. 1984. Survey of animal drugs with carcinogenic properties. Food Addit. Contam. 1:81–87.

Sooltan, J. R. A., G. C. Mead, and A. P. Norris. 1987. Incidence and growth potential of *Bacillus cereus* in poultry meat products. Food Microbiol. 4:347–351.

Sordillo, L. M., and L. A. Babiuk. 1991. Controlling acute *Escherichia coli* mastitis during the periparturient period with recombinant bovine interferon gamma. Vet. Microbiol. 28:189–198.

Speer, V. C. 1982. Antibiotics—the final word. P. 8 in Swine Health—1982 Production Symposium. Des Moines, Iowa: National Pork Producers Council.

Spika, J. S., S. H. Waterman, G. W. Soo Hoo, M. E. St. Louis, R. E. Pacer, S. M. James, M. L. Bisset, L. W. Mayer, J. Y. Chiu, B. Hall, K. Greene, M. E. Potter, M. L. Cohen, and P. A. Blake. 1987. Chloramphenicol-resistant *Salmonella newport* traced through hamburger to dairy farms: A major persisting source of human salmonellosis in California. N. Engl. J. Med. 316:565–570.

Standberg, E., and G. E. Shook. 1989. Genetic and economic responses to breeding programs that consider mastitis. J. Dairy Sci. 72:2136–2142.

Stark, B. A., and J. M. Wilkenson. 1988. Probiotics Theory and Applications. Marlow, United Kingdom: Chalcombe Publications.

Stear, M. J., S. Bath, J. Mackie, C. Dimmock, S. C. Brown, F. W. Nicholas, and B. Morris. 1985. The bovine major histocompatibility system and disease resistance. Pp. 173–178 in Characterization of the Bovine Immune System and the Genes Regulating Expression of Immunity with Particular Reference to Their Role in Disease Resistance, W. C. Davis, J. N. Shelton, and C. W. Weems, eds. Pullman, Washington: Washington State University.

Steele, J. H., and G. W. Beran. 1992. Perspectives in the uses of antibiotics and sulfonamides. Pp. 3–33 in CRC Handbook, Series in Zoonoses: Antibiotics, Sulfonamides, and Public Health. Boca Raton, Florida: CRC Press.

Stern, N. J. 1981. Recovery rate of *Campylobacter fetus* ssp. *jejuni* on eviscerated pork, lamb and beef carcasses. J. Food Sci. 46:1291–1293.

Stern, N. J., S. S. Green, N. Thaker, D. J. Krout, and J. Chiu. 1984. Recovery of *Campylobacter jejuni* from fresh and frozen meat and poultry collected at slaughter. J. Food Prot. 47:372–374.

Stern, N. J., and J. E. Line. 1992. Comparison of three methods for recovery of *Campylobacter* spp. from broiler carcasses. J. Food Prot. 55:663–666.

St. Georgiev, V. 1998. Infectious Diseases in Immunocompromised Hosts. Washington, D.C.: CRC Press.

Stokstad, E. L. R., T. H. Jukes, J. Pierce, A. C. Page, Jr., and A. L. Franklin. 1949. The multiple nature of the animal protein factor. J. Biol. Chem. 180:647–654.

Stribling, J.H. 1992. What's holding up animal drug approval? J. Am. Vet. Med. Assoc. 200(12), 1806–1808.

Strugnell, R., A. Cockayne, and C. W. Penn. 1990a. Molecular and antigenic analysis of treponemes. Crit. Rev. Microbiol. 17:231–250.

Strugnell, R., D. Maskell, N. Fairweather, D. Packard, A. Cockayne, C. Penn, and G. Morgan. 1990b. Stable expression of foreign antigens from the chromosome of *Salmonella typhimurium* vaccine strains. Gene 88:57–63.

Strugnell, R. G. Dougan, S. Chatfield, I. Charles, N. Fairweather, J. Tite, J. L. Li, J. Beeseley, and M. Roberts. 1992. Characterization of a *Salmonella typhimurium* are strain expressing the P.69 antigen of *Bortedella pertussis*. Infect. Immunol. 60:3994–4002.

Swann, M. M. 1969. Report of Joint Committee on the Use of Antibiotics in Animal Husbandry and Veterinary Medicine. Cmnd. 4190. London: Her Majesty's Stationery Office.

Swanson, J. C. 1995. Farm animal well-being and intensive production systems. J. Anim. Sci. 73(9):2744–2751.

Swarm, R. L., G. K. S. Roberts, A. C. Levy, and L. R. Hines. 1973. Observation in the thyroid gland in rats following the administration of sulfamethoxazole and trimethoprim. Toxicol. Appl. Pharmacol. 24(3):351–363.

Tauxe, R. V. 1986. Antimicrobial Resistance in Human Salmonellosis in the United States. J. Anim. Sci. 62(Suppl. 3):65–73.

Tauxe, R. V., J. Vandepitte, G. Wauters, S. M. Martin, V. Goossens, P. De Mol, R. Van Noyen, and G. Thiers. 1987. *Yersinia enterocolitica* infections and pork: the missing link. Lancet 1:1129–1132.

Tauxe, R. V., S. D. Holmberg, and M. L. Cohen. 1989. The epidemiology of gene transfer in the environment. Pp. 377–403 in Gene Transfer in the Environment. Levy and Miller, eds. New York: McGraw-Hill.

Tay, S. C. K., R. A. Robinson, and M. M. Pullen. 1989. *Salmonella* in the mesentric lymph nodes and fecal contents of slaughtered sows. J. Food Prot. 52:202–203.

Taylor, J. P., and J. N. Perdue. 1989. The changing epidemiology of human brucellosis in Texas, 1977–1986. Am. J. Epidemiol. 130(1):160–165.

Telzak, E. E., M. S. Greenberg, L. D. Budnick, T. Singh, and S. Blum. 1991. Diabetes mellitus—a newly described risk factor for infection from *Salmonella enteritidis*. J. Infect. Dis. 164(3):538–541.

Tengerdy, R. P., M. M. Mathias and C. F. Nockels. 1981. Vitamin E, immunity and disease resistance. Adv. Exp. Med. Biol. 135:27–42.

Tengerdy, R. P., D. L. Meyer, L. H. Lauerman, D. C. Lueker and C. F. Nockels. 1983. Vitamin E-enhanced humoral antibody response to *Clostridium perfringens* type D in sheep. Br. Vet. J. 139:147–152.

Ternstrom, A., and G. Molin. 1987. Incidence of potential pathogens on raw pork, beef and chicken in Sweden. J. Food Prot. 50:141–146.

Thapar, M.K., and E.J. Young. 1986. Urban outbreak of goat cheese brucellosis. Pediatr. Infect. Dis. 5(6):640–643.

Thompson, J. W. 1942. A history of livestock raising in the United States, 1607–1860. Washington, D.C.: U.S. Department of Agriculture.

Threlfall, E. J. 1992. Antibiotics and the selection of food-borne pathogens. Appl. Bacteriol. Symp. Ser. 21:96S–102S.

Threlfall, E. J., F. J. Angulo, and P. G. Wall. 1998. Ciprofloxacin-resistant *Salmonella typhimurium* DT104 [letter]. Vet. Rec. 142(10):255.

Threlfall, E. J., J. A. Frost, L. R. Ward, and B. Rowe. 1996. Increasing spectrum of resistance in multidrug resistant *Salmonella typhimurium*. Lancet 347:1052–1053.

Tillett, H. E., J. de Louvois, and P. G. Wall. 1998. Surveillance of outbreaks of waterborne infectious disease: categorizing levels of evidence. Epidemiol. Infect. 120(1):37–42.

Tokumaru, M., H. Konuma, M. Umesako, S. Konno, and K. Shinagawa. 1991. Rates of detection of *Salmonella* and *Campylobacter* in meats in response to the sample size. Intl. J. Food Microbiol. 13:41–46.

Tollefson, L. 1996. FDA reveals plans for antimicrobial susceptibility monitoring. J. Am. Vet. Med. Assoc. 208(4):459–460.

Tomasz, A. 1994. Multiple-antibiotic-resistant pathogenic bacteria: A report on the Rockefeller University Workshop. N. Engl. J. Med. 330:1247–1251.

Toner, M. 1994. Rwandans' Nightmare: Drug-resistant diseases. *Atlanta Journal Constitution*. August 7. Pp. 1 & 14.

Torres, O. R., R. Z. Korman, S. A. Zahler, and G. M. Dunny. 1991. The conjugative transposon Tn925: enhancement of conjugal transfer by tetracycline in *Enterococcus faecalis* and mobilization of chromosomal genes in *Bacillus subtilis* and *E. faecalis*. Mol. Gen. Genet. 225(3):395–400.

Tribble, L. F. 1991. Feeding growing-finishing pigs. Pp. 509–516 in Swine Nutrition. E. R. Miller, D. E. Ullrey, and A. J. Lewis, eds. Stoneham, Mass.: Butterworth-Heinemann.

Tscheuschner, I. 1972. Anaphylaktische reaction auf penicillin nach genuss von schweinefleisch. (Penicillin anaphylaxis following pork consumption.) Z. Haut. Geschlechtskr. 47:591–592.

Turek, P., H. Gorzova, and D. Mate. 1989. Microbiological surface contamination of swine after slaughter processing and cooling. Folia Veterinaria 33:131–139.

U.S. Department of Agriculture. 1996. Agricultural Statistics 1996. U.S. Department of Agriculture, Washington, D.C.

U.S. Congress, Office of Technology Assessment. 1991. U.S. Dairy Industry at a Crossroad: Biotechnology and Policy Choices—Special Report, OTA–F–470. U.S. Government Printing Office, Washington, D.C.

van den Bogaard, A., N. London, C. Driessen, and E. Stobberingh. 1997. Fluoroquinolone usage in animals and resistance in human faecal *E. coli*. P. 37 in Abstracts of the 37th Interscience Conference on Antimicrobial Agents and Chemotherapy, Sept. 28–Oct. 1, Toronto, Canada. Washingtion, D.C.: American Society for Microbiology.

VanArsdall, R. N., and K. E. Nelson. 1983. Characteristics of farmer cattle feeding. Agric. Econ. Rep. 503:41.

Van den Bogaard, A. E. J. M. 1993. A veterinary antibiotic policy: a personal view on the perspectives in the Netherlands. Vet. Microbiol. 35:303–312.

Veringa, E., and J. Verhoef. 1985. Influence of subinhibitory concentrations of clindamycin on the phagocytosis of *Staphylococcus aureus*. P. 127 in The Influence of Antibiotics on the Host-Parasite Relationship, Vol. 2. D. Adam, H. Hahn, and W. Opferkuch, eds. Berlin, Germany: Springer-Verlag.

Vickers, H.R., L. Bagratuni, and S. Alexander. 1958. Dermatitis caused by penicillin in milk. Lancet 1:351–352.

Vorster, S. M., M. R. Greebe, G. L. Nortje, and M. L. van der Walt. 1991. Incidence of food-borne bacterial pathogens in meat in the Pretoria erea. S. Afr. J. Food. Sci. Nutr. 3:51–54.

Wade, M. A., and A. P. Barkley. 1992. The economic impacts of a ban on subtherapeutic antibiotics in swine production. Agribusiness 8(2):93–107.

Walawski, K., M. Duniec, and U. Czarnik. 1993. Association between the M blood group system and differentiation of mastitis-susceptibility indices of cows. Genetica Polonica 34:56–63.

Wall, P. G., D. Morgan, K. Lamden, M. Griffin, E. J. Threlfall, L. R. Ward, and B. Rowe. 1995. Transmission of multi-resistant strains of *Salmonella typhimurium* from cattle to man. Vet. Rec. 136(23):591–592.

Wall, P. G., D. Morgan, K. Lamden, M. Ryan, M. Griffin, E. J. Threlfall, L. R. Ward, and B. Rowe. 1994. A case control study of infection with an epidemic strain of multiresistant *Salmonella typhimurium* DT104 in England and Wales. Commun. Dis. Rep. CDR Rev. 4(11):130–135.

Walser, M. M., and R. B. Davis. 1975. *In vitro* characterization of field isolates of *Pasteurella multocida* from Georgia turkeys. Avian Dis. 19(3):525–532.

Walton, J. R. 1985. Zoonoses. Pig News Info. 6:21–24.

Walton, J. R. 1986. Impact of antibiotic resistance in animal production on public health. J. Anim. Sci. 62(Suppl. 3):74–85.

Wang, C., and P. M. Muriana. 1994. Incidence of *Listeria* in packages of retail franks. J. Food Prot. 57:382–386.

Wang, G. H., K. T. Yan, X. M. Feng, S. M. Chen, A. P. Lui, and Y. Kokubo. 1993. Isolation and identification of *Listeria monocytogenes* from retail meats in Beijing. J. Food Prot. 55:56–58.

Warner, C. M., D. L. Meeker, and M. F. Rothschild. 1987. Genetic control of immune responsiveness: A review of its use as a tool for selection for disease resistance. J. Anim. Sci. 64:159.

Webster, C. D. 1991. Vitamins are important in fish diets. Ky. Fish Farming 4(2):4–5.

Wegner, T. N., J. D. Schuh, F. E. Nelson, and G. H. Stott. 1976. Effect of stress on blood leucocyte and milk somatic cell counts in dairy cows. J. Dairy Sci. 59:949–956.

Weinack, O. M., G. H. Snoeyenbos, C. F. Smyser, and A. S. Soerjadi. 1981. Competitive exclusion of intestinal colonization of *Escherichia coli* in chicks. Sites of bacterial attachment. Avian Dis. 25: 696–705.

Weiss, W. P., J. S. Hogan, K. L. Smith, and K. H. Hoblet. 1990. Relationships among selenium, vitamin E and mammary gland health in commercial dairy herds. J. Dairy Sci. 73:381–390.

Wenger, J. D., B. Swaminathan, P. S. Hayes, S. S. Green, M. Pratt, R. W. Pinner, A. Schchat, and C. V. Broome. 1990. *Listeria monocytogenes* contamination of turkey franks: evaluation of a production facility. J. Food Prot. 53:1015–1019.

WHO (World Health Organization). 1997. The medical impact of the use of antimicrobials in food animals: report of a WHO meeting, Berlin, Germany, Document No. WHO/EMC/ZOO/97.4.

WHO (World Health Organization). 1998. Infectious diseases kill over 17 million people a year: WHO warns of a global crisis. In statement on The World Health Report 1996: Fighting disease, Fostering Development. [Online]. Available: http://www.who.org/whr.1996/press1.htm. [1998, April 6].

Wicher, K., R. E. Reisman, and C. E. Arbesman. 1969. Allergic reaction to penicillin present in milk. J. Am. Med. Assoc. 208(1):143–145.

Wiedemann, B. 1993. Monitoring of resistant organisms in man and identification of their origin. Vet. Microbiol. 35:275–284.

Wilcock, B. P., and H. J. Olander. 1978. Influence of oral antibiotic feeding on the duration and severity of clinical disease, growth performance, and pattern of shedding in swine inoculated with *Salmonella typhimurium*. J. Am. Vet. Med. Assoc. 172:472–477.

Wilson, L.L. 1993. Special-fed Veal Calves: Overview of Production Methods and Drug Needs. Vet. Human Toxicol. 35(Suppl. 2): 29–32.

Wilson, R. C. 1994. Antibiotic residues and the public health. Chapter 5 in Animal Drugs and Human Health. L. M. Crawford and D. A. Franeo, eds. Lancaster, Pennsylvania: Technomic Publishing Company, Inc.

Witte. 1998. Medical consequences of antibiotic use in agriculture. Science 279:949–1096.

Witte, W., and I. Klare. 1995. Glycopeptide-resistant *Enterococcus faecium* outside hospitals: A commentary. Microbial Drug Resist. 1:259–263.

Wokatsch, R., and J. Bockemuhl. 1988. Serovars and biovars of *Campylobacter* strains isolated from humans and slaughterhouse animals in northern Germany. J. Appl. Bacteriol. 64:135–140.

Wray, C., S. Furniss, and C. L. Benham. 1990. Feeding antibiotic-contaminated wastemilk to calves—effects on physical performance and antibiotic sensitivity of gut flora. Br. Vet. J. 146(1):80–87.

Wray, C., I. M. McLaren, and Y. E. Beedell. 1993. Bacterial resistance monitoring of *Salmonella* isolated from animals, national experience of surveillance schemes in the United Kingdom. Vet. Microbiol. 35:313–319.

Yadava, R., M. Prasad, and K. G. Narayan. 1988. Dynamics of contamination of pork with *Salmonella* in a pork processing plant. Indian J. Anim. Sci. 58:66–665.

Yarabioff, Y. 1990. Incidence and recovery of *Listeria* from chicken with a pre-enrichment technique. J. Food Prot. 53:555–557.

Zimmerman, D. R. 1986. Role of subtherapeutic levels of antimicrobials in pig production. J. Anim. Sci. 62(Suppl. 3):6–17.

Zimmerman, M. C. 1958. Penicillinase treatment of 52 patients with allergic reaction to penicillin. Antibiotics Annual. Pp. 312–320.

Ziv, G. 1986. Therapeutic use of antibiotics in farm animals. Pp. 8–29 in Agricultural Uses of Antibiotics. W. A. Moats, ed. Washington, D.C.: American Chemical Society.

About the Authors

James R. Coffman is provost at Kansas State University. During his long-standing tenure there he has held numerous professorships and administrative positions, including dean of the College of Veterinary Medicine, head of the Department of Surgery and Medicine, and director of the Veterinary Teaching Hospital. Coffman holds bachelor's, master's, and doctorate of veterinary medicine degrees from Kansas State University. He is a diplomate of the American College of Veterinary Internal Medicine. Coffman's areas of research and expertise include equine medicine and laminitis research. He lends his experience and service to many national organizations, professional societies, editorial boards, and university committees.

George W. Beran is distinguished professor and program chair of preventive medicine in the Department of Microbiology, Immunology and Preventive Medicine of the College of Veterinary Medicine at Iowa State University. Beran serves as chair of several organizations and programs including the Food Safety Research Program of the Food Safety Consortium at Iowa State University. He is currently a member of the National Research Council's Board on Science and Technology for International Development proposal review panel and of the National Advisory Committee for Microbiological Criteria for Foods. Beran holds a doctorate in veterinary medicine, a Ph.D. in medical microbiology, and a Ph.D. in humane letters from Iowa State University, the University of Kansas, and Silliman University in the Philippines, respectively. He is a diplomate of the American College of Veterinary Preventive Medicine and of the American College of Epidemiology.

Harvey R. Colten is dean and vice president for medical affairs, Northwestern University Medical School. Prior to this he was pediatrician-in-chief at St. Louis Children's Hospital and Barnes Hospital, both in St. Louis, Missouri. Colten was also the Harriet B. Spoehrer Professor and chairman of the Department of Pediatrics, as well as professor of molecular microbiology at the Washington University School of Medicine. After receiving his undergraduate degree from Cornell University and his M.D. from Case Western Reserve University in Ohio, Colten received an honorary master's degree from Harvard University when he was appointed professor of pediatrics at the Harvard Medical School. He is an active member of numerous committees and boards, including the National Academy of Sciences Institute of Medicine. Colten's research interests include the regulation of acute-phase gene expression and genetic deficiencies of proteins important in pulmonary diseases, autoimmunity, and inflammation.

Connie Greig is owner and operator of Little Acorn Ranch, a 200-head Simmental seedstock operation in Iowa. Greig currently holds the positions of vice-chairman of the National Cattlemen's Beef Association's Animal Health Committee and of chairman of the Iowa Cattlemen's Beef Association's Industry Issues Committee. She has been an active spokesperson for animal care, animal welfare, and animal health issues as related to the food-animal industry. Greig completed undergraduate work and received a degree in English from the University of Iowa.

Jean Halloran is director of the Consumer Policy Institute, a division of Consumers Union. Her 20 years of experience in the public health sector have enabled her to touch a variety of issues, including food safety, pesticides, biotechnology, hazardous pharmaceuticals, sustainable agriculture, and toxic air pollution. In 1979 and 1980, she was on the staff of President Carter's Council on Environmental Quality, for which she helped prepare an Executive Order on export of hazardous products. Halloran obtained her undergraduate degree with honors in English literature from Swarthmore College in Pennsylvania.

Dermont Hayes is a professor in the Department of Economics, professor in charge of the Meat Export Research Center at Iowa State University, and head of the Trade and Agricultural Policy Division at the Center for Agricultural and Rural Development. He completed his undergraduate degree with honors in agricultural economics from University College in Dublin, Ireland. Continuing his education at the University of California at Berkeley, he received a master's degree in agricultural economics and a Ph.D. in international trade. His research interests include food safety, livestock modeling, demand analysis, commodity markets, and agricultural and trade policy.

John B. Kaneene is a professor of epidemiology and director of the Population Medicine Center at the College of Veterinary Medicine at Michigan State University. His research interests include molecular epidemiology of emerging and re-emerging enteric zoonotic diseases; epidemiology of antibiotic resistance in animal and human populations; risk assessment modeling as it relates to foodborne pathogens; epidemiology and prevention of drug residues in foods of animal origin; and development, implementation, and evaluation of disease surveillance systems. Kaneene's undergraduate studies in mathematics and his degree in veterinary medicine were completed at the University of Khartoum in Sudan. He received a master's of public health and a Ph.D. in epidemiology from the University of Minnesota.

Kristin McNutt is president of Consumer Choices, Inc., and editor of *Consumer Magazines Digest*. After securing an undergraduate degree in chemistry from Duke University, she studied nutrition and received a master's degree from Columbia University Physicians and Surgeons. McNutt completed Ph.D. work in biochemistry at Vanderbilt University. Her extensive educational background also includes a doctorate law degree in the DePaul College of Law. She served on the National Research Council Board on Agriculture Committee on Designing Foods and participated in the "More and Better Foods" project, in collaboration with the Academy of Scientific Research and Technology. McNutt is member of the Food and Drug Administration Food Advisory Committee.

David Meeker is associate professor of animal science at Ohio State University and coordinator of the Ohio Pork Industry Center, which coordinates expertise from various disciplines to facilitate the profitable and environmentally responsible production of wholesome pork. Until 1996 he served as vice-president of research and education for the National Pork Producers Council, where for 11 years he directed growth of staff and programs in production, marketing, economics, animal health, education, and research. He received B.S., M.S., and Ph.D. degrees in animal science from Iowa State University. In 1994 he received an M.B.A. in agribusiness from Iowa State. He has studied pork production abroad and served on several U.S. Department of Agriculture advisory committees.

Stephen C. Nickerson is professor and director of the Mastitis Research Laboratory Hill Farm Research Station. Nickerson's research and teaching areas emphasize bovine mastitis and lactation physiology. His educational background includes an undergraduate degree in animal science from the University of Maine and master's and Ph.D. degrees in dairy science from Virginia Polytechnic Institute and State University.

Thomas Seay is medical director of OnCare Southeast and chairman of the cancer committee at St. Joseph's Hospital in Atlanta, Georgia. He has been a staff physician and assistant professor at Emory University Hospital. Seay's research interests include molecular immunology and oncogene point mutation frequency in development of myelogenous leukemia. At the University of Georgia, Seay obtained an undergraduate degree in microbiology. He furthered his studies at East Tennessee State University, where he completed Ph.D. work in biomedical sciences. Seay holds M.D. from the James A. Quillen College of Medicine.

R. Gregory Stewart is currently the director of the poultry business unit of Bayer Corporation in Watkinsville, Georgia. Previously, he was president of Southern Veterinary Services, Inc., in St. Louis, Missouri. He received undergraduate degrees from the University of Florida and continued his education at the University of Georgia, where he obtained a master's degree in poultry science, a Ph.D. in medical microbiology, and a D.V.M. Stewart served two consecutive terms (1992–1996) on a National Research Council's Panel on Animal Health and Veterinary Medicine. Stewart's other experience includes teaching, research, and management positions.

Index

A

Accountability for drug use, 4, 5, 6, 27, 46, 62, 81, 98-99, 174, 178
Administration regimens. *See also* Subtherapeutic antibiotic use
  and antibiotic resistance, 31, 33, 72, 151, 163-164
  combinations of drugs, 160, 163-164, 197
  gradient approach, 72, 157-158
  in rotation, 31, 33, 72, 160
  routes, 34-37, 82, 83, 85, 103
  subtherapeutic doses, 71-72, 151
  therapeutic doses, 157, 158
Aerococcus viridans, 59
Aeromonas spp., 130-131
  A. hydrophila, 127, 128-129, 132-135
  A. liquefaciens, 59
  A. salmonicida, 59
Agalactia, 43
AGRICOLA, 14
Agricultural Marketing Service, 110-111
Agricultural Research Service, 89, 139, 174, 190
Alabama, 30
Allergenicity of antibiotics, 6, 69, 82, 84-85, 144
American Feed Industry Association, 13
American Sheep Industry Association, 60

American Veal Association, 60
American Veterinary Medical Association, 13, 63-64
Amoxicillin, 42, 45, 52, 54
Ampicillin, 42, 52, 54, 146, 162, 164, 165, 166, 167, 172
Amprolium, 32, 33, 57
Anaplasmosis, 44, 50
Animal and Plant Health Inspection Service (APHIS), 139, 162, 174, 190
Animal Drug Availability Act (ADAA), 6, 10, 99-100, 107
Animal health industry, economics of subtherapeutic drug use, 180, 186
Animal Health Institute (AHI), 81,148, 149, 171
Animal management practices
  and antibiotic resistance, 9, 150-153, 159, 160
  aquaculture, 58, 206
  beef cattle, 50, 67, 191, 206
  behavioral stress, 193
  biosecurity techniques, 197-199
  dairy cattle, 44, 64-65, 191-192, 197, 199, 201, 203-205
  fly control, 50, 199
  heat stress management, 190-193
  immune-function enhancers, 200-202
  intensive management and confinement operations, 31

moisture management, 39, 199-200
nutrition, 50, 192, 202-206
overcrowding, 193
pasture management, 50
poultry, 61, 191, 192-193
probiotics (direct-fed microbial), 195-197
recommendations, 11, 208-209
sheep, 54-55
subtherapeutic drug-use alternatives, 181,
    182, 189-190
swine, 41, 181, 191, 197-198, 206
vaccination, 193-195
Animal Medicinal Drug Use Clarification Act
    (AMDUCA), 5, 10, 97-99, 107
Anthelmintic, 54, 55-56, 82
Antibiotic drug use. *See also* Ban on
    subtherapeutic antibiotic use;
    Subtherapeutic antibiotic use
animal management alternatives to, 9, 190-
    202
applications, 2, 4, 19, 28, 71
for aquaculture, 59
for beef cattle, 52, 175
benefits, 1-2, 4, 13, 21, 25, 29, 68, 72, 73-
    75, 107, 174-175
case studies, 166-176
concerns, 15, 24, 25-26, 142-143, 155
in dairy industry, 45, 46, 47-48, 52, 119-120
disease eradication and, 190, 206
genetics and, 207-208
growth promotion with, 28, 31, 34, 51-53,
    81, 153-154
hazards (potential), 6, 75-81
history, 20-22, 153-154
illegal, 182
issues, 19-26
literature review, 3, 14, 15-19
magnitude of, 24-25
for minor species, 56, 57
multidrug therapy, 147-148
nutrition and, 202-206
in poultry industry, 18, 32, 175
recommendations, 10, 177-178
in sheep industry, 55
in swine industry, 41-42, 175
therapeutic, 13, 28, 72-73, 103, 153-161
trends, 25
in veal industry, 53, 54
Antibiotic drugs. *See also specific drug*
allergenicity in humans, 6, 69, 82, 84-85,
    144

availability concerns, 4, 7, 10, 24, 81, 107,
    143, 148-149, 176-177
bactericidal, 147-148
bacteriostatic, 147-148
banned, 77, 78, 83-84, 97, 101-102
cell division targets, 147
defensins, 147
DNA gyrase inhibitors, 147
endotoxin blockers, 146
human last line of defense, 35, 168-169,
    175
identifying and screening new drugs, 145-
    148
mechanisms of action, 28, 143-145, 154-
    155
metabolism modifiers administered with,
    146
nonsystemic, 82
over-the-counter availability, 4, 6, 46, 65,
    81, 182, 186
protein secreton inhibitors, 147
protein synthesis inhibitors, 146-147
residues in foods, 14, 21, 63, 116-117, 118
synthetic, 146, 163, 168
systemic, 82
toxicity to humans, 6, 77, 81-82, 83-84, 144
Antibiotic resistance
administration regimen and, 31, 33, 72,
    151, 160, 162, 163-164
animal management practices and, 150-153,
    159
age of animal population and, 166
assessment methods, 8-9, 170
and availability of drugs, 4, 7, 9, 24, 81,
    107, 143, 148-149, 168-169
causes, 69, 70, 81, 86
cross-genera transfer, 152-153
cross-resistance, 178
data availability, 69, 70, 73
definition of, 7-8, 21, 166, 170, 171, 176
development and transmission, 7, 76-77, 78,
    79, 150, 151-153, 155-156, 161, 168,
    171, 172, 176
economic factors, 150, 182-183
fluoroquinolone controversy, 166, 168-175,
    182-183
food-borne pathogens, 2, 8, 23, 70-71, 86,
    87, 138, 140, 155, 166, 168, 171, 172
and human health risk, 2, 4, 7, 9, 13, 21,
    22-26, 69, 70, 76-78, 79, 86-87, 138,
    143, 150, 155, 160, 161-166, 168, 172

literature review, 3, 22
mechanisms of action, 146, 151, 154-155, 169
multidrug, 21, 23-24, 78, 79, 80, 107, 138, 149, 152, 153, 154, 159, 162, 170, 176, 183
nonpathogenic bacteria, 8-9, 176, 196
plasmid transfer, 22, 152-153, 169
productivity effects, 43
recommendations, 10, 177-178
regulatory and approval process and, 7, 9, 166, 168-176
reservoirs of bacteria, 79, 80, 87, 153, 155, 159, 160, 161, 166, 168, 169, 172
selection pressures, 77, 150, 154, 169, 176
sentinel organisms, 172, 174, 177
Subtherapeutic drug use and, 7, 18, 79, 81, 150, 151, 154, 156, 160
therapeutic doses and, 7, 72-73, 79, 150-151, 156, 158, 160-161, 169, 176
tracking emergence of, 7, 10, 70, 140, 157, 160, 162-166, 168, 172, 173-174, 176, 177
trends, 78-81, 161-166, 183, 196
vancomycin-like, 18, 22, 152-153
veterinary clinical implications, 161-166, 176-177
virginiamycin controversy, 175-176
Antioxidant therapy, 202-206
Antiparasitic drugs, 2, 14, 41-42, 45, 51, 58
Antiprotozoal compounds, 31, 33, 59, 82
Antiseptics, topical
literature, 14
uses, 1, 12
AOAC INTERNATIONAL, 112, 125, 126
Apramycin, 42, 164, 165, 167
Aquaculture industry
compassionate INADs, 94
drug use in, 2, 13, 58-60, 94, 101, 119, 149. *See also* Fish and shellfish
growth and structure, 56-58
management strategies, 58, 206
quality assurance, 58
residues in fish and shellfish, 119
Arcobacter spp., 127, 128-129
Arizona, 192
Arkansas, 30
Arsanilate, 32
Arsanilate sodium, 43
Arsenical compounds, 14, 31, 33, 34, 38, 116-117, 118

Arsenilic acid, 42, 43
Association of American Feed Control Officials, 197
Atrophic rhinitis, 43
Avian influenza, 31, 33, 61, 206
Avian leukosis, 207
Avoparcin, 18, 79, 166, 168, 171
Azithromycin, 170

B

Bacillus cereus, 128-131, 134-135
Bacitracin, 21, 32, 38, 39, 42, 52, 57, 75, 82
Bacterial hemorrhagic septicemia, 59
Bacterial infections
categories of, 71
stress and, 71
Bactericides, uses, 2, 12
Bambermycin, 32, 42, 82
Ban on subtherapeutic antibiotic use
consumer costs, 181-182, 183-184
economics analysis, 180-186
effect of, 15, 18, 180-184
extra-label, 107
fluoroquinolones, 107
and management practices, 181, 182
measurement of costs, 180-182
petitions for, 156-157
recommendations, 15
total vs. partial, 182-183
Banned drugs, 77, 78, 83-84, 97, 101-102
Beef cattle production. *See also* Meat
and antibiotic resistance, 162, 167, 169
breeding programs, 207
disease prevention, 50, 51-53, 159, 175, 180
economics, 25, 51, 180, 181, 182, 184, 185, 187
growth promotion, 50, 51, 53, 56, 154
history and growth, 48-49, 102
management strategies, 50, 67, 191, 206
microbiological hazards, 75, 130-131
quality assurance program, 67-68
residues in slaughtered animals, 83
specialty producers, 181
structure of industry, 30, 49
therapeutic drug use, 51-53, 74, 180, 182
trends in drug use, 25, 50-51
vaccinations, 50, 53
Beef Quality Assurance program, 67-68

Behavioral stress, management of, 193
Beta-carotene, 204-205
Beta-lactam antibiotic residues, 84, 119, 120, 123, 143, 144. *See also* Penicillin
Biosecurity measures, 35, 159, 197-199
BIOSIS, 14
Bison, 56
Blackhead, 33
Bloat, 2, 13
Bluetongue, 50, 55
Bodo spp., 59
Bordetella spp., 194
  B. avium, 31
  B. pertussis, 194
Bovine leukocyte adhesion deficiency, 207
Bovine lingual antimicrobial peptide, 147
Bovine lymphocyte antigen, 207-208
Bovine respiratory syncytial virus, 45
Bovine somatotropin, 2, 13, 48
Bovine viral diarrhea, 45
Breeding, 40, 44, 47, 48, 49
  for disease resistance, 35, 206-208
Brucella spp., 127
  B. melitensis, 136
Brucellosis, 45, 50, 53, 72, 136, 190, 206
Buquinolate, 32

C

California, 54, 98, 136, 191
Campylobacter spp.
  antibiotic-resistant, 159-160, 166, 170, 171, 172, 196
  C. coli, 127
  C. fetus, 74
  C. jejuni, 23, 127, 130-135, 197
  food-borne illness in humans, 86, 127-135, 137
  vaccination against, 194
Campylobacteriosis, 23
Canada, 104-105, 164, 165
Carbadox, 43
Carbenicillin, 162
Carcinogenic compounds, 6, 33, 82, 84, 102
Catfish Farmers of America, 60
Ceftiofur, 25, 52
Ceftiofur sodium, 34
Center for Drug Evaluation and Research, 174
Center for Food Safety and Applied Nutrition, 174

Center for Veterinary Medicine, FDA, 2, 13, 33, 88. *See also* Regulatory and approval process
  criticisms of policies of, 95-96
  extra-label use policy, 5, 96-99, 142
  Office of New Animal Drug Evaluation, 89
  Office of Surveillance and Compliance, 89
  organizational structure, 5, 89, 90
  practices and procedures, 91-92, 100, 107
  residue monitoring, 112-113, 114, 123, 126
  responsibilities, 5, 10, 89, 112, 173-174, 197
  trends in drug approvals, 94, 101, 169
Centers for Disease Control and Prevention, 22, 85-86, 88, 127, 130, 133, 139, 140, 170, 174
Cephalosporins, 77, 161, 162
Cephalothin, 162, 165
Cephapirin, 45
Chemical residues in animals, 58, 61, 161
Chemotherapeutic compounds, 43
Chickens. *See* Poultry
Chilodonella spp., 59
Chloramphenicol, 77, 78, 83-84, 97, 119, 120, 162, 163, 164, 165, 166, 167, 172
Chlortetracycline, 21, 32, 42, 52, 55, 57, 75, 154, 158
Cholera, 31, 41, 190
Chromium, 205-206
Ciprofloxacin, 169, 170, 172-173
Classes of food-animal drugs, 2, 12
Clean Water Act, 139
Cleidodiscus spp., 59
Clenbuterol, 116-117, 118
Clinton administration, 91-92, 100, 138-139, 195-196
Clopindol, 32
Clostridium spp.
  in beef cattle, 50, 53, 130-131
  C. botulinum, 128-129
  C. perfringens, 39, 40, 43, 55, 128-135
  in poultry, 39-40, 134-135
  resistant strains, 39-40
  in sheep, 55, 132-133
  in swine, 43, 128-129
  vaccination against, 194
Cloxacillin, 45
Coccidia, resistant, 31, 33
Coccidiosis, 31, 39, 44, 54, 56
Coccidiostats, 31, 32, 33, 34, 38, 39, 45, 51, 56, 57, 82

Codex Alimentarius Commission, 114
Codex Committee on Residues of Veterinary
    Drugs in Foods, 106
Colemon Natural Beef, 181
Colibacillosis, 55
Coliform plasmid transfer, 22
Colisepticemia, 72
Colony stimulating factors, 200-202
Colorado, 54
Committee on Drug Use in Food Animals
    charge to, 2, 13-14
    process, 3
Competitive exclusion products, 39, 196-197
Compliance Policy Guides, 63
Consumer
    concerns, 13, 21-22, 69
    costs of ban on subtherapeutic antibiotic
        use, 181-182, 183-184
    education, 175, 178
Continuing education programs, 67
Copper, 205, 206
Corynebacterium bovis, 204
Cost of medications, 31, 35, 36-37, 51
Costia spp., 59
Council on Agriculture and Science
    Technology (CAST) report, 15, 16, 18,
    21, 75, 160, 182
Coxiella burnetti, 127
Cryptosporidium parvum, 127
Culicoid control, 50
Cysticercus spp., 127
Cytidine monophosphate-KDO synthetase, 146
Cytokines, 29, 195, 200, 202

D

Dactylogyrus spp., 59
Dairy industry. *See also* Drug residues in milk
    antibiotic drug use, 45, 46, 47-48, 52, 119-
        120, 162
    breeding programs, 208
    disease control, 44, 45-47, 52, 162, 191,
        197
    economics, 25, 45-46
    food-borne pathogens from, 75
    heat stress management, 191-192
    history and growth of, 44, 102
    human health risks, 46-47, 162-163
    integration of, 30, 44
    management strategies, 44, 64-65, 191-192,
        197, 199, 201, 203-205

production enhancers, 2, 13, 48, 52, 205-206
prophylactic treatments, 45, 197
quality assurance program, 46, 63-67, 119,
    122
therapeutic treatments, 45-47, 51-53
Databases, 14, 67, 98, 99, 120, 140, 176, 177
Decoquinate, 54, 57
Delaney Clause, 102
Denmark, 168
Dequinate, 32
Development of new drugs. *See also*
    Regulatory and approval process
    approval process and, 5, 9-10, 91, 96, 99-
        100, 101-103, 106-109, 114, 143, 149,
        166
    ban on subtherapeutic antibiotics and, 186
    corporations, number of, 101
    costs, 96, 99, 101, 103, 106-107, 149
    efficacy requirements, 5, 94, 95, 99-100,
        103, 104, 108, 175
    environmental evaluation, 96, 101, 175
    field trials, 94-95, 99-100, 108
    food safety requirements, 83, 100-103, 104,
        114
    identifying and screening new compounds,
        145-148
    incentives for, 9, 175
    length of time for, 91-92, 103
    for minor species, 101
    recommendations, 10, 177, 178
    target-animal safety studies, 95, 103, 104
Diarrhea, 50, 52. *See also* Scours
Diethylstilbestrol, 82, 97, 102
Dihydroseptomycin, 52
Dimetridazole, 97
Direct-fed microbial products, 195-197
Disease control. *See also* Therapeutic drug use;
    Subtherapeutic drug use; Vaccination
    in beef cattle, 50, 51-53
    breeding programs, 207-208
    culling, 47-48, 206
    in dairy industry, 44, 45-47, 52, 162
    eradication programs, 55, 60-61, 190, 206
    in poultry, 31-33, 34, 38-40, 60-61, 158-
        159, 169-170, 171-172, 175, 180, 206
    prophylactic treatments, 45
    in sheep, 55-56
    spontaneous recovery, 47, 48
    in swine, 41-42, 43, 74, 75, 158-159, 163,
        175, 180, 190, 206
Drug Importation Act, 88

Drug residues in foods. *See also* Drug residues
    in milk
  action levels, 114
  administration route and, 82, 85, 103
  anabolic compounds, 50
  analytical methods, 111-112, 113-115, 119,
      123, 140, 141
  carcinogenic, 82
  Compound Evaluation System, 116
  defined, 112
  exposure potential, 113, 116
  in fish and seafood, 58, 119, 140
  foreign standards, 104-105
  human health risks from, 6, 50, 81-86, 87,
      100-103, 116
  maximum residue levels, 82, 114
  in meat and poultry, 33, 41, 51, 83, 115-119
  microbial contamination risks compared,
      85-86, 87
  monitoring and enforcement, 67, 84, 111,
      113-114, 115-119, 123, 140, 141
  pharmacokinetics in diseased animals and,
      140-141
  recommendations, 141
  regulatory and approval process, 82, 100-
      103, 107, 110-111, 114-115
  risk assessment, 100-103, 116, 117
  safe levels, 114
  screening, 6, 65-66, 111-112
  surveillance testing, 115-116, 123-124, 140
  standard setting, 84, 105-106, 108-109,
      111-113
  target tissue sites, 113-114, 117
  tolerance levels, 104-105, 108, 111, 114,
      117, 119
  toxicity, 81-82, 103, 112-113
  tracking, 41, 113-115
  violations, 83, 115, 116-117, 118, 183
Drug residues in milk
  analytical methods, 119, 122, 124-126
  controversies, 125-126
  database program, 120
  monitoring and enforcement, 120, 124-125
  Pasteurized Milk Ordinance, 63, 64, 66,
      119, 121-122, 123, 125, 126
  testing for, 65-66, 122-124, 125-126
  tracking, 46
  violation rates, 120-121
Duck, 57
Dysentery, 75
Dystocia, 44

E

Echinococcus multilocularis, 194
Economics issues
  antibiotic resistance, 150
  cost of medications, 31, 35, 36-37, 51
  drug development costs, 96, 99, 101-103,
      106-107, 149
  food-animal production, 1, 4, 21, 24-25, 75
  food-borne illnesses, 38, 138
  subtherapeutic drug use, 179-187
  testing for residues, 125
Economic Research Service, USDA, 13
Ectoparasites, 31, 50
Edwardsiella ictaluri, 59
Efrotomycin, 25, 42
Egg Products Inspection Act, 111
Eimeria, 39, 194
Endectocides, 51
Endotoxins, 146
Enforcement of regulations
  product labeling, 96-97
  recommendations, 141
  residues in foods, 115
  responsibility for, 84
Enteric septicemia, 59, 73
Enteritis, 44, 54, 57, 127, 164, 165
Enterococcus spp., 74, 79, 152-153
Enterotoxemia, 47, 55
Enzootic abortion, 55
Epididymitis, 55
Epistylis spp., 59
Erysipelas, 31, 41, 43
Erysipelothrix rhusiopatheae, 75, 128-129, 194
Erythromycin, 32, 42, 45, 52, 55, 75, 82, 160,
      162
Escherichia coli
  in cattle, 130-131, 193, 201
  compounds available for treating infections,
      35, 163-164
  drug-resistant, 22, 39, 153, 155, 156, 159,
      163-164, 165, 166, 169, 174, 196
  enterotoxigenic, 196
  immune function mediators and, 201
  in meat and meat products, 128-133
  monitoring, 140
  nonpathogenic, in gut flora, 39
  nutrition and, 203
  O157:H7 strain, 72, 74, 127, 128-135, 138,
      155, 193, 194
  in poultry, 35, 39, 134-135, 153, 194, 196
  scours, 43

in swine, 43, 128-129, 194
    vaccinations, 193, 194
Estradiol, 53
Estradiol/progesterone, 53
Estradiol/testosterone, 53
Estrus synchronizers, 51, 55
European Economic Community, 104, 105, 106
Extra-label use of drugs, 5, 10, 67, 92, 96-99,
    107, 140, 142

F

Farm Bill of 1990, 13
Federal Food, Drug, and Cosmetic Act, 5, 88,
    93, 96, 111
    Food Additives Amendment, 102 n.2
Federal Insecticide, Fungicide, and Rodenticide
    Act, 111
Federal Meat Inspection Act (FMIA), 111
Federal Security Agency, 88
Feed
    poultry, 34
Fish and shellfish, drug residues in, 119, 140
Florida, 98, 192
Fluoroquinolones, 25, 32, 35, 107, 160, 166,
    168-175, 182-183
Fly control, 50, 55
Food and Agriculture Organization, 106
Food and Drug Administration (FDA), 73, 130.
        See also Center for Veterinary Medicine
    Bureau of Veterinary Medicine, 89, 96
    Compliance Policy Guides, 63
    food safety responsibilities, 138, 139, 140
    Grade A Pasteurized Milk Ordinance, 63,
        64, 66, 121-122
    history, 88
    milk safety program, 119, 120, 123
    monitoring activities, 5, 85-86, 115, 119
    Office of Seafood, 119
    Officer of the Commissioner, 174
    quinolone policy, 170
    residue standard setting and enforcement,
        84, 99, 111
Food Animal Residual Avoidance Databank
    (FARAD) project, 5, 67, 98, 99
Foodborne Diseases Active Surveillance
    Network, 140
Food-borne pathogens, 126-127. *See also*
    Microbial contamination of food
    antibiotic resistance in, 8, 70-71, 86, 87,
        138, 140, 171

determination of, 71, 127-133
    hazardous organisms, 73-74, 75, 126-127
    outbreaks of illness, 22-23, 25-26, 85-86,
        122, 133, 136-137, 146, 155, 172
    selection of, 80
    sentinel organisms, 127, 136-137, 172
    surveillance barriers, 71
Food handling, 7, 8, 139, 172
FoodNet, 140
Food poisoning. *See* Food-borne pathogens
Food safety, responsibility for, 98, 139, 195-
    196
Food Safety and Quality national initiative, 98
Food Safety Inspection Service (FSIS), 5, 63,
    83, 85, 86, 88, 111, 112, 113, 115, 116,
    117, 127, 130, 141, 174
Foot-and-mouth disease, 50
Foot rot, 44
Formalin, 59, 94
France, 164, 165, 166
Fungi, 31
Fungicides, 2, 12, 33, 59
Furamazone, 52
Furazolidone, 33, 165, 167
Furunculosis, 59

G

Gaffkemia, 59
Gastroenteritis, 43
Gastrointestinal diseases, 50
Geese, 56
Genetic selection strategies, 35, 207-208
Gentamycin, 32, 42, 52, 83, 162, 165, 169
Gentamycin sulfate, 34
Georgia, 30
Germany, 38, 166, 169, 170
Goats, 56, 57, 83, 101, 102, 149
Gonadotropins, 55
Good laboratory practice (GLP) regulations, 89,
    95
Grade A Pasteurized Milk Ordinance (PMO),
    63, 64, 66, 119, 121-122, 123, 125
Gram-negative bacteria, 146
Growth promotion and feed efficiency
    with antibiotics, 28, 31, 34, 51-53, 81, 153-
        154
    in beef cattle, 50, 51-53, 56, 154
    in dairy cattle, 52
    in minor species, 57
    in poultry, 31, 34, 38, 56, 154

in sheep, 55-56
with steriodal and nonsteroidal estrogenic
  agents, 29, 31
in swine, 42-43, 154
Grub control, 57
Guidelines
  definition, 95-96
  dosage, 10
  testing, 100,108, 123, 126
Gyrodactylus spp., 59

H

Halofuginone, 116-117, 118
Hazard Analysis and Critical Control Points,
  62, 68, 137, 139
Heat stress management, 190-193
Helminth control, 42
Hemophilus piscium, 59
Hemophilus pleuropneumonia, 43
Hemorrhagic enteritis, 31
Hetacillin, 45
Hill Farm Research Station, 199
Histomonas influenza, 155
Histomoniasis, in poultry, 33
Hospital-acquired (nosocomial) bacterial
  infections, 22, 24, 69
Human health risks
  animal-to-human transfer of disease, 78, 79,
    80, 86-87, 143, 161-162, 168, 171, 172
  antibiotic resistance and, 2, 4, 7, 9, 13, 21,
    22-26, 69, 70, 76-78, 79, 86-87, 138,
    150, 154-155, 160, 161-166, 168, 172
  carcinogens, 82
  cases of disease, 3, 22-23
  from dairy cattle, 46-47
  hospital-acquired infections compared, 22,
    24, 69
  magnitude of threat, 2, 3, 9, 23-24, 70, 77-
    78, 86
  manure exposure and, 79, 87
  mathematical model, 18
  from poultry, 38-40
  regulatory and approval process and, 100-
    103
  from residues in food, 81-86, 100-103, 116
  sensitive populations, 8, 9, 25-26, 70
  steroid growth promoters, 50
  of subtherapeutic antibiotic use in animals,
    18, 75, 76, 150, 160
  toxicity of antibiotics, 6, 77, 81-82, 83-84

I

Icthyopthirius spp., 59
Identification of treated animals, 65
Immunostimulants, 200-202
Imported foods, 140
Infectious bovine rhinotracheitis, 45, 53
Influenza, 31, 33
Injection site tissue damage, 67
Insecticides and insecticidal ear tags, 51
Inspection at slaughter, 75
Institute of Medicine (IOM), 15, 17, 18, 150,
  156
International Conference on Harmonization,
  104
International Meeting on Nucleic Acid
  Vaccines for Prevention of Infectious
  Diseases, 195
Ionophores, 2, 12
  antiprotozoals, 33
  coccidiostats, 31, 32, 33
  for growth promotion, 50, 56
Iowa, 40
Ipronidazole, 33, 97
Irradiation of food, 71, 175
Iron, 206
Israel, 192
Ivermectin, 57, 116-117, 118

J

Japan, 104, 105
Joint Expert Committee on Food Additives,
  106

K

Kanamycin, 162, 165

L

Labels/labeling, drug, 65, 67, 96, 100
Lactobacillus spp., 39-40, 196
Laminitis, 44
Lasalocid, 32, 52, 56
Leptospira interrogans, 127
Leptospirosis, 43, 45, 53, 72, 74
Levamisole, 116-117, 118
Lice, 43
Lincoln, Abraham, 88

Lincomycin, 38, 39, 42, 82, 162
Lincosaminides, 160
Listeria spp., 127
   L. monocytogenes, 75, 128-135
Literature review
   databases, 14
   major reports, 3, 15-19, 22
Litter, water activity of, 39
Liver abscesses, 50, 75, 180
Louisiana State University, 199
Lyme disease, 70

M

Maduramycin, 32
Manure, environmental exposure to, 79, 80,
   159, 161, 166
Marek's disease, 31, 34, 207
Mange, 43, 55
Mastitis, 43, 44, 45, 46, 47, 52, 162, 191-192,
   199-200, 201, 203-205, 208
Meat
   bacterial contamination, 74, 75, 127-137
   drug residues in, 47, 63, 64, 83, 85, 113,
     115-119
   inspection, 111
Melengestrol, 53
Methicillin, 162
Metritis, 43, 44, 45, 205
Microbial contamination of food. *See also*
   Food-borne pathogens; *specific*
   pathogens
   costs of, 138
   illness determinants, 131-133
   magnitude and severity of threat, 69, 86, 87,
     137-138
   meat and meat products, 127-136, 141
   milk and other dairy products, 121-122,
     133, 136
   poultry, 35, 38-40, 75, 134-135
   prevention, 71, 195-196
   recommendations, 141
   residue risks compared, 85-86, 87
   risk assessment, 140
   routes of, 127
   surveillance and monitoring of, 85-86, 138,
     139, 140, 141
Milk. *See also* Drug residues in milk
   pathogen contamination, 121-122, 133, 136,
     163-164

Milk and Dairy Beef Quality Assurance
   Program, 63
Milk and Dairy Beef Residue Prevention
   Protocol, 63, 66, 123
Minnesota, 137
Minor species. *See also individual species*
   drug use in, 5, 56, 57, 149
   veal calves as, 54
Mite control, 55
Moisture management, 39, 199-200
Monensin, 32, 52, 57
Monitoring
   antibiotic resistance in pathogens, 7, 70,
     140, 157, 160, 162-166, 168, 174, 176
   disease outbreaks, 85-86
   drug residues in food, 5, 6, 34, 71, 86, 113-
     114, 115, 124-125, 140
   microbial contamination, 86
Monogenetic trematodes, 59
Montana, 54
Morantel tartrate, 118
Morocco, 39
Mosquito control, 50
Mutagens, 6, 82, 84
Mycobacterium spp., 127, 194
Mycoplasma spp., 194
   M. galisepticum, 33, 60
   M. meleagridis, 60
   M. synovia, 33, 60

N

Nalidixic acid, 165, 168, 169, 173
Narasin, 32
National Antimicrobial Monitoring System,
   174
National Antimicrobial Susceptibility
   Monitoring Program, 140
National Aquaculture Association, 60
National Broiler Council, 60, 61
National Cattlemen's Association, 51
National Cattlemen's Beef Association, 60, 67
National Committee for Clinical Laboratory
   Standards (NCCLS), 170, 171
National Conference on Interstate Milk
   Shipments (NCIMS), 119, 120, 123,
   125
National Drug Residue Milk Monitoring
   Program, 120
National Food Safety Initiative, 139-140

National Institutes of Health (NIH), 195
National Mastitis Council, 125
National Milk Producers Federation, 60,
      63-64
National Pork Producers Council (NPPC), 60,
      61, 62, 63
National Poultry Improvement Plan, 60-61
National Research Council, 2, 13, 16, 205
National Residue Program, 115
National Surveillance for Antibiotic Resistance
      in Zoonotic Enteric Pathogens, 174
National Turkey Federation, 60
   Chemical Residue Avoidance Program, 61
National Turkey Improvement Plan, 60
National Veterinary Services Laboratory, 162
Necrotic enteritis, 39
Nematode control, 45
Neomycin, 32, 42, 52, 55, 57, 82, 83, 162, 164,
      165, 166, 167
Nequinate, 32
Netherlands, 166, 170, 171
Newcastle disease, 31, 61
Nicarbazin, 32
Nitrarsone, 33
Nitrofurans, 25, 33, 35, 82, 84, 97, 102, 164
Nitrofurazone, 82, 165
Nitroimidazole, 82, 84, 102
Nonpathogenic bacteria, 8-9, 176
Nonsteroid growth promoters, 14
North Carolina, 30, 40, 98
Nourseotricin, 153
Novobiocin, 32, 45, 57, 82, 162
Nutrition, 11, 30, 50, 192, 202-206

O

Office of Science and Technology Policy, 140
Office of Technology Assessment, 22, 76
Oleandomycin, 32, 42, 82
Organochlorine and organophosphate
      compounds, 14, 116-117, 118
Ormetoprin, 59
Over-the-counter antibiotic sales, 4, 6, 46, 65,
      81, 182, 186
Overcrowding, management of, 193
Oxazolidinones, 146
Oxolinic acid, 119
Oxytetracycline, 32, 33, 42, 45, 52, 53, 55, 59,
      75, 94, 154

P

Parainfluenza type 3, 45, 53
Parvovirus, 43
Pasteurella spp., 194
   P. multocida, 35, 39
   pneumonia, 43
Pasteurellosis, 169
Pathogens. *See also* Antibiotic resistance;
      Food-borne pathogens; Microbial
      contamination of food; *specific*
      pathogens
   adaptation to environment, 76-77
   animal-to-human transfer, 78, 79, 80, 86-
      87, 143, 161-162
   eradication of, 35
Pathogen Reduction Task Force, 85-86, 130
Penicillin, 18, 20, 21, 32, 38, 39, 42, 45, 51-53,
      55, 57, 81, 82, 83, 85, 117, 119, 143,
      144, 148, 154, 155, 156, 161, 162, 163-
      164, 166, 169
Pennsylvania, 204
Peptide production enhancers, 2, 13
Pfisteria, 101
Pheasant, 57
Phenothiazine, 57
Pinkeye, 44, 50
Pirlimycin, 45
Poison Control Center, 95
Porcine stress syndrome, 207
Pork Quality Assurance (PQA) program, 61-63
Poultry and poultry products
   drug residues in, 33, 83, 115-119
   microbial contamination, 35, 38-40, 75,
      134-135, 168
Poultry production
   and antibiotic resistance, 18, 32, 153, 158,
      162, 167, 168, 169-170, 171-172
   breeding programs, 207
   Clostridium infections, 39-40
   concerns, 35
   cost of medications, 35, 36-37
   day-old-chick vaccination, 31, 34
   disease control, 31-33, 34, 38-40, 60-61,
      158-159, 169-170, 171-172, 175, 180,
      206
   drug approval process, 103
   drug use history and trends, 31-34, 35, 169-
      170
   economics of, 25, 30-31, 181, 184, 185,
      186-187

Escherichia coli infections, 35, 39, 196
feed and nutrition, 30, 34
growth promotion, 1, 31, 34, 38, 56, 154
history and growth of industry, 29-30, 102
integration of industry, 30-31, 33, 49
management practices, 61, 191, 192-193
quality assurance program, 34, 60-61
routes of drug administration, 34-37
Salmonella infections, 38-39, 158, 162, 167, 197, 206
vaccinations, 31, 33, 40
water medication, 34-35
withdrawal period, 33, 34, 38
Poultry Products Inspection Act (PPIA), 111
Prevention of bacterial infections, 71-72. *See also* Prophylactic treatments; Subtherapeutic antibiotic use
Probiotics, 39-40, 195-197
Production enhancers, in dairy industry, 48
Production of food animals. *See also* Animal management practices; *individual industries*
intensiveness, 21, 29
size of industry, 101, 102
trends, 27, 29
Productivity effects of antibiotic resistance, 43
Prophylactic use of drugs
in beef industry, 50, 180
in dairy industry, 45, 197
immune function mediators, 200
in poultry industry, 31, 33, 34
risk-benefit analysis, 71-72
Propionibacterium acnes, 202
Pseudomonas spp., 59
Pseudorabies, 43
Psoroptis ovis, 199
Pure Food and Drug Act, 88

Q

Quail, 57
Quality assurance programs, 27-28
aquaculture, 58
beef, 67-68
certification, 62, 68, 119
dairy, 63-67, 119
Hazard Analysis and Critical Control Points, 62, 68
incentives for participants, 66
objectives and focus, 60, 68
pork, 61-63

poultry, 34, 60-61
record-keeping, 4, 65, 66, 67
residue screening, 112
VCPR and, 5, 28, 54, 56, 64, 67, 97, 98-99
Quinolones, 147, 159-160, 197
Quinoxaline di-*N*-oxides, 82, 84

R

Rabbits, 57
Rabies, 70, 72
Recombinant bovine somatotropin, 2, 13, 48
Recommendations
animal management research, 11, 208-209
antibiotic development and use, 10, 177, 178
antibiotic resistance surveillance, 11, 177-178
consumer education, 178
database, 177
food animal identification, 178
monitoring and enforcement, 141
nutrition research, 11, 208-209
regulatory and approval process, 10, 107-109, 177
vaccination research, 11, 209
Records, treatment, 4, 65, 66, 67
Regulations, 89, 94-95, 96, 97, 106
Regulatory and approval process. *See also individual statutes and agencies*
antibiotic resistance and, 166, 168-176
carcinogenic drugs, 82
compassionate INAD, 94
continuing education programs, 67
direct-fed microbial products, 196-197
dispute settlement, 93, 108
drug development perspectives, 5, 91, 96, 99-100, 101-103, 106-109, 114, 143, 149, 166
efficacy requirements, 6, 94, 95, 99-100, 103, 104, 107, 108
enforcement policies, 96-97
environmental evaluation, 96, 101, 104
extra-label usage, 5, 67, 92, 96-99, 107, 140, 142
field trials, 94-95, 99-100, 108
flexibility in, 91, 108
food-safety research program, 96
guidelines for meeting criteria, 95-96
history, 88

human drug application process compared, 95, 97, 103, 104, 107
human health risks and, 82, 100-103
investigational new animal drug (INAD) application, 89-90, 92, 93, 94, 108
IR4 program, 54
length of, 5, 24, 91, 93, 103, 106-107
monitoring activities, 5, 89
New Animal Drug Application (NADA), 89, 92, 93, 114
organizational structure, 88-89, 90
panel approach, 105-106
preapproval process, 89-91, 92-93, 94-95
quality of sponsor applications, 94
recommendations, 10, 107-109, 177
redirected drug use, 95
redundancy in, 95, 103
reforms needed, 95-96, 99, 107-108
residues in foods, 83, 100-103, 104-106, 107, 108-109, 112, 114
restructuring, 5, 9-10, 91-100, 107, 143
socioeconomic and political pressures, 96, 143
target-animal safety studies, 95, 104
trends in approvals, 94, 101-102
worldwide harmonization of, 104-106, 109, 143
Reindeer, 57
Reinfection and cross-infection of animals, 159
Research barriers, 20, 56
Residues. *See* Drug residues in food
Resistance, defined, 77. See also Antibiotic resistance
Respiratory disease complex, 50, 53
Respiratory infections, 44, 50, 52, 54, 55
Rifamycin, 77
Robenidine, 32
Rockefeller University, 80
Roosevelt, Theodore, 88
Roxarsone, 32, 33, 43
Rumen foaming, 2, 13

S

Sales of animal drugs, 103
Salmonella spp., 127
animal-to-human transfer, 162-163, 171, 172
in cattle, 162, 167, 169
drug-resistant, 22, 23, 136, 150, 156, 158, 159, 162, 163, 164-166, 167, 169, 171, 172-173, 174, 196

DT-104 strain, 23, 72, 73-74, 138, 149, 155, 170, 172-173
in meat and meat products, 128-133, 162
moisture conditions and, 39
monitoring, 140
in poultry and poultry products, 31, 134-135, 158, 162, 167, 193, 194, 206
reservoirs, 155
S. dublin, 136, 164
S. enteritidis, 136, 164, 165, 194, 206
S. gallinarum, 31, 60-61
S. heidelberg, 163
S. javiana, 136
S. newport, 162-163
S. oranienburg, 136
S. pullorum, 31, 60
S. typhimurium, 136, 155, 159, 164-166, 167, 194
in sheep, 167
in swine, 162, 167
vaccinations, 193
virulence and pathogenicity, 38, 72, 73-74, 138, 150, 155, 159, 196
Salmonellosis
economic impacts, 38
in humans, 23, 38, 70, 73-74, 78, 81, 86, 136
in poultry, 38-39
in swine, 74
Salinomycin, 32
Sanitation, 61, 63
satA-gene-mediated streptogramines, 79
Scours, 43, 44
Screening for drug residues in food, 6, 65-66, 111-112, 145-148
analytical approaches, 111-112
confirmatory methods, 112
Screwworm control, 55
Scyphidia spp., 59
Selection pressures, 77, 150, 154, 169, 176
Selenium, 203, 204, 205, 206
Sentinel Site Study, 86, 130
Septicemia, 146
Sheep production
antibiotic resistance, 167
disease control, 55-56
drug use in, 55-56, 101, 149
economics, 25
growth of industry, 54, 102
management strategies, 54-55
microbiological hazards, 75, 132-133
residues in slaughtered animals, 83

Shigella sp., 86, 127, 130
Shipping fever, 55
Slaughtered animals
    residues in, 83
    test subjects, 90
South Dakota, 54
Spain, 171
Specific-pathogen-free stock, 35, 206
Spectinomycin, 32, 42
Squab, 56
Staphylococcus spp.
    multidrug resistant, 153
    S. aureus, 35, 46-47, 128-131, 134-135,
        201, 203, 205
Sterile packaging, 71, 175
Steroid anabolic growth promoters, 2, 12-13,
    14, 50, 53
Storage of drugs, 65
Streptococcus
    antibiotic resistance, 162
    infections, 43
    S. agalactiae, 162
    S. faecalis, 196
    S. suis, 74
Streptomycin, 21, 32, 42, 45, 52, 55, 57, 82,
    144, 158-159, 162, 163-164, 165, 166,
    172
Streptothricin, 153
Stress, and bacterial infection, 71, 159, 180,
    202
Subtherapeutic antibiotic use. *see also* Ban on
    subtherapeutic antibiotic use
    administration strategies, 71-72, 151, 157
    and antibiotic resistance, 7, 18, 79, 81, 150,
        151, 154, 156, 179
    criticisms of, 156
    definition of, 4, 15, 28, 180
    economic analysis, 107, 179-187
    human health risks, 18, 75, 76, 150, 160
    importance, 68, 154, 157
    low therapeutic dose distinguished from, 51
    mechanism of action, 77, 154, 157
    substitutes for, 182, 189-190
    swine, 41, 42-43
    trends, 25
    uses, 4, 28, 42-43, 68
Sulfa drugs, 14, 81, 94, 120, 145-146, 148, 160
Sulfabromomethazine, 52
Sulfacetamide, 84
Sulfachloropyrazine, 32, 43, 52, 84
Sulfadimethoxine, 52, 84, 120

Sulfaethoxypyridazine, 43, 52
Sulfamethazine, 32, 43, 50, 52, 63, 84
Sulfamethoxazole, 78, 163-164, 165, 166
Sulfamethoxine, 32, 52, 59
Sulfamyxin, 32
Sulfanilamide, 84
Sulfanitran, 32
Sulfaquinoxaline, 32, 57, 84
Sulfathiazole, 43, 84
Sulfonamides, 32, 33, 51, 52, 54, 55, 84, 116-
    117, 118, 165, 172
Surveillance testing, drug residues in foods,
    115-116, 123-124, 140
Surveys of food-borne illness, 133-137
Swann Committee Report, 15, 16, 156
Sweden, 166
Swine production. *See also* Pork
    antibiotic resistance, 43, 158-159, 160-161,
        162, 163, 167, 168
    breeding programs, 207
    disease control, 41-42, 43, 74, 75, 158-159,
        163, 175, 180, 190, 206
    economics, 25, 40, 75, 181, 182, 185, 186,
        187
    growth and metabolic performance, 42-43,
        154
    integration of industry, 30, 40-41, 49
    management systems, 41, 181, 191, 197-
        198, 206
    microbiological hazards, 128-129
    residues in slaughtered animals, 83, 85
    size of industry, 40, 102
    slaughter rejection, 75, 76
    therapeutic drug use, 182

T

Testing feed quality, 61
Testing for drug residues
    analytical methods, 111-112, 113-115, 119,
        123, 140
    in milk, 122-124, 125-126
    toxicity, 112-113
    unresolved issues, 125-126
Tetracycline, 18, 21, 32, 38, 42, 50, 51-53, 78,
    81, 82, 83, 120, 152-153, 156, 159, 160,
    162, 164, 165, 166, 167, 172
Texas, 54, 136
Thailand, 170
Therapeutic drug use
    administration regimen, 34-35, 157

and antibiotic resistance, 7, 72-73, 79, 150-
    151, 156, 157, 158-159, 160-161, 176
in beef cattle, 51-53, 180
in dairy cattle, 45-47
definition, 180
economics of, 74
low-dose, 51, 189
minimal inhibitory concentration (MIC),
    150-151, 166, 176
in poultry, 34-35
reduction strategies, 188-189
regulation of, 182
risk—benefit assessment, 72-73, 74, 75,
    179
Thiabendazole, 57
Tiamulin, 42
Tilmicosin, 52, 160
Tobromycin, 169
Topical drugs, 1, 12, 82
Toxic shock syndrome, 146
Toxic Substances Control Act, 111
Toxicity of food-animal drugs, 81-82, 83-84,
    103, 112-113, 144
Toxoplasma gondii, 127
Toxoplasmosis, 72
Tracking
    antibiotic resistance, 7, 70, 140, 157, 160,
        162-166, 168, 174, 176
    drug residues in food, 113-115
Trenbolone, 53
Trends
    in antibiotic resistance, 78-81
    in drug use, 31-34, 50-51
Tricaine methanesulfonate, 59
Trichinella spiralis, 127
Trichodina spp., 59
Trimethoprim, 146, 160, 163, 164, 165, 166,
    167, 172
Triple sulfonamides, 162, 165
Trypanosomiasis, 207
Tuberculosis, 31, 50, 72, 190, 206
Turkeys. *See* Poultry
Tylosin, 32, 33, 38, 42, 50, 52, 75, 82

U

United Egg Producers, 60
United Kingdom, 75, 155, 164, 168, 170, 171,
    172
United States and Canada Free Trade
    Agreement, 104-105

University of California at Davis, 98
University of Florida, 98
U.S. Department of Agriculture, 2
    Bureau of Chemistry, 88
    Cooperative State Research, Education, and
        Extension Service, 98, 139
    food safety responsibilities, 138, 140, 174
    National Agriculture Library, 14
    Pathogen Reduction Task Force, 85-86, 130
    residue monitoring and enforcement
        responsibilities, 111, 114-115
    Residue Monitoring Program, 67, 83, 84
U.S. Department of Health and Human
    Services, 88, 90
U.S. Environmental Protection Agency, 88,
    111, 139
U.S. Fish and Wildlife Service, 119
U.S. Public Health Service, 88, 90, 119, 121,
    122
U.S. Trout Farmers Association, 60

V

Vaccinations, 127
    beef cattle, 50, 53, 193
    dairy cattle, 45, 193
    eradication of disease, 206
    mutations introduced by, 194
    nucleic acid, 195
    pathogen targets, 193-194
    poultry, 31, 33, 35, 40, 193, 194
    research recommendations, 11, 209
    sheep, 55
    swine, 41, 43, 194
Vancomycin, 18, 22, 79, 152-153, 166, 168
Veal production, 53-54, 101, 102, 163, 181
Veterinarian-client-patient relationship
    (VCPR), 5, 28, 54, 56, 64, 67, 97, 98-99
Veterinary feed directive drugs, 100
Vibrio spp., 127
Vibriosis, 55
Virginiamycin, 32, 38, 39, 42, 79, 82, 175-176
Vitamin A, 204-205
Vitamin E, 203, 204, 205, 206

W

Water
    medication, 2, 34-35, 58
    quality and availability, 192

Withdrawal
    diets, 34
    intervals, 99
    times, 33, 38, 67, 83, 84, 90, 96, 97, 99,
        113, 117, 126, 161
World Health Organization (WHO), 17, 18, 78,
    106
Worms, 31, 33, 43, 50, 55, 56, 57
Wyoming, 54

Y

Yersinia spp., 74
    Y. enterolitica, 127, 128-131

Z

Zeranol, 53, 55-56
Zinc, 205, 206
Zoalene, 32
Zoonotic disease transfer, 8, 18, 69-70, 72, 74,
    87, 150-151, 154, 160, 162-163, 176
Zoothamnium spp., 59